Teaching Atlas of Nuclear Medicine

Teaching Atlas of Nuclear Medicine

edited by

Kevin J. Donohoe, M.D.
Division of Nuclear Medicine
Beth Israel Deaconess Medical Center
Boston, Massachusetts

and

Annick D. Van den Abbeele, M.D.
Division of Nuclear Medicine
Dana-Farber Cancer Institute
Boston, Massachusetts

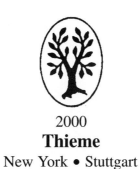

2000
Thieme
New York • Stuttgart

Thieme New York
333 Seventh Avenue
New York, NY 10001

Editor: Jane E. Pennington
Editorial Director: Avé McCracken
Editorial Assistant: Todd Warnock
Developmental Manager: Kathleen P. Lyons
Director, Production and Manufacturing: Anne Vinnicombe
Production Editor: Janice G. Stangel
Marketing Director: Phyllis Gold
Sales Manager: Ross Lumpkin
Chief Financial Officer: Seth S. Fishman
President: Brian D. Scanlan
Cover Designer: Kevin Kall
Compositor: Alexander Graphics, Inc., and Graphic World, Inc.
Printer: Maple-Vail Book Manufacturing Group

Library of Congress Cataloging-in-Publication Data

Teaching atlas of nuclear medicine/edited by Kevin J. Donohoe, Annick Van den Abbeele.
    p.   cm.
    Includes bibliographical references and index.
    ISBN 0-86577-775-6
    1. Radioisotope scanning—Atlases. I. Donohoe, Kevin J. II. Van den Abbeele, Annick,
1953-
    [DNLM: 1. Radionuclide Imaging—Atlases. 2. Radionuclide Imaging—Case Report.
WN 17 T253 1999]
RC78.7.R4 T43 1999
616.07'575 21—dc21

                                99-040822

Important note: Medical knowledge is ever-changing. As new research and clinical experience broaden our knowledge, changes in treatment and drug therapy may be required. The authors and editors of the material herein have consulted sources believed to be reliable in their efforts to provide information that is complete and in accord with the standards accepted at the time of publication. However, in view of the possibility of human error by the authors, editors, or publisher of the work herein, or changes in medical knowledge, neither the authors, editors, publisher, nor any other party who has been involved in the preparation of this work, warrants that the information contained herein is in every respect accurate or complete, and they are not responsible for any errors or omissions or for the results obtained from use of such information. Readers are encouraged to confirm the information contained herein with other sources. For example, readers are advised to check the product information sheet included in the package of each drug they plan to administer to be certain that the information contained in this publication is accurate and that changes have not been made in the recommended dose or in the contraindications for administration. This recommendation is of particular importance in connection with new or infrequently used drugs.

Some of the product names, patents, and registered designs referred to in this book are in fact registered trademarks or proprietary names even though specific reference to this fact is not always made in the text. Therefore, the appearance of a name without designation as proprietary is not to be construed as a representation by the publisher that it is in the public domain.

Printed in the United States of America

5 4 3 2 1

TNY ISBN 0-86577-775-6
GTV ISBN 3-13-108611-4

To my mother and father, who have given me knowledge
and a sense of humor.
To my mentors Dennis Patton and Tim Woolfenden, who have
shown me how to teach and explore.
And to Mary, who has given me her love and support.

Kevin J. Donohoe, M.D.

To my parents Nelly and Karel Gerard Van den Abbeele,
my sister Karyn,
my brothers Eric and Michel,
and their families,
for giving me the roots as well as the wings,
for inspiring the best,
and for their endless encouragement, love, and support.

Annick D. Van den Abbeele, M.D.

CONTENTS

V. SCINTIGRAPHY OF NEOPLASTIC DISEASE

A. Lymphoma
Annick D. Van den Abbeele

B. Breast
Frank Bradley

C. Neuroendocrine
Christopher P. Fey and Annick D. Van den Abbeele

D. Antibody Scintigraphy
Milos Janicek, Christopher P. Fey, and Annick D. Van Den Abbeele

E. Positron Imaging of Tumors
Hossein Jadvar and Alan J. Fischman

VI. INFLAMMATION IMAGING
Kevin J. Donohoe

A. Soft Tissue Inflammation

VII. IMAGING IN ACQUIRED IMMUNODEFICIENCY SYNDROME
Nayer Nikpoor, Rachel Powsner, and Victor Lee

VIII. RENAL SCINTIGRAPHY
Finn Mannting

IX. BILIARY SCINTIGRAPHY
Kevin J. Donohoe

X. LYMPHOSCINTIGRAPHY

A. Lymphedema
Annick D. Van den Abbeele

B. Sentinel Node
Rachel Powsner

CONTRIBUTORS

Frank Bradley, M.D.
Department of Radiology
Beth Israel Deaconess Medical Center
Boston, Massachusetts

Puneet Chandak, M.D.
Division of Nuclear Medicine
Department of Radiology
Brigham and Women's Hospital
Boston, Massachusetts

Leonard Connolly, M.D.
Associate Director, Resident/Fellow Training
Joint Program in Nuclear Medicine
Division of Nuclear Medicine
Children's Hospital
Boston, Massachusetts

Kevin J. Donohoe, M.D.
Division of Nuclear Medicine
Beth Israel Deaconess Medical Center
Boston, Massachusetts

Laura Drubach
Division of Nuclear Medicine
Children's Hospital
Boston, Massachusetts

Christopher P. Fey, M.D.
Clinical Fellow
Division of Nuclear Medicine
Brigham and Women's Hospital
Boston, Massachusetts

Alan Fischman, M.D., Ph.D.
Director
Division of Nuclear Medicine
Massachusetts General Hospital
Boston, Massachusetts

B. Leonard Holman, M.D., Ph.D. (deceased)
Chairman, Department of Radiology
Brigham and Women's Hospital
Boston, Massachusetts

Hossein Jadvar, M.D., Ph.D.
Clinical Fellow
Joint Program in Nuclear Medicine
Harvard Medical School
Boston, Massachusetts

Milos Janicek, M.D., Ph.D.
Division of Nuclear Medicine
Dana-Farber Cancer Institute
Boston, Massachusetts

Victor Lee, M.D.
Division of Nuclear Medicine
Boston Medical Center
Boston, Massachusetts

Finn Mannting, M.D., Ph.D.
Director
Division of Nuclear Medicine
Brigham and Women's Hospital
Boston, Massachusetts

Nayer Nikpoor, M.D.
Division of Nuclear Medicine
Brigham and Women's Hospital
Boston, Massachusetts

Rachel Powsner, M.D.
Acting Director
Division of Nuclear Medicine
Boston Medical Center
Boston, Massachusetts

CONTRIBUTORS

Jac D. Scheiner, M.D.
Clinical Assistant Professor
Department of Diagnostic Imaging
Brown University School of Medicine
Providence, Rhode Island

S. Ted Treves, M.D.
Director, Resident/Fellow Training
Joint Program in Nuclear Medicine
Chief, Division of Nuclear Medicine
Children's Hospital
Boston, Massachusetts

Annick D. Van den Abbeele, M.D.
Director
Division of Nuclear Medicine
Dana-Farber Cancer Institute
Boston, Massachusetts

FOREWORD

This collection of 169 cases makes a definite contribution to the nuclear medical literature. Like most attempts at problem-based learning, it challenges the reader to test herself or himself while acquiring new knowledge. Novice and master clinician alike should approach each case as follows:

Read the Clinical Presentation and Techniques sections
Examine the images and interpret them
State the clinical question as it should have been posed by the referring physician
Compare your image interpretation and differential diagnosis with that of the
    authors
Study the Discussion and Pearls/Pitfalls sections
Call up the Suggested Readings on Medline to determine your interest

From this exercise, the reader will be provided with a systemic review of current nuclear medical practice.

A casebook, unlike a textbook, is meant to be worked with, not referred to. Working with this one should be looked upon as a challenge and, in this case, as a joy as well.

Go to it!

S. James Adelstein, M.D., Ph.D.
Harvard Medical School
Joint Program in Nuclear Medicine

PREFACE

The *Teaching Atlas of Nuclear Medicine* has been carefully constructed to provide the concise information needed for the interpretation of Nuclear Medicine images. Rather than attempt to include all possible image presentations for all possible diseases, this Atlas focuses on the common presentations of many diseases, and utilizes this information as a tool to understand how images are affected by normal physiology and by disease. The reader should then be able to apply that knowledge to any clinical situation. This is a much more efficient process than memorizing all possible image patterns expected to be seen in all diseases.

Individual cases are presented in a manner similar to how a study would be presented in clinical practice or during a board exam. A brief clinical presentation is provided, followed by the images. The reader should try to approach the images as they normally would in any clinical situation. From the technical aspects of the imaging procedure to a differential diagnosis of the findings, all reasons for why the scans appear as they do should be considered.

Pertinent technical aspects of each study follow the images to further elucidate the type of study obtained, if not initially obvious. This information is followed by a differential diagnosis and then by the final diagnosis. A brief discussion section is provided to outline why the images appear as they do, and to discuss the specific image findings that should have helped make the final diagnosis.

In many cases the diagnosis may be difficult. If the reader does not arrive at the same diagnosis as the author, he or she should not be discouraged, but rather should understand what the important normal and abnormal findings are, and the physiology behind those findings. An understanding of the physiology behind the image is an important tool to acquire. It can be used for interpretation of images that appear later in the book as well as later in the reader's career.

A concise listing of possible pearls and pitfalls that may be encountered with the imaging procedure are also provided. The reader should consider their relevance to the specific case, including how the pearls may have assisted image interpretation and how the pitfalls may make an accurate diagnosis more difficult.

We have attempted to make the book challenging for the reader, and also fun. We hope the skills acquired in reading this book will not only provide you with the tools necessary to pass a board exam or to recognize a specific disease process on a specific scan, but will also provide you with an understanding of physiologic imaging that can be applied even as imaging technology evolves. It is the understanding of the physiology behind the images that will serve you in the years to come.

Kevin J. Donohoe, M.D.
Annick D. Van den Abbeele, M.D.

Section I

Skeletal Scintigraphy

Case 1

Clinical Presentation

37-year-old woman presenting with acute-onset low back pain.

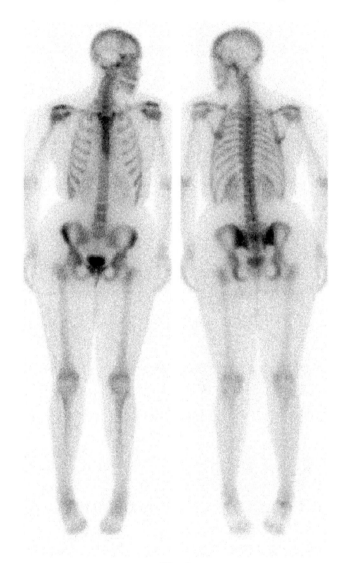

Fig. A

Technique

- 20 mCi technetium-99m–labeled methylene diphosphonate (MDP) intravenously.
- Whole-body or spot images of the skeleton obtained approximately 3 hours after tracer administration.
- Emphasize the importance of oral hydration to improve soft tissue and bladder clearance.

Image Interpretation

Whole-body views (Fig. A) demonstrate normal tracer distribution throughout the bony skeleton.

Differential Diagnosis

False negative bone scans are rare, but may be seen in:

- Multiple myeloma
- Any bony lesion that has not yet provoked an osteoblastic response (e.g., very early disease)
- Attenuation (e.g., soft tissue) over a focal abnormal site of uptake

Diagnosis and Clinical Follow-up

Because no focal abnormalities were noted, pain was thought to be muscular.

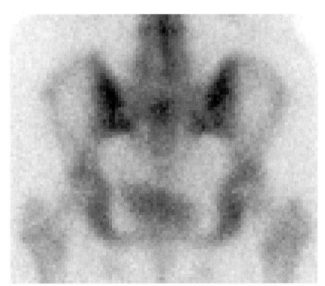

Fig. B

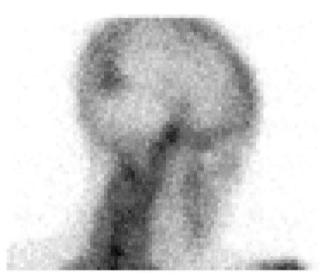

Fig. C

Discussion

Bone scans are one of the most frequently ordered studies in nuclear medicine. The superb sensitivity of the bone scan for detecting osteoblastic activity associated with bone repair makes it an excellent primary screening test for malignancies that metastasize to bone and for the diagnosis of bony trauma not apparent on plain radiographic studies. The low specificity and the high sensitivity of bone scans mean that additional studies, such as plain film, computed tomography (CT), magnetic resonance imaging (MRI), and possibly biopsy, are often warranted when abnormalities are noted, particularly when metastatic disease is a concern.

In benign disease, the bone scan is performed more often as a secondary study after other imaging studies are negative and a high suspicion of bone disease remains. As mentioned, abnormalities noted on bone scan are nonspecific, and correlation with other information, such as history, physical exam, and previously acquired anatomic imaging studies, is often necessary to determine the cause and significance of any abnormal bone tracer uptake.

Suggested Readings

Datz FL. *Gamuts in Nuclear Medicine*. 2nd ed. Norwalk, CT: Appleton & Lange, 1987.

Harbert JC. The musculoskeletal system. In: Harbert JC, Eckelman WC, Neumann RD, eds. *Nuclear Medicine Diagnosis and Therapy*. New York: Thieme, 1996, p. 801.

Case 2

Clinical Presentation

64-year-old man with a history of prostate cancer diagnosed 2 years ago now presenting with prostate-specific antigen (PSA) elevated to 25 ng/mL.

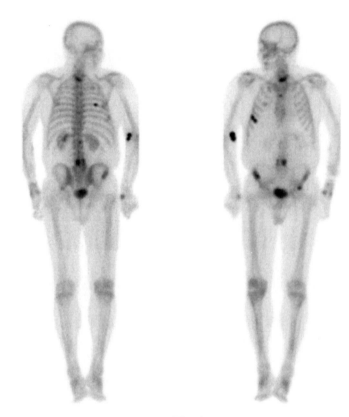

Fig. A

Technique

- 20 mCi technetium-99m–labeled methylene diphosphonate (MDP) intravenously.
- Whole-body or spot images of the skeleton obtained 3 hours after tracer administration.
- Emphasize the importance of oral hydration to improve soft tissue and bladder clearance.

Image Interpretation

Whole-body views (Fig. A) show foci of intense tracer uptake in the pelvis, spine, and ribs. Partial infiltration of the injection is noted in the right antecubital fossa.

- *(continued)* Local metastatic disease in the pelvis or sacrum may be obscured by tracer in the urinary bladder. If the bladder cannot be emptied completely, having the patient sit on the detector, or taking single photon emission computed tomography (SPECT) or lateral views may allow separation of tracer activity concentrated in the urinary bladder from bony structures. Catheterization of the urinary bladder, particularly in patients with bladder outlet obstruction, can lead to urosepsis and therefore should not be done routinely.

- Hyperostosis frontalis interna in the skull may resemble metastatic disease without straight anterior views demonstrating the bilateral, symmetrical nature of the tracer uptake.

- Diffuse metastatic uptake in the hemipelvis or in any other bone may resemble Paget's disease. Radiographic correlation should always be obtained if this pattern of uptake is present.

- The usefulness of bone scans in patients with PSA of less than 8 ng/mL is unclear. They may serve as useful baselines, particularly in patients with severe degenerative disease or other known bone pathology.

- The workup of equivocal abnormalities noted on bone scan depends on several factors, including the prior probability of disease and information obtained from the patient and the referring physician. Not every abnormality noted on bone scan needs radiographic correlation.

Differential Diagnosis

Despite the non-specificity of focal abnormal bony uptake of bone tracers, certain *patterns* of uptake are practically pathognomonic. Multiple sites of uptake may be seen in several diseases, but the pattern of uptake noted in this case is likely secondary to metastatic disease.

Diagnosis and Clinical Follow-up

Tracer uptake is consistent with prostate cancer metastic to the skeleton. Subsequent radiographs of the spine and pelvis demonstrated blastic lesions consistent with metastatic prostate cancer.

Discussion

If the initial workup of prostate cancer includes an elevated PSA (above 8 to 20 ng/mL), bone pain, or histologically aggressive tumor, the bone scan is the most cost-effective tool for diagnosing metastasis to bone. On the other hand, if the PSA is less than 8 and other evidence of metastasis is lacking, the bone scan may not be warranted.

Prostate cancer is almost always associated with an aggressive osteoblastic response, causing obvious focal uptake in sites of metastatic disease. The tumor can initially spread through local lymphatics or hematogenously through Batson's plexus to the pelvis and spine and throughout the axial skeleton. Spread to the appendicular skeleton outside regions occupied by red marrow is rare, but not unheard of, in cases of advanced metastatic disease.

Prostate cancer may also be associated with urinary tract obstruction, from either tumor obstruction at the prostate, unrelated prostatic hypertrophy, or local pelvic nodal metastases. Abnormal amounts of tracer retention in the ureters or renal pelvis should be mentioned in the dictated report, and the patient should be questioned about symptoms of obstruction. It is not uncommon that back pain thought to be caused by bony metastasis is subsequently found to be caused by urinary tract obstruction discovered on the bone scan.

Suggested Readings

Freitas JE, Gilvydas R, Ferry JD, et al. The clinical utility of prostate-specific antigen and bone scintigraphy in prostate cancer follow-up. *J Nucl Med* 32:1387–1390, 1991.

Fuse H, Nagakawa O, Seto H, et al. Bone marrow scintigraphy in the diagnosis of bone metastasis in prostate cancer. *Int Urol Nephrol* 26:53–61, 1994.

Harbert JC. The musculoskeletal system. In: Harbert JC, Eckelman WC, Neumann RD, eds. *Nuclear Medicine Diagnosis and Therapy*. New York: Thieme, p. 801, 1996.

Klein EA. An update on prostate cancer. *Cleve Clin J Med* 62:325–338, 1995.

Case 3

Clinical Presentation

43-year-old woman with a history of breast cancer diagnosed 5 years earlier presenting with elevated serum calcium and alkaline phosphatase on routine follow-up.

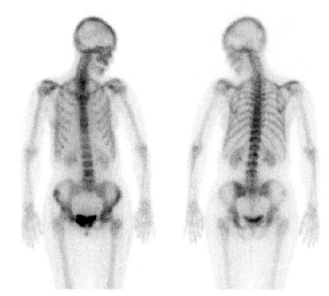

Fig. A–Baseline

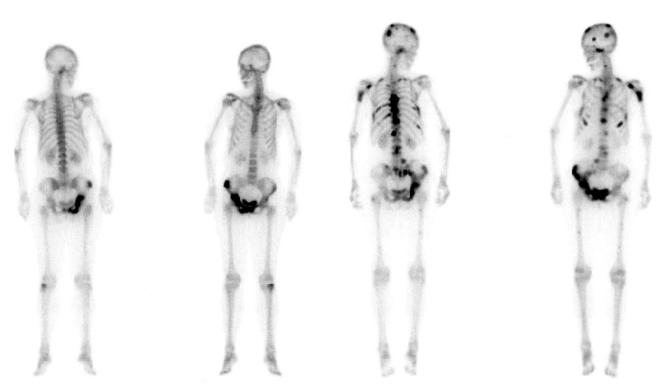

Fig. B–16 months later   **Fig. C–28 months later**

PEARLS/PITFALLS

- Soft tissue should be carefully evaluated for the possibility of liver uptake (Fig. D, posterior; Fig. E, anterior) or hemithorax asymmetry (Fig. F, posterior; Fig. G, anterior) suggesting metastatic spread to the liver or pleural effusion.

- Isolated sternal lesions may represent metastasis in up to 76% of patients with breast cancer.

- Focal lesions on adjacent ribs are most often caused by trauma, but chest wall invasion of locally recurrent disease should also be considered.

- Lesions noted in weight-bearing areas, such as the femurs, should be radiographed to rule out impending pathologic fracture.

- Therapy with samarium-153 or strontium-89 should be considered in patients with bone pain and avid tracer uptake in bony lesions.

- Following therapy, particularly hormone therapy, healing bony lesions noted on previous scans can demonstrate more intense tracer uptake. This "flare response" should not be mistaken for worsening disease.

- Anterior chest wall uptake may appear asymmetrical and irregular because of previous mastectomy, surgical trauma, or differences in soft tissue attenuation. A surgical history and oblique views may help if rib lesions are being considered.

- When to do a bone scan in the workup for breast cancer is subject to debate. Scans in stage I or stage II disease are often negative but may serve as a useful baseline in patients with degenerative disease.

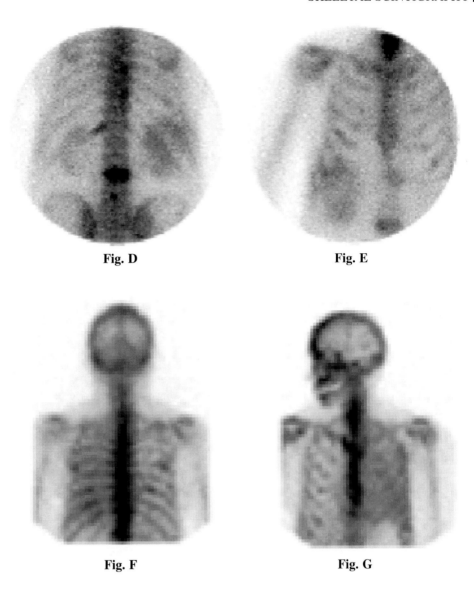

Fig. D   Fig. E

Fig. F   Fig. G

Technique

- 20 mCi technetium-99m–labeled methylene diphosphonate (MDP) intravenously.
- Whole-body or spot images of the skeleton obtained 3 hours after tracer administration.
- Emphasize the importance of oral hydration to improve soft tissue and bladder clearance.

Image Interpretation

The images demonstrate the progression of findings over approximately 2.5 years. Figure A, at baseline, shows right anterior iliac crest focal uptake and the possibility of pubic symphysis involvement. Figure B, 16 months later shows more extensive involvement of the pelvis. Figure C, 28 months later shows progressive disease throughout the axial skeleton, left humerus, and faint focal abnormalities in the femora as well.

Differential Diagnosis

- Metastatic neoplastic disease
- Paget's disease (more likely to be considered on earlier images)
- Fibrous dysplasia (more likely to be considered on earlier images)
- Trauma (not as likely when multiple sites of uptake are seen on later images)

Diagnosis and Clinical Follow-up

Metastatic breast cancer with progression of disease.

Discussion

Routine bone scanning during the primary workup of breast cancer is probably not warranted unless there are signs or symptoms that suggest the possibility of metastatic disease.

If the patient has a history of arthritis or other disease involving bone but shows no signs or symptoms of bone metastasis, the benefit of a bone scan is more controversial. The low specificity of the bone scan makes it likely that abnormalities will be detected, in which case a decision must be made concerning the extent to which these abnormalities are to be pursued. Plain film correlation is usually sufficient to diagnose changes secondary to arthritis or previous trauma. Although it is recognized that metastatic disease may be superimposed on arthritic changes, the number of missed lesions does not warrant more extensive testing of all sites of arthritis detected on bone scan.

Suggested Readings

Kwai AH, Stomper PC, Kaplan WD. Clinical significance of isolated scintigraphic stenal lesions in patients with breast cancer. *J Nucl Med* 29:324–328, 1988.

Ohtake E, Murata H, Maruno H. Bone scintigraphy in patients with breast cancer: Malignant involvement of the sternum. *Radiat Med* 12:25–28, 1994.

Case 4

Clinical Presentation

65-year-old man presenting with non–small cell lung carcinoma. A bone scan was obtained for staging.

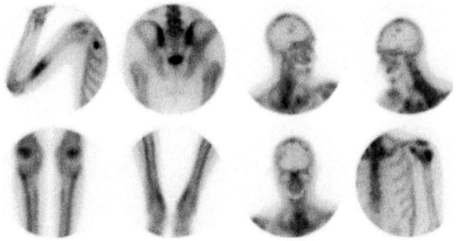

Fig. A

Technique

- 20 mCi technetium-99m–labeled methylene diphosphonate (MDP) intravenously.
- Whole-body or spot images of the skeleton obtained 3 hours after tracer administration.
- Emphasize the importance of oral hydration to improve soft tissue and bladder clearance.

Image Interpretation

Selected spot views (Fig. A) show focal increased activity in the right distal humerus, the left proximal humerus, the skull, and a right upper rib anteriorly. Also noted is diffusely increased activity in the femora and tibiae bilaterally in a "train track" cortical pattern.

Differential Diagnosis

- Metastatic lung cancer
- Lung disease (causing hypertrophic osteoarthropathy) and concommitant trauma or osteomyelitis at sites of focal bony uptake.

Diagnosis and Clinical Follow-up

The findings were thought to be secondary to non–small cell lung cancer with bony metastases and hypertrophic osteoarthropathy (HPO) of the lower extremities.

PEARLS/PITFALLS

- It is not uncommon to see HPO with lung tumors (Fig. B) and in patients with known lung cancer or other malignancies that are known to have spread to the lung.

- Look for asymmetrical tracer uptake in the lung fields. Malignant pleural effusion or focal tumor uptake of tracer may be seen.

- As with all bone scans, careful review of soft tissue uptake should be performed including both kidneys. The patient in Figure B had previously undetected hydronephrosis and horseshoe kidney.

- ^{18}FDG is more accurate for staging lung cancer than computed tomography (CT).

- Areas of decreased tracer uptake due to lytic lesions are more difficult to see than areas of increased uptake.

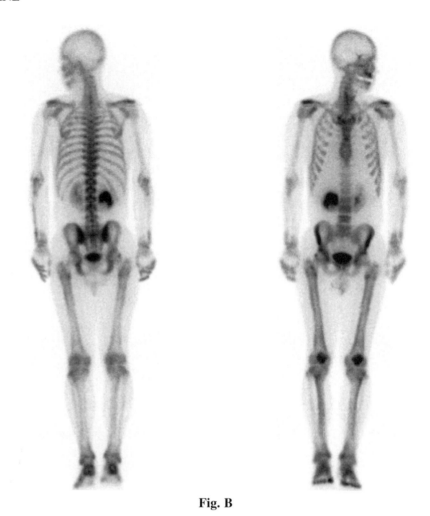

Fig. B

Discussion

Lung cancer does not always show the intensity of the osteoblastic response seen with breast or prostate cancer. Irregular tracer uptake and areas of decreased activity surrounded by osteoblastic activity at the periphery can be seen, as in the skull shown in Figure A. Bone scans should always be surveyed for foci of both decreased and increased uptake.

With prostate and breast cancer, metastases are most likely seen in the axial skeleton, but with lung cancer, metastases can also be seen in the peripheral skeleton.

Suggested Readings

Knight SB, Delbeke D, Stewart JR, et al. Evaluation of pulmonary lesions with FDG-PET. Comparison of findings in patients with and without a history of prior malignancy. *Chest* 109:982–988, 1996.

Patz EF Jr, Lowe VJ, Goodman PC, et al. Thoracic nodal staging with PET imaging with 18FDG in patients with bronchogenic carcinoma. *Chest* 108:1617–1621, 1995.

Sazon DA, Santiago SM, Soo Hoo GW, et al. Fluorodeoxyglucose-positron emission tomography in the detection and staging of lung cancer. *Am J Respir Crit Care Med* 153:417–421, 1996.

Steinert HC, Hauser M, Allemann F, et al. Non–small cell lung cancer: Nodal staging with FDG PET versus CT with correlative lymph node mapping and sampling. *Radiology* 202:441–446, 1997.

Worsley DF, Celler A, Adam MJ, et al. Pulmonary nodules: Differential diagnosis using 18F-fluorodeoxyglucose single-photon emission computed tomography. *AJR Am J Roentgenol* 168:771–774, 1997.

Case 5

Clinical Presentation

31-year-old woman in otherwise good health presenting with back pain. The patient was referred to a neurologist after a lumbar spine lesion was noted on plain films.

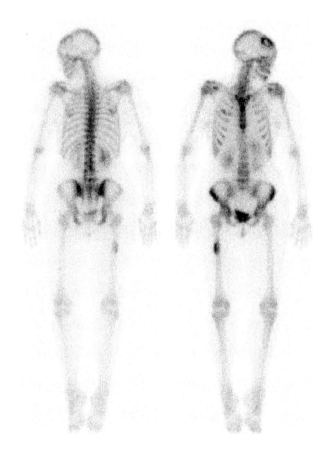

Fig. A

Technique

- 20 mCi technetium-99m–labeled methylene diphosphonate (MDP) intravenously.
- Whole-body or spot images of the skeleton obtained 3 hours after tracer administration.
- Emphasize the importance of oral hydration to improve soft tissue and bladder clearance.

Image Interpretation

Whole-body bone images (Fig. A) show three relatively obvious lesions and two more subtle abnormalities. Areas of increased tracer uptake are noted in the skull, the anterior aspect of the right approximately third rib, and the right femur. The

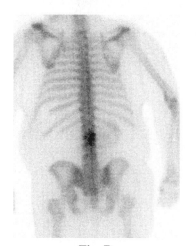

Fig. B

skull lesion has a central area of decreased activity. More subtle findings include a focus of decreased activity in the right side of the lower lumbar spine and an irregular contour of the left kidney.

Differential Diagnosis

- Renal cell carcinoma with bony metastases
- Osteomyelitis (hematogenous spread to multiple bony sites is not common in adults)
- Polyostotic Paget's disease (atypical appearance for Paget's, particularly in skull and femur)
- Concommitant, unrelated bony lesions such as:
  Stress reaction (in femur)
  Trauma (in femur and spine)
  Craniotomy (commonly causes a rim of increased uptake with central photopenia)

Diagnosis and Clinical Follow-up

Computed tomography (CT) scan and magnetic resonance imaging (MRI) demonstrated a large left renal mass. Biopsy revealed renal cell carcinoma. Embolization of the femur and lumbar metastatic lesions was performed with some relief. The patient was referred to an outside institution for follow-up.

Discussion

Bone metastases from renal carcinoma may not demonstrate the marked osteoblastic response seen with breast and prostate metastases. It is common to see areas of little tracer uptake surrounded by a ring of osteoblastic response, as in the skull lesion of this patient. Less than 5% of bone scans performed during the staging workup of renal carcinoma patients are positive. Therefore, the bone scan is more likely to be done during the workup of a symptomatic lesion that was noted on plain film.

Many patients with renal cell carcinoma have already had a nephrectomy by the time the bone scan is obtained. A nephrectomy may be performed with or without removal of one of the lower ribs. Figure B shows a common bone scan appearance in another patient with a history of previously diagnosed renal cell carcinoma. A kidney and an ipsilateral lower rib are missing secondary to nephrectomy.

It should not be assumed that a missing kidney or rib is the result of surgery, however. The patient should be questioned about a surgical history to rule out a nonfunctioning kidney or aggressive metastatic lesion to the rib. Because renal cell carcinoma can be multifocal, careful attention should also be paid to the renal contour on the side contralateral from the known primary tumor.

Suggested Reading

Jacobson AF. Bone scanning in metastatic disease. In: Collier DB, Fogelman I, Rosenthall L, eds. *Skeletal Nuclear Medicine.* St. Louis: Mosby, pp. 87–123, 1996.

Case 6

Clinical Presentation

72-year-old man with a history of metastatic prostate cancer referred for pain in the left shoulder and lower neck.

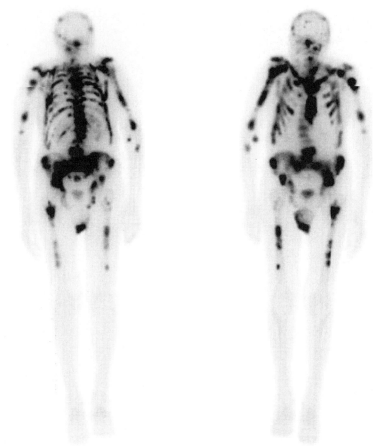

Fig. A

Technique

- 20 mCi technetium-99m–labeled methylene diphosphonate (MDP) intravenously.
- Whole-body or spot images of the skeleton obtained 3 hours after tracer administration.
- Emphasize the importance of oral hydration to improve soft tissue and bladder clearance.

Image Interpretation

Whole-body views (Fig. A) show intense tracer uptake throughout the axial skeleton and proximal portions of the appendicular skeleton. Little uptake is noted in the soft tissues, including the kidneys. A small amount of tracer is noted in the urinary bladder.

Differential Diagnosis

- Widespread, confluent axial skeleton metastases (superscan)

Diagnosis and Clinical Follow-up

Disseminated prostate cancer. Patient previously had received strontium-89 therapy with little improvement in his pain. He was therefore scheduled for external beam therapy to the neck and left shoulder.

Discussion

A bone scan with disseminated, intense uptake is often called a *superscan*. The definition of a superscan is not agreed on universally, however, and the term does not relate to a specific set of findings on bone scintigraphy. Generally, an image is considered a superscan when there is markedly increased uptake in the skeleton that causes diminished soft tissue activity. Faint tracer activity may still be seen in the kidneys and bladder, even when confluent, intense uptake in the axial skeleton is present. As in this case, some superscans show tracer uptake that is heterogeneous enough to identify individual lesions, particularly with the newer cameras that offer better resolution.

Superscans that result from metastatic disease (usually prostate cancer) are characterized by involvement of the axial skeleton (red marrow) as opposed to the appendicular skeleton. Occasionally, these lesions are diffuse and confluent, and the scan may, at first, appear normal. The abnormal increased uptake can be identified by noting the unusually clear appearance of the bony structures, the paucity of soft tissue uptake, and the abrupt cutoff of increased tracer uptake in the proximal, compared with the distal, portions of the appendicular skeleton (Fig. B).

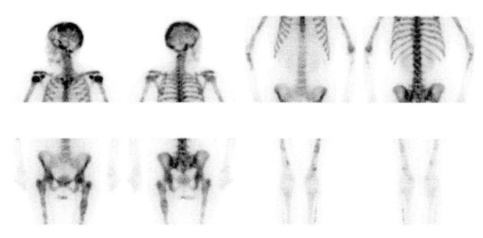

Fig. B

In addition to metastatic disease, hyperparathyroidism or other metabolic diseases that cause rapid bone turnover which may result in a superscan. Metabolic disease, as distinguished from metastatic disease, affects all the bones of the skeleton, resulting in increased tracer uptake evenly throughout the axial and appendicular portions of the skeleton (Fig. C).

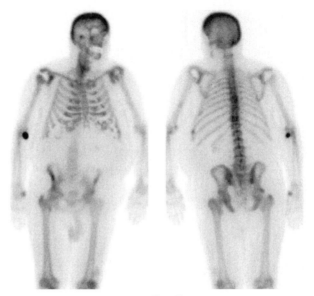

Fig. C

Suggested Readings

Constable AR, Cranage RW. Recognition of the superscan in prostatic bone scintigraphy. *Br J Radiol* 54:122–125, 1981.

Massie JD, Sebes JI. The headless bone scan: An uncommon manifestation of metastatic superscan in carcinoma of the prostate. *Skeletal Radiol* 17:111–113, 1988.

Ohashi K, Smith HS, Jacobs MP. "Superscan" appearance in distal renal tubular acidosis. *Clin Nucl Med* 16:318–320, 1991.

Sy WM. Bone scan in primary hyperparathyroidism. *J Nucl Med* 15:1089–1091, 1974.

Sy WM, Patel D, Faunce H. Significance of absent or faint kidney sign on bone scan. *J Nucl Med* 16:454–456, 1975.

Case 7

Clinical Presentation

93-year-old man presenting with a history of colon cancer.

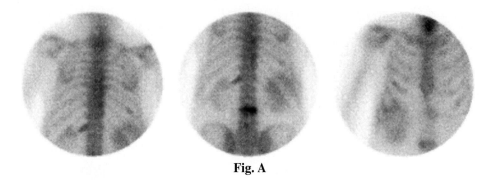

Fig. A

Technique

- 20 mCi technetium-99m–labeled methylene diphosphonate (MDP) intravenously.
- Whole-body or spot images of the skeleton obtained 3 hours after tracer administration.
- Emphasize the importance of oral hydration to improve soft tissue and bladder clearance.

Image Interpretation

Three selected spot views (Fig. A) demonstrate tracer uptake in the lumbar spine, a lower left costovertebral junction, and the right upper quadrant of the abdomen.

Differential Diagnosis

(uptake in the right upper quadrant of the abdomen):

- Hepatic metastasis
- Soft tissue tracer uptake secondary to metastatic calcification, superimposed on liver
- Prior radiocolloid scan
- Colloid formation during radiopharmaceutical preparation
- Hepatic necrosis
- Metastatic calcification in the liver

Diagnosis and Clinical Follow-up

The bony abnormalities were secondary to metastatic colon cancer. The uptake in the right upper quadrant was secondary to metastatic disease in the liver.

- The symmetry of tracer distribution in the soft tissues of the abdomen and chest should be reviewed on all studies. Faint uptake in the liver or in a pleural effusion may be caused by metastatic disease.

- The metastatic soft tissue uptake in this case could be mistaken for asymmetrical renal uptake. Asymmetry of uptake in the region of the liver should be carefully reviewed before it is dismissed.

Discussion

Bone scans are insensitive for soft tissue metastases, yet all scans should include a survey of the soft tissues, especially when the patient is referred for staging of metastatic disease. Uptake noted in the soft tissues on bone scan can be the first indication of metastatic disease.

Suggested Readings

Peller PJ, Ho VB, Kransdorf MJ. Extraosseous Tc-99m MDP uptake: A pathophysiologic approach. *Radiographics* 13:715–734, 1993.

Petersen M. Radionuclide detection of primary pulmonary osteogenic sarcoma: A case report and review of the literature. *J Nucl Med* 31:1110–1114, 1990.

Pickhardt PJ, McDermott M. Intense uptake of technetium-99m-MDP in primary breast adenocarcinoma with sarcomatoid metaplasia. *J Nucl Med* 38:528–530, 1997.

Case 8

Clinical Presentation

78-year-old male with a history of colon cancer presenting with knee pain.

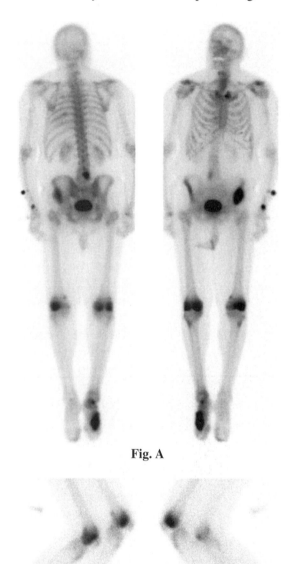

Fig. A

Fig. B

Technique

- 20 mCi technetium-99m–labeled methylene diphosphonate (MDP) intravenously.
- Whole-body or spot images of the skeleton obtained 3 hours after tracer administration.
- Emphasize the importance of oral hydration to improve soft tissue and bladder clearance.
- Lateral spot views of the knees were obtained.

Image Interpretation

Whole-body (Fig. A) and spot views of the knees (Fig. B) show mildly increased activity posteriorly in approximately the eighth right rib and intense, focally increased tracer uptake in the lumbar spine at approximately L4 and L5, in the region of the anterior iliac crest on the left, in the distal femora bilaterally, and in the midfoot on the right. The injection site is noted at the intravenous access in the left distal forearm.

Differential Diagnosis

- Metastatic disease
- Trauma
- Degenerative joint disease
- Paget's disease
- Fibrous dysplasia
- Avascular necrosis (of knees)
- Skin contamination (particularly at the foot)

Diagnosis and Clinical Follow-up

The rib abnormality was diagnosed as secondary to recent open thoracotomy and biopsy of a lung mass. Computed tomography (CT) scan showed the left iliac crest uptake was in the soft tissues and was consistent with myositis ossificans. (Patient had a history of previous surgical procedure in this area.) On CT, the lumbar spine was read as degenerative disease. Magnetic resonance imaging (MRI) of the lumbar spine later demonstrated marrow abnormalities consistent with metastatic disease in the same location as the bone scan abnormality. It is important to note that the knee findings were largely confined to the distal femora and did not involve the tibial surfaces, decreasing the likelihood of degenerative disease. On MRI, the knees showed osteonecrosis. The right foot lesion was biopsied and was demonstrated to be secondary to metastatic colon cancer.

Discussion

Several important points are illustrated by this study. First, bone scans are very sensitive for abnormalities but are not very specific. The rib abnormality was caused by trauma, the pelvis abnormality was benign, the knee abnormalities were secondary to ischemia, and the spine and foot abnormalities were secondary to malignant disease. The bone uptake at any of these sites could be caused by a variety of diseases. The pattern of bone uptake may suggest a particular disease, but the scintigraphic findings must be correlated with other tests as well as with history and physical exam.

Second, the CT scan directed at the bone scan finding in the lumbar spine was read as consistent with degenerative disease. It is clear from the intensity and focus of the uptake on bone scan, however, that the finding is not typical of degenerative disease. If the physician reading the CT scan had also looked at the bone scan, he or she might have been less likely to dismiss the reported bone scan findings when the CT scan showed changes typical of degenerative disease in the same region of the spine.

The final point is that, although it is always a good idea to try to relate all findings to one disease process, if there is any question of the cause of a number of abnormalities noted on a single bone scan, the abnormalities should all be pursued individually rather than diagnosing the cause of one abnormality and attributing the same disease process to the others.

Suggested Readings

Bordy Z, Pasztarak E, Bansagi G, et al. Soft-tissue involvement by adenocarcinoma imaged during bone scintigraphy. *Clin Nucl Med* 22:508, 1997.

Drane WE. Myositis ossificans and the three-phase bone scan. *AJR Am J Roentgenol* 142:179–180, 1984.

Nisolle JF, Delaunois L, Trigaux JP. Myositis ossificans of the chest wall. *Eur Respir J* 9:178–179, 1996.

Stuckey SL. Colonic adenocarcinoma metastatic to bone with gross heterotopic bone formation. Bone scan appearance with correlative imaging. *Clin Nucl Med* 21:396–397, 1996.

Sud AM, Wilson MW, Mountz JM. Unusual clinical presentation and scintigraphic pattern in myositis ossificans. *Clin Nucl Med* 17:198–199, 1992.

Case 9

Clinical Presentation

51-year-old woman presenting with leiomyosarcoma.

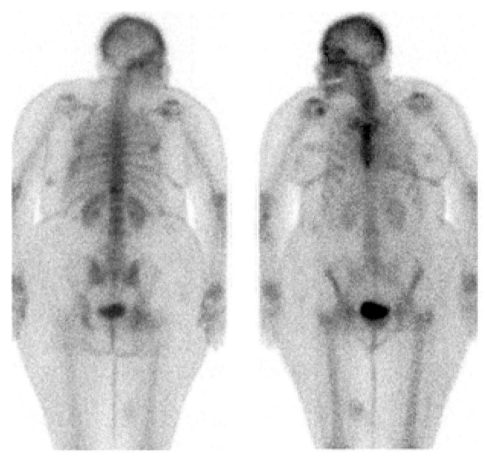

Fig. A

Technique

- 20 mCi technetium-99m–labeled methylene diphosphonate (MDP) intravenously.
- Whole-body or spot images of the skeleton obtained 3 hours after tracer administration.
- Emphasize the importance of oral hydration to improve soft tissue and bladder clearance.

Image Interpretation

Whole-body anterior and posterior views (Figs. A and B) show tracer uptake in the right shoulder but also in the soft tissues of the right thigh medially and the right and left flanks.

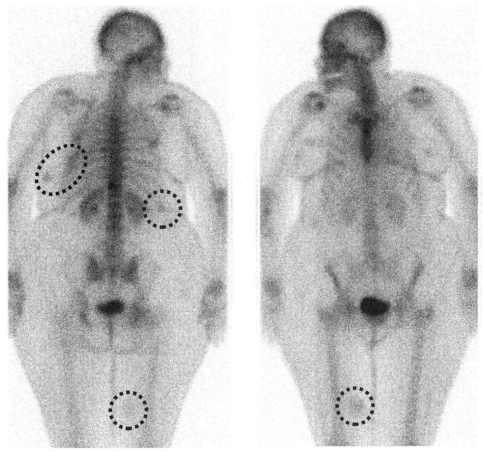

Fig. B

Differential Diagnosis

- Soft tissue metastases
- Cellulitis
- Soft tissue trauma
- Primary soft tissue tumor
- Skin contamination
- Soft tissue abcess

Diagnosis and Clinical Follow-up

Computed tomography (CT) scan (Figs. C and D) demonstrates disseminated disease, including a $7 \times 7 \times 3$ cm soft tissue mass in the posterior aspect of the left chest wall and in the soft tissues of the right flank, lateral to the kidney. There were also numerous nodules in the lungs and axillae.

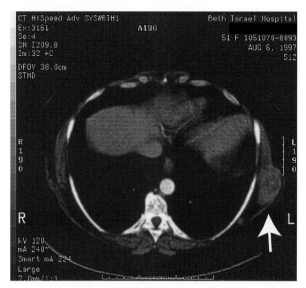

Fig. C

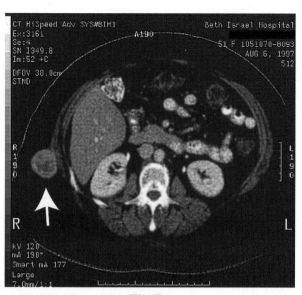

Fig. D

Discussion

Uptake of bone radiopharmaceuticals in soft tissue metastasis is important and should be reported when detected with bone scanning. Bone tracer uptake in soft tissues is not very sensitive, however, as illustrated by this patient, in whom only the largest soft tissue metastases were noted. The majority of the lesions in the lungs, abdomen, and axillae were not detected.

Suggested Reading

Peller PJ, Ho VB, Kransdorf MJ. Extraosseous Tc-99m MDP uptake: A pathophysiologic approach. *Radiographics* 13:715–734, 1993.

Case 10

Clinical Presentation

68-year-old woman presenting with low back pain.

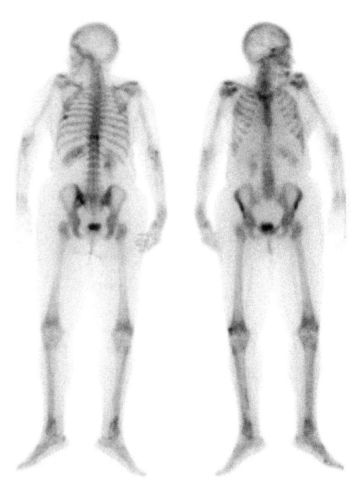

Fig. A

Technique

- 20 mCi technetium-99m–labeled methylene diphosphonate (MDP) intravenously.
- Whole-body or spot images of the skeleton obtained 3 hours after tracer administration.
- Emphasize oral hydration to improve soft tissue and bladder clearance.

Image Interpretation

Whole-body images demonstrated increased focal uptake in a left rib and in the spine at approximately T-10. A focus of *decreased* uptake is noted in the inferior aspect of the left sacroiliac (SI) joint with adjacent increased activity in the upper portion of the left SI joint.

Differential Diagnosis

- Metastatic disease (e.g., lung, thyroid, or renal cancer or multiple myeloma; less likely to be seen with prostate or breast cancer)
- Attenuation artifact (keys or coins in pocket, jewelry, pacemaker overlying chest wall)
- Prosthetic joint (hip, knee)
- Avascular necrosis
- Prior surgery (e.g., rib resection)
- Early osteomyelitis
- Bone infarct from sickle cell disease
- Benign tumor (e.g., hemangioma)
- Bone cyst
- Pixel overflow
- Camera defect (e.g., crystal, photomultiplier tube, or collimator defect)

Diagnosis and Clinical Follow-up

The diagnosis was metastatic lung cancer. Computed tomography scan showed multiple nodules in the lungs and liver. Lytic lesions were also noted in the spine and left SI joint.

Discussion

As noted before, focal cold defects noted on bone scans can have many causes, from malignant to benign to artifactual. The malignancies that most commonly warrant bone scanning—prostate and breast cancer—rarely cause cold defects because of the intense osteoblastic response often associated with these tumors. Even if plain radiographs demonstrate "lytic" lesions (in tumors other than multiple myeloma), the bone scan is likely to demonstrate an area of increased tracer uptake caused by osteoblasts attempting to repair the bony injury.

Suggested Readings

Bataille R, Chevalier J, Rossi M, Sany J. Bone scintigraphy in plasma-cell myeloma. A prospective study of 70 patients. *Radiology* 145:801–804, 1982.

Berruti A, Piovesan A, Torta M, et al. Biochemical evaluation of bone turnover in cancer patients with bone metastases: Relationship with radiograph appearances and disease extension. *Br J Cancer* 73:1581–1587, 1996.

Kagan AR, Steckel RJ, Bassett LW. Diagnostic oncology case study: Lytic spine lesion and cold bone scan. *AJR Am J Roentgenol* 136:129–131, 1981.

Otsuka N, Fukunaga M, Morita K, Ono S, Nagai K. Photon-deficient finding in sternum on bone scintigraphy in patients with malignant disease. *Radiat Med* 8:168–172, 1990.

Weingrad T, Heyman S, Alavi A. Cold lesions on bone scan in pediatric neoplasms. *Clin Nucl Med* 9:125–130, 1984.

Case 11

Clinical Presentation

51-year-old man recently diagnosed with hepatoma and presenting with low back pain.

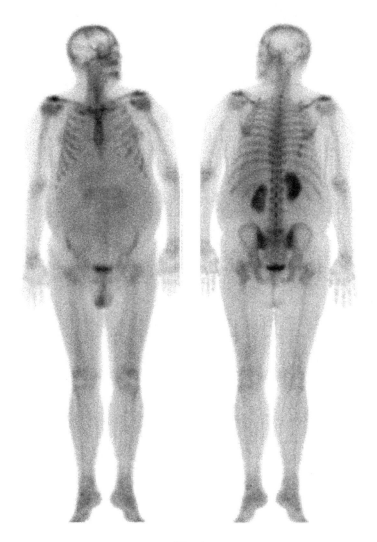

Fig. A

Technique

- 20 mCi technetium-99m–labeled methylene diphosphonate (MDP) intravenously.
- Whole-body or spot images of the skeleton obtained 3 hours after tracer administration.
- Emphasize oral hydration to improve soft tissue and bladder clearance.

Image Interpretation

Whole-body images demonstrate diffuse tracer uptake in the abdomen. Slightly more intense uptake is noted in the region of the left lobe of the liver. Also seen are two foci of increased activity in approximately the eighth and ninth right ribs posteriorly and uptake at approximately L5.

Differential Diagnosis

• Nonspecific uptake within hepatic tumor
• Ascites (or other exudative effusion)
• Renal failure (although this would also cause diffuse soft tissue uptake throughout the extremities)

Diagnosis and Clinical Follow-up

The diagnosis was hepatoma with ascites. The diffuse uptake in the abdomen is secondary to ascites. Bony remodeling at L5 may be related to the cause of the lower back pain. Follow-up radiographs were not obtained because the back pain improved spontaneously.

Discussion

Diffuse uptake of tracer in a body cavity, such as the pleural space or the abdominal cavity, is often secondary to tracer accumulation in an effusion. The tracer is more likely to accumulate in an exudative effusion caused by malignancy, but exudates can also be seen with inflammatory processes.

Suggested Reading

Kida T, Hujita Y, Sasaki M, Inoue J. Accumulation of 99mTc methylene diphosphonate in malignant pleural and ascitic effusion. *Oncology* 41:427–430, 1984.

Case 12

Clinical Presentation

71-year-old woman with history of breast cancer. Bone scan requested to assess bony metastasis.

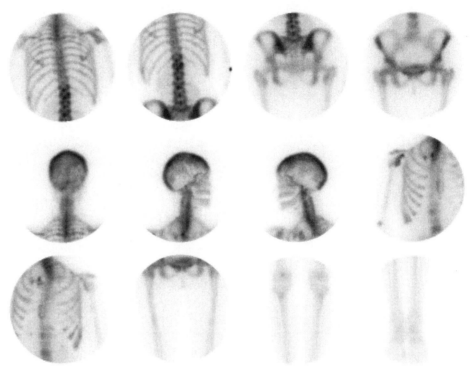

Fig. A

Technique

- 20 mCi technetium-99m–labeled methylene diphosphonate (MDP) intravenously.
- Whole-body or spot images of the skeleton obtained 3 hours after tracer administration.
- Emphasize oral hydration to improve soft tissue and bladder clearance.

Image Interpretation

Multiple spot images of the skeleton demonstrated abrupt decreased tracer activity in the upper thoracic region down to approximately T11. Increased activity is noted throughout the remainder of the axial skeleton.

Differential Diagnosis

- Radiation therapy
- Prosthetic implant

- Attenuation artifact
- Electrical burn
- Severe vascular disease

Diagnosis and Clinical Follow-up

Disseminated breast cancer with metastases throughout the spine and ribs was documented on computed tomography scan and magnetic resonance imaging. The patient had received previous radiation therapy to the thoracic region of the spine.

Discussion

Radiation therapy should be considered as a cause of diminished bony tracer uptake, particularly when the pattern of diminished uptake approximates the size and location of a known radiation port. When considering the frequency with which bone scans are obtained in patients who have had radiation therapy, however, it is not often we see diminished tracer uptake. In this patient, visualization of the radiation port was certainly enhanced by the surrounding disseminated disease. What we are seeing as an area of "diminished" activity may actually be one of the few skeletal regions where the bony metastatic disease has responded to therapy.

Suggested Readings

Ahluwalia R, Morton KA, Whiting JH Jr, Menzel-Anderson C, Datz FL. Scintigraphic appearance of bone during external beam irradiation. *Clin Nucl Med* 19:385–387, 1994.

Cox PH. Abnormalities in skeletal uptake of 99Tcm polyphosphate complexes in areas of bone associated with tissues which have been subjected to radiation therapy. *Br. J Radiol* 47:851–856, 1974.

Israel O, Gorenberg M, Frenkel A, et al. Local and systemic effects of radiation on bone metabolism measured by quantitative SPECT. *J Nucl Med* 33:1774–1780, 1992.

King MA, Casarett GW, Weber DA. A study of irradiated bone. I. histopathologic and physiologic changes. *J Nucl Med* 20:1142–1149, 1979.

King MA, Weber DA, Casarett GW, Burgener FA, Corriveau O. A study of irradiated bone. Part II. Changes in Tc-99m pyrophosphate bone imaging. *J Nucl Med* 21:22–30, 1980.

Case 13

Clinical Presentation

37-year-old woman with a history of sickle cell disease and a hip prosthesis presenting with increasing right hip pain.

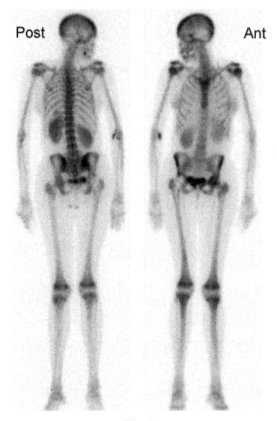

Fig. A

Technique

- If osteomyelitis is suspected, acquire blood flow and blood pool images of the area of interest. Flow is obtained during tracer injection. Images are collected for 1 minute at approximately 1 second per frame. Blood pool images are obtained immediately after flow images and must be obtained within 10 minutes after tracer injection.
- If osteomyelitis is not suspected, the imaging technique is no different from that used in standard bone imaging (see Case 1).

Image Interpretation

The bone image (Fig. A) shows slight irregularity in the ribs posteriorly and relatively increased tracer concentration in the metaphyses of the long bones. Also noted on the posterior image are relatively large kidneys and a suggestion of tracer concentration in a small, infarcted spleen, just above the left kidney. A right hip prosthesis is also noted.

PEARLS/PITFALLS

- Tracer uptake in an infarcted spleen may be very slight and difficult to distinguish from the kidney below.

- Increased uptake on bone scan is not specific for infarct or osteomyelitis and may be caused by a number of conditions described previously. Correlative imaging with gallium, radiolabeled white blood cells, or magnetic resonance imaging (MRI) is often needed.

- The appearance of bony lesions varies from decreased activity in acute infarct to increased tracer activity in infarcts undergoing repair. Knowledge of the history of the disease is important in scan interpretation.

- Small acute infarcts in areas subject to AVN may not be seen adequately with the bone scan. When in doubt, the patient should be referred for MRI.

Differential Diagnosis

(multiple bony foci of increased and decreased activity):

- Sickle cell disease
- Metastatic disease to the bone (particularly multiple myeloma, lung cancer, renal cancer, thyroid cancer)
- Attenuating artifact in a patient with osteoblastic metastasis (pacemaker, belt buckle, coins in pocket, prosthesis)
- Decreased bony activity secondary to radiation therapy in a patient with bony metastatic disease
- Multifocal osteomyelitis
- Photomultiplier tube defects (incorrect photopeak, faulty photomultiplier tube)

Diagnosis and Clinical Follow-up

The patient had known sickle cell disease. No follow-up was obtained.

Discussion

Bone scans in patients with sickle cell disease can show several characteristic findings. In this patient, expansion of the red marrow resulted in increased tracer uptake in the metaphyseal regions of the long bones. Tracer uptake in an infarcted spleen was also noted just above the kidney on the left, as was decreased tracer activity in the right hip secondary to the presence of a hip prosthesis. Avascular necrosis (AVN) of the hip is a frequent complication of sickle cell disease, occurring in as many as 41% of patients.

Depending on the age of the patient, it is not uncommon to see tracer uptake in old infarcted areas and decreased uptake in acutely infarcted areas, as seen in the selected spot views of Figure B. Regions with active bone repair at sites of old infarcts, healing ischemic lesions, or osteomyelitis are difficult to distinguish on bone scintigraphy alone. Correlative imaging with gallium-67 citrate or indium-111–labeled white blood cells is often necessary to diagnose concurrent osteomyelitis.

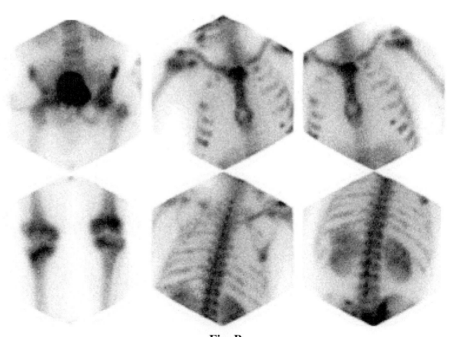

Fig. B

Suggested Readings

Heck LL, Brittin GM. Splenic uptake of both technetium-99m diphosphonate and technetium-99m sulfur colloid in sickle cell beta degrees thalassemia. *Clin Nucl Med* 14:557–563, 1989.

Kahn CE Jr, Ryan JW, Hatfield MK, et al. Combined bone marrow and gallium imaging. Differentiation of osteomyelitis and infarction in sickle hemoglobinopathy. *Clin Nucl Med* 13:443–449, 1988.

Mandell GA. Imaging in the diagnosis of musculoskeletal infections in children. *Curr Probl Pediatr* 26:218–237, 1996.

Milner PF, Kraus AP, Sebes JI, et al. Sickle cell disease as a cause of osteonecrosis of the femoral head. *N Engl J Med* 325:1476–1481, 1991.

Ware HE, Brooks AP, Toye R, et al. Sickle cell disease and silent avascular necrosis of the hip. *J Bone Joint Surg Br* 73:947–949, 1991.

Case 14

Clinical Presentation

54-year-old man with history of sickle cell disease complaining of pain in his left thigh. A bone scan and radiographs of the femur were obtained to assess bone infarct versus osteomyelitis.

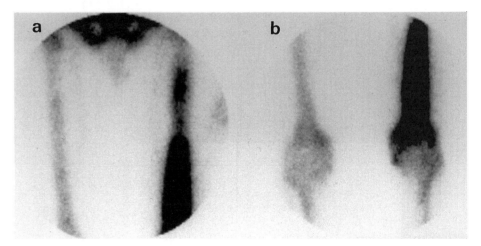

Figs. A, B

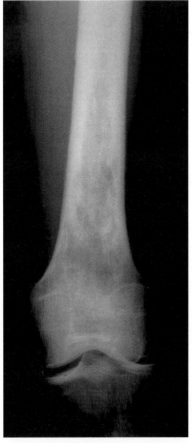

Fig. C

Technique

- 24 mCi technetium-99m-methylene diphosphonate (MDP) administered intravenously.
- Low-energy all-purpose collimator.
- Energy setting is 20% centered at 140 keV.
- Planar views of the lower extremities obtained 3 to 4 hours after tracer injection.

Image Interpretation

Anterior spot views of the left midshaft (Fig. A) and distal left femur (Fig. B) reveal diffuse intense tracer uptake involving the femoral shaft and the lateral and medial femoral condyles. There is no extension of tracer activity to the tibia. An anteroposterior radiograph of the left distal femur (Fig. C) demonstrates diffuse sclerosis in most of the femoral shaft. There is also periosteal thickening, endosteal scalloping, and fluffy calcifications in the distal femur.

Differential Diagnosis

- Bone/bone marrow infarction
- Osteomyelitis

Diagnosis and Clinical Follow-up

The diagnosis was bone infarction. Fine needle aspiration of the left femur was consistent with sickle cell disease. No organisms were seen on special stains.

Discussion

Patients with sickle cell anemia are susceptible to infarction in the bone and bone marrow. If the involvement is primarily in the bone marrow space, the bone scan may be normal in the acute phase but typically shows increased tracer uptake during the healing phase. An alternative approach is to perform bone marrow scanning with technetium-99m sulfur colloid, which is very sensitive for the detection of bone marrow infarction, specifically following the acute event. Affected areas fail to accumulate tracer and are seen as a cold or photon-deficient area on technetium-99m sulfur colloid scan.

Suggested Readings

Burke TS, Tatum JL, Fratkin MJ. Radionuclide bone imaging findings in recurrent calcaneal infarction in sickle cell disease. *J Nucl Med* 29:411–413, 1988.

Kim HC, Alar A, Russell MO, et al. Differentiation of bone and bone marrow infarcts from osteomyelitis in sickle cell disorders. *Clin Nucl Med* 14:249–254, 1989.

Van Zanten TEG, Stratuis Van EPS Lw, Golding RP, et al. Imaging the bone marrow with magnetic resonance during a crisis and in chronic forms of sickle cell disease. *Clin Radiol* 40:486–489, 1989.

Case 15

Clinical Presentation

52-year-old man presenting with elevated alkaline phosphatase on routine physical exam. He was asymptomatic and had no history of malignancy.

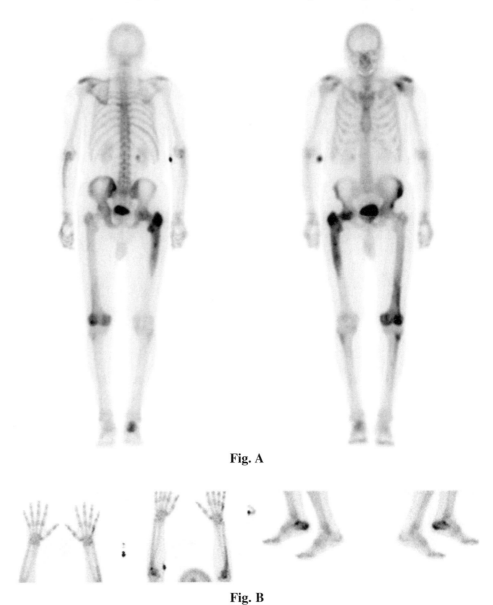

Fig. A

Fig. B

Technique

- 20 mCi technetium-99m–labeled methylene diphosphonate (MDP) intravenously.
- Whole-body or spot images of the skeleton should be obtained 3 hours after tracer administration.
- Emphasize the importance of oral hydration to improve soft tissue and bladder clearance.

PEARLS/PITFALLS

- Correlative imaging, such as with plain radiographs, should always be obtained. Despite the typical scintigraphic appearance of Paget's disease, other diseases, such as osteosarcoma, can show a similar appearance.

- Serum alkaline phosphatase levels do not necessarily reflect the extent of disease activity noted on bone scan.

- Uptake in an entire (anterior and posterior elements) vertebral body is a clue that the cause is more likely to be Paget's disease rather than metastatic disease.

- Focal progression of symptoms should also be followed with radiographs to rule out the development of osteosarcoma.

Image Interpretation

Whole-body (Fig. A) and spot images (Fig. B) demonstrate increased tracer uptake diffusely in the proximal right femur, the distal left femur, the left hemipelvis, the left scapula, the proximal left ulna, and the right calcaneus. More focal increased tracer uptake is noted at the level of approximately T7 and the left proximal tibia.

Differential Diagnosis

(intense tracer uptake occupying a large area in one or more bones):

- Paget's disease
- Primary bone tumor
- Fibrous dysplasia
- Intensely osteoblastic metastases (e.g., prostate, breast cancer)

Diagnosis and Clinical Follow-up

Radiographs demonstrated Paget's disease. The patient remained stable. Repeat bone scan obtained almost 3 years later (Fig. C), when the patient returned with increased symptoms of sciatica, demonstrated markedly decreased tracer uptake at sites previously demonstrating avid tracer uptake. The patient was subsequently diagnosed with spinal stenosis.

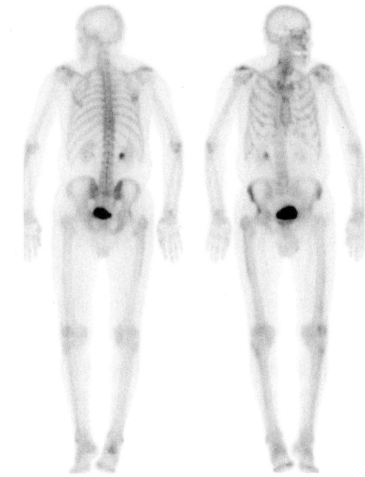

Fig. C

Discussion

The bone scan is the most sensitive imaging study available for the diagnosis of Paget's disease and is characterized by marked uptake at sites of active disease. Serial bone scintigraphy is seldom performed, and therefore the scintigraphic evolution of Paget's disease has not been well-documented.

Suggested Reading

Fogelman I, Ryan PJ. Bone scanning in Paget's disease. In: Collier BD, Fogelman I, Rosenthall L, eds. *Skeletal Nuclear Medicine*. New York: Mosby, pp. 171–181, 1996.

Case 16

Clinical Presentation

74-year-old man presenting with prostate cancer. A bone scan was requested to rule out metastasis.

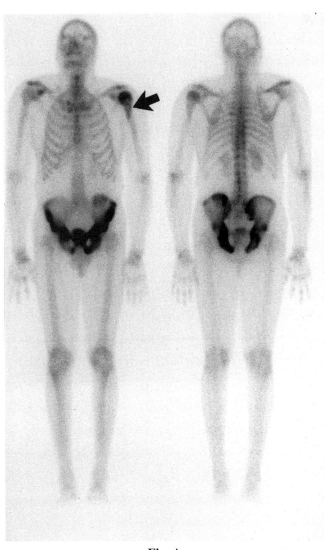

Fig. A

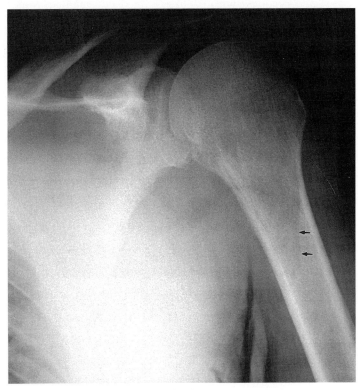

Fig. B

Technique

- 24 mCi technetium-99m–labeled methylene diphosphonate (MDP) administered intravenously.
- Low-energy high-resolution collimator.
- Energy setting is 20% centered at 140 keV.
- Imaging for whole-body planar image in anterior and posterior projections obtained 3 to 4 hours after tracer injection. Camera speed is 10 cm/min.

- Changes occurring over a short period of time on follow-up bone scans might not be due to Paget's disease, and other pathologies should be considered.

- To rule out fracture in a bone already involved with Paget's disease, magnetic resonance imaging is more useful than a bone scan.

- If malignant change is suspected in a patient with known Paget's disease, radiographic investigation is required.

- Sarcomatous changes in a bone already involved with Paget's disease may be photopenic; gallium scan often shows increased tracer uptake in the photopenic region.

- The sharp margin of tracer uptake in the humerus in the case presented here is suggestive of Paget's disease rather than infection.

Image Interpretation

Whole-body planar images (Fig. A) in the anterior (left) and posterior (right) projections show heterogeneous increased tracer uptake throughout the pelvis. There is also increased tracer uptake in the left proximal humerus with sharp lower margin (*arrow*). An anteroposterior radiograph (Fig. B) of the left shoulder shows a radiolucent area in the proximal humerus beginning in the head and ending in a wedge-shaped edge (blade of grass) suggestive of the osteolytic stage of Paget's disease (*arrows*).

Differential Diagnosis

- Paget's disease
- Tumor
- Fracture
- Osteomyelitis

Diagnosis and Clinical Follow-up

The diagnosis was Paget's disease. No clinical follow-up was available for this patient.

Discussion

Paget's disease is often an incidental finding on bone scans. The increased uptake is seen in both the early resorptive, or lucent, phase and the proliferative, or sclerotic, phase. The incidence of malignant transformation in pagetoid bone is low. When the patient complains of pain in the involved bone, however, further evaluation for malignant transformation is warranted.

Suggested Readings

Serafini AN. Paget's disease of bone. *Semin Nucl Med* 6:47–58, 1976.

Smith J, Botet JF, Yeh DSJ. Bone sarcomas in Paget's disease: A study of 85 patients. *Radiology* 152:583–590, 1984.

Case 17

Clinical Presentation

63-year-old man with a history of prostate cancer presenting with increasing alkaline phosphatase and left chest wall pain.

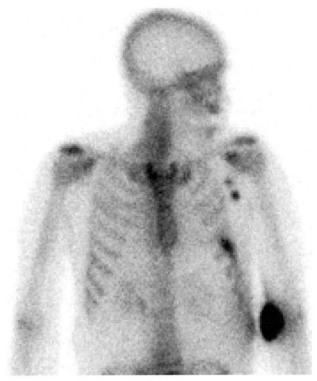

Fig. A

Technique

- 20 mCi technetium-99m–labeled methylene diphosphonate (MDP) intravenously.
- Whole-body or spot images of the skeleton obtained 3 hours after tracer administration.
- Emphasize importance of oral hydration to improve soft tissue and bladder clearance.

Image Interpretation

The selected anterior view of the chest (Fig. A) shows increased tracer uptake in the left axilla and in a left rib laterally. A large area of infiltrated tracer is seen in the left antecubital region.

Differential Diagnosis

(focal soft tissue uptake of tracer):

PEARLS/PITFALLS

- Infiltration of the injected dose is easily diagnosed by imaging the injection site.

- If the infiltrated injection site is just out of the field of view, narrow angle scatter from the high activity in the injection site can be mistaken for tracer concentration in the superficial soft tissues of the body adjacent to the injection (as in the lower left ribs in Fig. A).

- Focal uptake in the lateral portions of the breasts can also be mistaken for axillary nodal uptake.

- Nodal uptake can also be caused by malignancy. Uptake in axillary nodes should be definitively demonstrated to be proximal to an infiltrated injection site before discounted as unimportant.

- Accumulation of tracer in axillary node secondary to infiltration at injection site.
- Contamination (clothing, skin surface, camera face, imaging table)
- Injection site
- Normal breast uptake
- Soft tissue injury (cellulitis, abcess, electrical burn)
- Adenocarcinoma metastatic to soft tissues (e.g., colon, lung)
- Primary soft tissue tumor (benign or malignant)
- Vascular calcification
- Previous intramuscular injections (e.g., demerol, iron dextran)

Diagnosis and Clinical Follow-up

There was infiltration of tracer injection with subsequent tracer migration to the ipsilateral axillary lymph node. The rib abnormality was found to be secondary to a lytic metastatic lesion.

Discussion

Soft tissue uptake of tracer is occasionally seen in bone scans for a number of reasons, including metastatic disease. One of the more common causes of soft tissue uptake is axillary nodal uptake secondary to lymphatic drainage from an infiltrated tracer injection. This is usually easily identified when the injection site is imaged. If no infiltrate is seen at the injection site or the injection site is in the contralateral arm, further investigation of the nodal uptake is warranted.

Suggested Reading

Datz FL. *Gamuts in Nuclear Medicine.* 2nd ed. Norwalk, CT: Appleton & Lange, 1987.

Case 18

Clinical Presentation

82-year-old woman presenting with lung cancer, hypercalcemia, and bone pain.

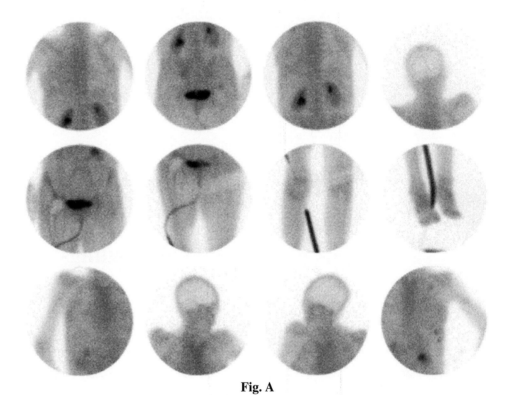

Fig. A

Technique

- 20 mCi technetium-99m–labeled methylene diphosphonate (MDP) intravenously.
- Whole-body or spot images of the skeleton obtained 3 hours after tracer administration.
- Emphasize importance of oral hydration to improve soft tissue and bladder clearance.

Image Interpretation

Spot views of the body (Fig. A) show minimal bone uptake and obvious urinary excretion of technetium-99m–labeled MDP.

Differential Diagnosis

(poor tracer uptake in bone):

- Incorrect radiopharmaceutical administered or incorrect preparation of bony tracer

PEARLS/PITFALLS

- Poor localization of radiotracer to bone (or any target organ) can occur for a number of reasons. When a bone scan or any other type of scan shows unusual distribution of the radiopharmaceutical, the cause should be investigated and the reason documented.

- If a patient has a known history of hypercalcemia or bone pain, however, consider questioning the patient about other medications prior to injecting the radiopharmaceutical.

- Even if some bone uptake of tracer is seen, the bone scan should still not be considered a reliable study to rule out metastatic disease during concurrent therapy with some bisphosphonates. It is possible that the phosphonate will preferentially diminish tracer uptake at sites of more active osteoblastic activity, decreasing the sensitivity of the bone scan for metastases.

- Some bisphosphonates, such as etidronate, clearly interfere with the bone scan; others may not. More investigation is needed, particularly of the newer agents.

- The time a patient needs to be off each of the bisphosphonates prior to the bone scan is not known.

- Medications interfering with bony uptake of tracer (e.g., etidronate)
- Iron overload
- Poor hydration

Diagnosis and Clinical Follow-up

Concurrent etidronate therapy was being performed at the time of the injection of the bone tracer. No other follow-up was available.

Discussion

Diffuse tracer distribution in the soft tissues with poor definition of bony structures is most commonly seen in dehydrated patients and occasionally when the radiopharmaceutical is not properly prepared and in patients with end-stage renal dysfunction. The marked lack of bone uptake demonstrated by this patient, however, is more than would be expected in dehydration, and the prominent appearance in the urinary collecting system makes renal failure unlikely.

Etidronate (used to treat bone pain or hypercalcemia) binds to the exposed hydroxyapatite crystal surface of bone. The overwhelming amount of therapeutic etidronate floods the available hydroxyapatite binding sites, preventing the tracer quantity of technetium-99m-MDP from localizing to bone. The radiolabeled MDP, therefore, diffuses throughout the soft tissues before it is excreted in the urine.

Suggested Readings

Koizumi M, Ogata E. Bisphosphonate effect on bone scintigraphy. *J Nucl Med* 37:401, 1996. Letter.

Koyano H, Schimizu T, Shishiba Y. The bisphosphonate dilemma [see comments]. *J Nucl Med* 36:705, 1995. Letter.

Pecherstorfer M, Schilling T, Janisch S, et al. Effect of clodronate treatment on bone scintigraphy in metastatic breast cancer [see comments]. *J Nucl Med* 34:1039–1044, 1993.

Case 19

Clinical Presentation

73-year-old woman presenting with pleuritic chest pain.

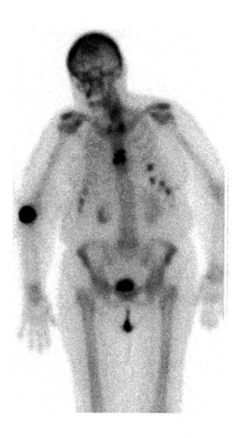

Fig. A

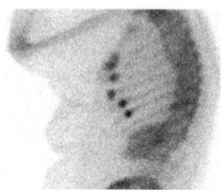

Fig. B

Technique

- 20 mCi technetium-99m–labeled methylene diphosphonate (MDP) intra-venously.

- Whole-body or spot images of the skeleton obtained 3 hours after tracer administration.
- Emphasize importance of oral hydration to improve soft tissue and bladder clearance.

Image Interpretation

Figure A is an anterior view of the upper bony skeleton demonstrating intense tracer uptake at the costochondral junctions of several lower ribs bilaterally and in the midsternum. Figure B is a left lateral view of the chest, confirming the location of the abnormalities in the ribs and sternum.

Differential Diagnosis

(adjacent focal abnormalites in adjacent ribs)

- Trauma
- Surgical resection
- Local extension of invasive chest wall lesion (usually associated with destruction of adjacent portions of the ribs)
- Pooling of tracer in underlying renal calyces (for T-11 and T-12 ribs posteriorly)

Diagnosis and Clinical Follow-up

The focal uptake in several adjacent ribs is most consistent with trauma. The symmetry of the abnormalities and the uptake in the sternum suggest the trauma was caused by a blow to the anterior aspect of the chest. This patient had a cardiorespiratory arrest in the emergency room several days prior to the study and cardiopulmonary resuscitation was performed in the emergency room.

Discussion

The pattern of uptake in bony abnormalities provides some information about the cause of the abnormalities. Focal uptake in several adjacent ribs in the absence of other findings suggests trauma.

Suggested Reading

Stomper PC, Kaplan WD. Clinical significance of isolated scintigraphic sternal lesions in patients with breast cancer. *J Nucl Med* 29:324–328, 1988.

Case 20

Clinical Presentation

55-year-old man with a history of benign prostatic hyperplasia (BPH), presenting with elevated prostate specific antigen (PSA).

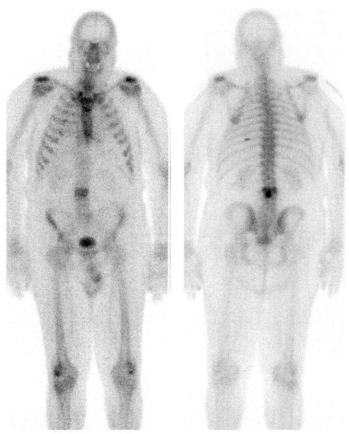

Fig. A

Technique

- 20 mCi technetium-99m–labeled methylene diphosphonate (MDP) intravenously.
- Whole-body or spot images of the skeleton obtained 3 hours after tracer administration.
- Emphasize importance of oral hydration to improve soft tissue and bladder clearance.

Image Interpretation

Anterior and posterior views of the vertebral whole body (Fig. A) demonstrate focally increased tracer uptake in the entire vertebral body of approximately L3. The left eighth rib also shows focal uptake posteriorly.

Differential Diagnosis

- Paget's disease
- Prostate cancer
- Osteomyelitis
- Primary bone tumor

Diagnosis and Clinical Follow-up

The radiograph demonstrates Paget's disease in the lumbar vertebra (Fig. B).

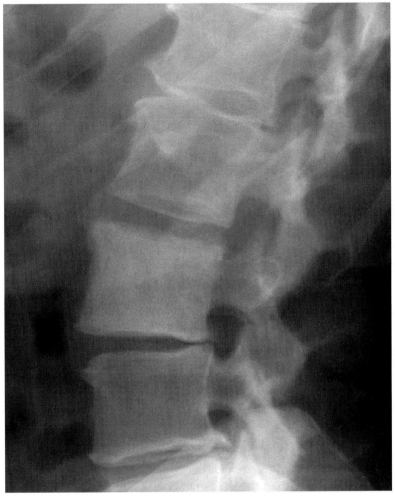

Fig. B

Discussion

The appearance of the "Mickey Mouse sign" (also known as the "champagne glass sign" or "T-sign") is very specific for the diagnosis of Paget's disease. As with any abnormal bone uptake, however, a plain radiograph should be obtained to confirm the diagnosis.

Suggested Readings

Estrada WN, Kim CK. Paget's disease in a patient with breast cancer [see comments]. *J Nucl Med* 34:1214–1216, 1993.

Van Heerden BB. Mickey Mouse sign in Paget's disease. *J Nucl Med* 35:924–925, 1994. Letter.

Case 21

Clinical Presentation

41-year-old man presenting with an abnormality in the head noted on gallium scan.

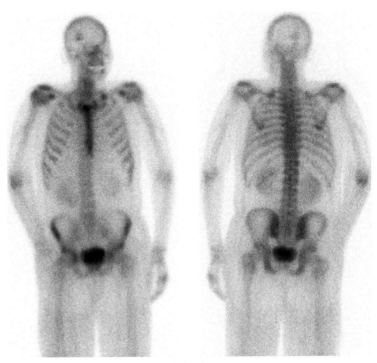

Fig. A

Technique

- 20 mCi technetium-99m–labeled methylene diphosphonate (MDP) intravenously.
- Whole-body or spot images of the skeleton obtained 3 hours after tracer administration.
- Emphasize importance of oral hydration to improve soft tissue and bladder clearance.

Image Interpretation

Tracer uptake is noted in the right side of the skull in the right anterior oblique view (Fig. A, left). The posterior view of the skull (Fig. A, right) suggests a faint lesion that may be related to the occipital abnormality noted on the gallium scan or that may be shine through of the lesion seen on the right in the anterior view.

Differential Diagnosis

(focal uptake in the head):

• Skull metastasis
• Brain neoplasm (e.g., meningioma)
• Cartilagenous rest
• Sinusitis
• Surface contamination
• Craniotomy site
• Brain abcess
• Fracture
• Infarct
• Bone island

Diagnosis and Clinical Follow-up

Computed tomography (CT) scan demonstrated 3-cm enhancing abscesses in the left occipitoparietal region and the right subinsular region of the brain. No bone involvement was noted.

The results of this study suggested that the occipital lesion noted on the gallium scan did not originate in the bone. They also revealed a second lesion that was likely to be on the right side of the head because it was seen better on the right anterior oblique view. The tracer uptake in this lesion was probably caused by the right insular lesion noted on CT scan.

Discussion

Visualization of abscesses with bone radiopharmaceuticals is uncommon. In this case, the gallium and the bone radiopharmaceuticals seemed to favor different abscesses and therefore caused some confusion as to the location of the two lesions. It is also possible that the patient developed the abscesses at different times, one prior to the gallium scan and the other just prior to the bone scan.

Suggested Readings

Malley MJ, Holmes RA. Serendipitous detection of intrarenal abscesses on technetium-99m MDP imaging while evaluating a foot ulcer. *Clin Nucl Med* 13:127–128, 1988.

Moallem A. Nonspecific tissue accumulation of diffusible radionuclide imaging agents in areas of inflammation. *Clin Nucl Med* 17:4–6, 1992.

Peller PJ, Ho VB, Kransdorf MJ. Extraosseous Tc-99m MDP uptake: A pathophysiologic approach. *Radiographics* 13:715–734, 1993.

Tamgac F, Baillet G, Alper E, et al. Extraskeletal accumulation of Tc-99m HMDP in a tuberculous cold abscess. *Clin Nucl Med* 20:1092, 1995.

Case 22

Clinical Presentation

36-year-old man with a history of intravenous (IV) drug abuse presenting with right hip and flank pain radiating down the right leg.

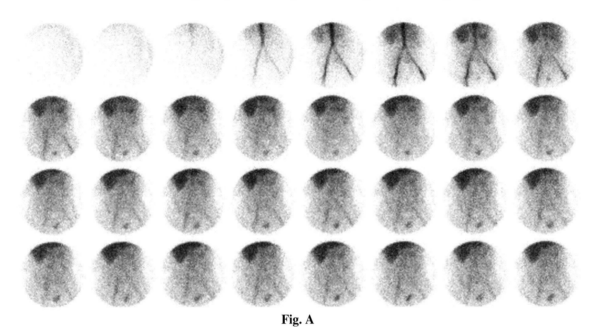

Fig. A

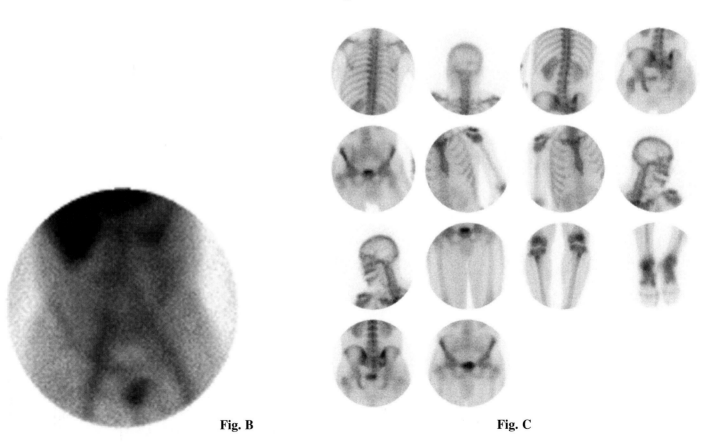

Fig. B   Fig. C

Technique

- 20 mCi technetium-99m–labeled-methylene diphosphonate (MDP) intravenously.
- Flow images of the hips obtained for 1.5 seconds per frame at the time of tracer injection.
- Blood pool image obtained for 3 minutes within 10 minutes of tracer injection.
- Whole-body or spot images of the skeleton obtained 3 hours after tracer administration.
- Emphasize importance of oral hydration to improve soft tissue and bladder clearance.

Image Interpretation

Anterior blood flow images (Fig. A) demonstrate symmetrical blood flow to both hips. Blood pool images (Fig. B) also show symmetrical tracer activity over the bony structures. Delayed images (Fig. C) show asymmetrical tracer activity in the sacroiliac (SI) joints with a prominent defect in tracer uptake in the right SI joint, with slightly increased tracer accumulation just above the defect.

Differential Diagnosis

(focal uptake in pelvis):

- Neoplastic disease (primary and metastatic)
- Osteomyelitis
- Urine contamination
- Trauma (surgical or accidental)
- Cellulitis (including decubitus ulcer)

Diagnosis and Clinical Follow-up

Gallium scan done following the bone scan (see Inflammation Imaging, Case 106) demonstrated an area of intense tracer concentration in the right SI joint that was more extensive than the area of abnormalities noted on bone scan. Magnetic resonance imaging (MRI) demonstrated local edema and bone destruction consistent with osteomyelitis.

Discussion

Three phase bone scintigraphy is highly sensitive and specific for osteomyelitis if the plain radiograph is normal. The pattern most commonly seen is increased activity in all three phases of the study. Flow images are more difficult to interpret when the area in question, such as the spine or pelvis, overlies major vessels or vascular structures.

Occasionally, subperiosteal abcess or other causes of local edema and increased tissue pressure at the site of infection will cause a decrease in blood flow, resulting in a defect in tracer activity, rather than a focus of increased activity. The flow and blood pool phases of this particular study, however, are negative because they were performed in the anterior projection rather than in the posterior projection. This study illustrates the importance of close communication with the referring physician and Nuclear Medicine technologist to assure the study is acquired optimally.

Suggested Readings

Schauwecker DS. The scintigraphic diagnosis of osteomyelitis. *AJR Am J Roentgenol* 158:9–18, 1992.

Schauwecker DS, Braunstein EM, Wheat LJ. Diagnostic imaging of osteomyelitis. *Infect Dis Clin North Am* 4:441–463, 1990.

Schauwecker DS, Park HM, Mock BH, et al. Evaluation of complicating osteomyelitis with Tc-99m MDP, In-111 granulocytes, and Ga-67 citrate. *J Nucl Med* 25:849–853, 1984.

Case 23

Clinical Presentation

29-year-old female runner with one-week complaint of pain in her lower legs. Bone scan requested to evaluate these symptoms.

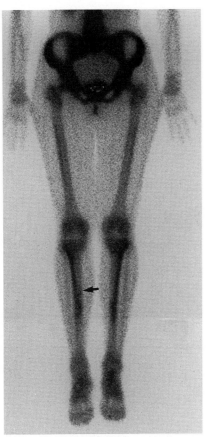

Fig. A

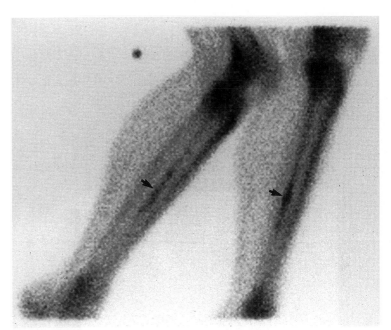

Fig. B

Technique

- Adult dose is 25 mCi technetium-99m methylene diphosphonate (MDP) administered intravenously.
- Low-energy high-resolution collimator.
- Energy setting is 20% centered at 140 keV.
- Imaging time 3 to 4 hours after tracer injection. Prior to the scan, the patient should be instructed to drink 2 quarts (8 cups) of fluids and to void frequently.

Image Interpretation

An anterior view of the pelvis and lower extremities (Fig. A) shows very mild irregular tracer uptake at the midportion of the right tibia (*arrow*). A spot lateral view of the tibia and fibula (Fig. B) shows moderately increased linear tracer uptake involving the middle-to-distal tibiae posteriorly (*arrows*).

PEARLS/PITFALLS

- It is important to obtain lateral views in patients who are complaining of lower limb pain; otherwise, the diagnosis of shin splints may be missed on the anterior and posterior views.

- If a lateral view is not obtained, the differentiation between shin splints and stress fracture may be difficult to make.

- The scintigraphic pattern of shin splints is not predictive of further injury unless there is a focal component to the tracer uptake.

- The clinical significance of shin splints is therefore quite different from that of a stress fracture because patients with shin splints can continue to exercise, as opposed to patients with stress fractures, who must refrain from exercising for at least 6 weeks to avoid complete fracture.

- Conventional radiographs usually do not show any abnormality.

Differential Diagnosis

- Shin splints
- Stress fracture
- Trauma

Diagnosis and Clinical Follow-up

The diagnosis was shin splints. No follow-up was available for this patient.

Discussion

The term "shin splint" is used to describe stress-related leg pain along the medial or posteromedial aspect of the tibia in athletes and is often seen bilaterally. The etiology is thought to be microperiosteal tears at points of periosteal stress. The periosteal stress is likely mediated by Sharpey's fibers through their connection to the bone. Bone scintigraphy is highly sensitive for the diagnosis of shin splints.

Suggested Reading

Pavlov H. Athletic injuries. *Radiol Clin North Am* 28:435–443, 1990.

Case 24

Clinical Presentation

40-year-old female without history of foot trauma. Noted increased pain in arch of her right foot during hiking.

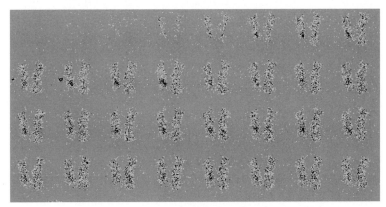

Fig. A   **Figs. B, C**

Technique

- 20 mCi technetium-99m–labeled methylene diphosphonate (MDP) administered intravenously.
- Flow images obtained at 2 seconds per frame for one minute at the time of tracer injection.
- Blood pool images obtained for 5 minutes immediately following flow images.
- Delayed images obtained 3 hours following tracer injection
- Low-energy all purpose collimator
- Energy window is 20% centered at 140 keV

Image Interpretation

Blood flow images (Figure A) demonstrate increased tracer flow to the right mid foot. Blood pool images (Figure B) show increased tracer accumulation in the right mid foot. Delayed images (Figure C) demonstrate focally increased tracer activity in the second metatarsal of the right foot.

Differential Diagnosis

- Stress fracture
- Stress reaction
- Trauma
- Metastasis (particularly lung cancer, renal cancer)
- Brown tumor
- Enchondroma

Diagnosis and Clinical Follow-up

Radiographs demonstrated a stress fracture in the second metatarsal of the right foot.

Discussion

Stress fracture often occurs when normal bone undergoes accelerated remodeling secondary to increased stress. The bone resorption associated with the remodeling may be more accelerated than new bone formation, subsequently weakening the bone. Continued stress may then result in bone fracture. As with many sites of trauma, the fracture is associated with local inflammatory changes which are demonstrated in the flow and blood pool phases of the three-phase bone scan. Delayed images should also clearly demonstrate the focus of bony remodeling.

Multiple views of the site of tracer uptake should be obtained if there is a question of the depth of penetration of the abnormality through the bone shaft, particularly when long bones are involved. If any view shows the tracer uptake involves less than 50% of the diameter of the bone, the diagnosis of stress reaction may be more appropriate.

Suggested Readings

Pavlov H. Athletic injuries. Radiol Clin North Am 1990; 28:435–43.

Pavlov H, Torg JS, Frieberger RH. The Roentgen examination of runner's injuries. Radiographics 1:17–37, 1981

Case 25

Clinical Presentation

44-year-old man presenting with right hip pain following a fall from a ladder. The plain radiograph of the hip was normal. A bone scan was ordered to further evaluate the symptoms.

ANT

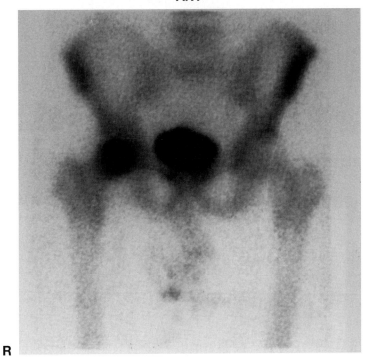

R   L

Fig. A

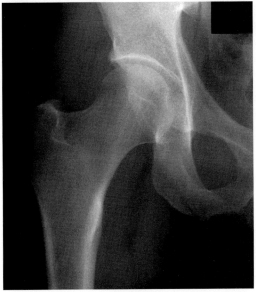

Fig. B

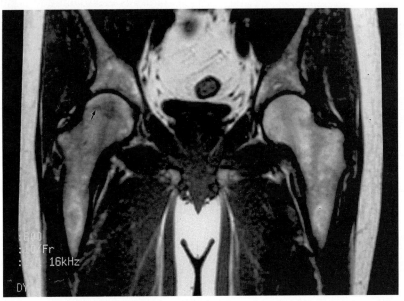

Fig. C

Technique

- 25 mCi of technetium-99m–labeled methylene diphosphonate (MDP) administered intravenously.
- Low-energy high-resolution collimator.
- Energy window is 20% centered at 140 keV.
- Imaging obtained 3 to 4 hours after radiotracer injection.

Image Interpretation

An anterior spot view of the pelvis (Fig. A) reveals focal intense radiotracer uptake in the head of the right femur. A plain radiograph of the same hip (Fig. B) is normal. T1-weighted image of the pelvis (Fig. C) shows abnormal linear gray signal intensity in the lateral aspect of the right femoral neck (the fracture line is shown with the *arrow*) with surrounding ill-defined gray signal intensities in the medullary cavity suggestive of edema or bone bruise.

Differential Diagnosis

- Fracture
- Avascular necrosis
- Malignancy
- Osteomyelitis

Diagnosis and Clinical Follow-up

The diagnosis was right femoral neck fracture. No follow-up was available for this patient.

Discussion

Plain radiographs remain the primary diagnostic procedure for the evaluation of skeletal trauma. The bone scan is more sensitive, however, and frequently positive early after the trauma, except with older patients. Focal activity at the site of injury is maximum 2 to 3 months after trauma, then progressively declines in an uncomplicated fracture, and returns to normal within 6 months to 2 years after the injury, depending on the location and the age of the patient.

Suggested Readings

Matin, P. The appearance of bone scan following fractures including immediate and long term studies. *J Nucl Med* 20:1227–1231, 1979.

Taylor A Jr, Datz FL, eds. *Clinical Practice of Nuclear Medicine*. New York: Churchill Livingstone, 1991.

Case 26

Clinical Presentation

67-year-old woman presenting with left ankle pain. A bone scan was requested to assess symptoms.

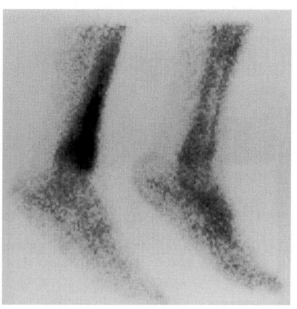

Fig. A

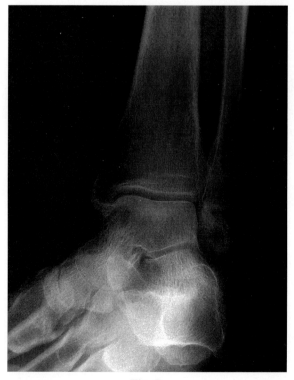

Fig. B

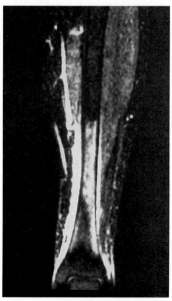

Fig. C

Technique

- 25 mCi of technetium-99m–labeled methylene diphosphonate (MDP) administered intravenously.
- Low-energy high-resolution collimator.
- Energy window is 20% centered at 140 keV.
- Imaging obtained 3 to 4 hours after tracer injection.

Image Interpretation

A lateral spot view of the left distal tibia and left ankle (Fig. A) reveals diffuse increased tracer uptake along the anterior cortex. A radiograph of the left ankle (Fig. B) shows a small ill-defined lucency in the distal tibial diaphysis. Magnetic resonance imaging (MRI) coronal inversion recovery image of tibia (Fig. C) shows bright signal intensities in the distal half of the tibia and surrounding soft tissue consistent with edema.

Differential Diagnosis

- Malignancy
- Fracture

Diagnosis and Clinical Follow-up

The diagnosis was stress fracture mimicking malignancy. The patient's ankle pain gradually subsided, and the follow-up plain radiograph 6 months later showed further evidence of healed stress fracture.

Discussion

The most common scintigraphic presentation of stress fracture is oval or fusiform tracer uptake parallel to the long axis of the involved bone. Diffuse or linear radiotracer uptake along the cortex is not uncommon, however.

Suggested Reading

Daries AM, Carter SR, Grimer RJ, et al. Fatigue fractures of the femoral diaphysis simulating malignancy. *Br J Radiol* 62:893–896, 1989.

Case 27

Clinical Presentation

73-year-old woman presenting with left hip pain after a fall. Initial radiographs of the hip were normal. A bone scan was requested to assess the left hip pain 3 days after the trauma.

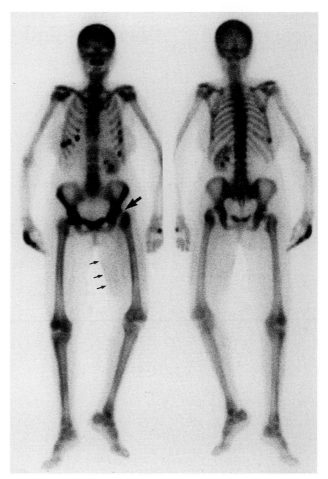

Fig. A

Technique

- 25 mCi technetium-99m–labeled methylene diphosphonate (MDP) administered intravenously.
- Low-energy high-resolution collimator.
- Energy window is 20% centered at 140 keV.
- Whole-body images obtained 4 hours after tracer injection at 10 cm/min.

Image Interpretation

Whole-body views in the anterior (left) and posterior (right) projections revealed a photopenic area in the neck of the left femur (*arrow*). There is mild to moderate soft tissue tracer uptake in the left thigh consistent with edema (shown with the small arrows). In addition, there are foci of increased tracer uptake in several anterior ribs bilaterally consistent with rib fractures. The right kidney is not visualized secondary to previous nephrectomy.

Differential Diagnosis

• Fracture
• Bone infarction (acute stage)
• Lytic lesion
• Osteomyelitis

Diagnosis and Clinical Follow-up

The diagnosis was left hip fracture. Plain radiographs of the left hip performed following the bone scan showed a fracture of the left femoral neck with slight displacement of the femoral shaft. The patient underwent surgery for total hip replacement.

Discussion

In patients above 65 years of age with clinical suspicion of fracture, the plain radiograph may fail to reveal a fracture and bone scan or magnetic resonance imaging (MRI) may be useful in diagnosing the fracture.

Suggested Reading

Taylor A Jr, Datz FL, eds. *Clinical Practice of Nuclear Medicine.* New York: Churchill Livingstone, 1991.

Case 28

Clinical Presentation

72-year-old woman with a history of systemic lupus erythematosus on steroid therapy complaining of right hip pain. A bone scan was ordered for further assessment of hip pain.

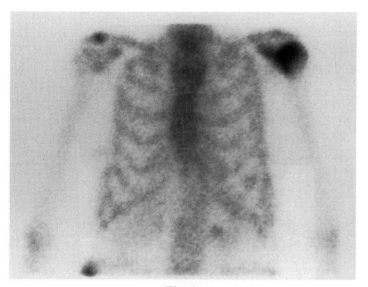

Fig. A

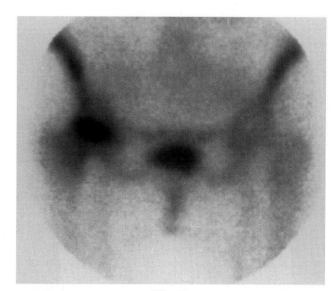

Fig. B

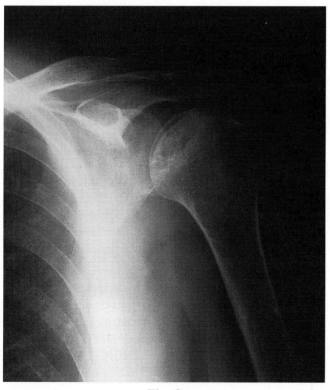

Fig. C

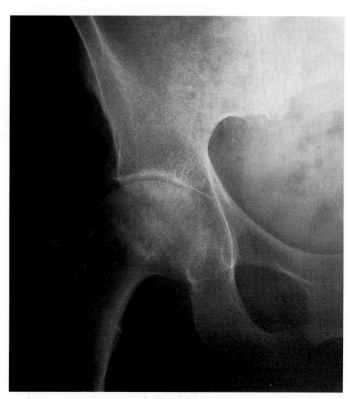

Fig. D

Technique

- 25 mCi technetium-99m–labeled methylene diphosphonate (MDP) administered intravenously.
- Low-energy high-resolution collimator.
- Energy window is 20% centered at 140 keV.
- Spot views obtained 3 to 4 hours after tracer injection (one million counts for axial skeleton and 0.5 million counts for extremities).

Image Interpretation

An anterior spot view of the chest including left shoulder (Fig. A) reveals intense focal increased uptake in the head of the left humerus. An anterior view of the pelvis (Fig. B) shows a focus of increased uptake in the right hip. An external rotation posterior oblique radiograph of the left shoulder (Fig. C) shows a sclerotic area in the humeral head with a thin lucent line beneath the cortex (crescent sign). There is slight collapse of the cortex. An anteroposterior radiograph of the right hip (Fig. D) shows a sclerotic area in the femoral neck with a thin lucent line underneath the cortex of the femoral neck superiorly (crescent sign). Slight flattening of the femoral head cortex is also noted.

Differential Diagnosis

- Avascular necrosis
- Trauma

Diagnosis and Clinical Follow-up

The diagnosis was osteonecrosis. No follow-up was available for this patient.

Discussion

There are numerous causes of bone necrosis. The appearance on skeletal scintigraphy is highly dependent on the time course of the process. With acute interruption of the blood supply, newly infarcted bone appears cold or photon deficient. In the postinfarction or healing phase, there is increased osteogenesis and increased tracer uptake at the margin of the infarcted area.

Suggested Readings

Kundel HL, Mitchell M, Steinberg ME, et al. Comparison of MR, CT, and radionuclide imaging of avascular necrosis of the hip using ROC curves. *Radiology* 153:137, 1984. Abstract.

Thickman D, Axel L, Kressel HY, et al. MR imaging of avascular necrosis of the femoral head. *Skeletal Radiol* 15:133–140, 1986.

Turner JH. Post-traumatic avascular necrosis of the femoral head predicted by preoperative Tc-99m antimony colloid scan. *J Bone Joint Surg Am* 65:787–796, 1983.

Case 29

Clinical Presentation

61-year-old woman with history of osteoporosis complaining of persistent low back pain.

POST

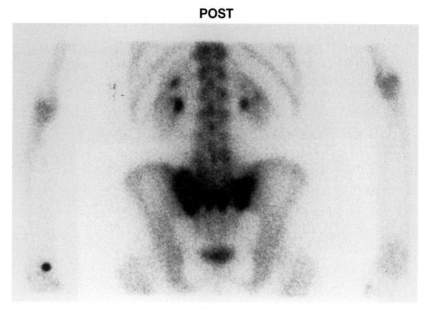

Fig. A

Technique

- 24 mCi technetium-99m–labeled methylene diphosphonate (MDP) administered intravenously.
- Low-energy high-resolution collimator.
- Energy window is 20% centered at 140 keV.
- Static views (0.5 million counts per view) obtained 3 to 4 hours after radiotracer injection.

Differential Diagnosis

- Fracture
- Metastatic disease
- Paget's disease

Image Interpretation

A posterior spot view of the pelvis reveals increased tracer uptake across the body of the sacrum and bilateral increased uptake in the sacral alae (Honda sign), called the "H type" insufficiency fracture.

PEARLS/PITFALLS

- Bone scan has been suggested for the early diagnosis of insufficiency fractures in the sacrum.
- Oblique and lateral sacral views are useful in the diagnosis of sacral and coccygeal insufficiency fractures.
- A full bladder can obscure the sacrum. If the patient is unable to empty the bladder, delayed images up to 24 hours after tracer injection is recommended.

Diagnosis and Clinical Follow-up

The diagnosis was sacral insufficiency fracture. No follow-up was available for this patient.

Discussion

The term "insufficiency fracture" is used to describe fractures that occur when normal or physiological stress is applied to abnormally weakened bones, such as in patients with osteoporosis.

Suggested Reading

Roub LW, Gumerman LW, Hanley EN, et al. Bone stress: A radionuclide imaging perspective. *Radiology* 132:431–438, 1979.

Case 30

Clinical Presentation

26-year-old man with a history of osteogenic sarcoma of the left proximal tibia status post–nonvascularized allograft at the site of the resected tibial tumor. A bone scan was performed to assess the allograft and rule out skeletal metastasis.

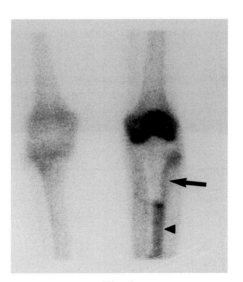

Fig. A

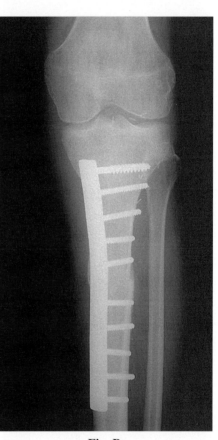

Fig. B

Technique

- 24 mCi of technetium-99m–labeled methylene diphosphonate (MDP) administered intravenously.
- Low-energy high-resolution collimator.
- Energy window is 20% centered at 140 keV.
- Static spot views (0.5 million counts per each view) should be obtained 3 to 4 hours after tracer injection.

Image Interpretation

Spot view of the left knee and proximal tibia (Fig. A) in the anterior projection 3 months after surgery shows no significant tracer uptake in the region of the nonvascularized allograft. There is increased tracer uptake in the femoral condyle, patella and distal end of the tibia adjacent to the allograft (*arrow head*) likely secondary to disuse osteoporosis. There is a mild linear tracer uptake at the left margin of the allograft (*arrow*) that most likely represents osteoblastic invasion from the host site (the so-called "osteoblastic creeping"). An anteroposterior radiograph of the knee and proximal part of the tibia (Fig. B) shows the proximal tibial allograft and its fixation hardware maintained in position. There is callus formation at the allograft–native bone site, indicating healing response.

Diagnosis and Clinical Follow-up

Findings were consistent with a status post–allogenic bone graft placement. There was no evidence of skeletal metastasis. No follow-up was available for this patient.

Discussion

Increased uptake generally indicates healing and viability of the bone, whereas decreased uptake is more difficult to interpret.

Suggested Readings

Dee P, Lambruschi PG, Hiebert JM. The use of Tc-99m MDP bone scanning in the study of vascularized bone implants: Concise communication. *J Nucl Med* 22:522–525, 1981.

Lipson RA, Dief H, Gregson ND, et al. Bone scanning in assessing viability of vascularized skeletal tissue transplants. *Clin Orthop* 160:279–289, 1981.

Lisbona R, Rennie WRJ, Daniel PK. Radionuclide evaluation of free vascularized bone graft viability. *AJR Am J Roentgenol* 134:387–388, 1980.

Case 31

Clinical Presentation

33-year-old man with history of chronic renal disease presenting with back pain. A bone scan was performed to evaluate any abnormality in the spine.

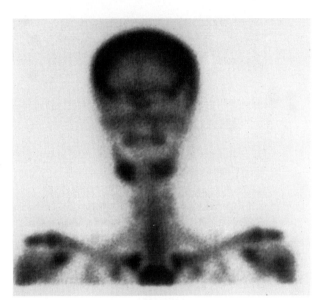

Fig. A

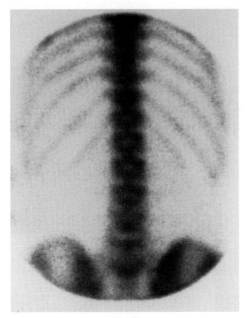

Fig. B

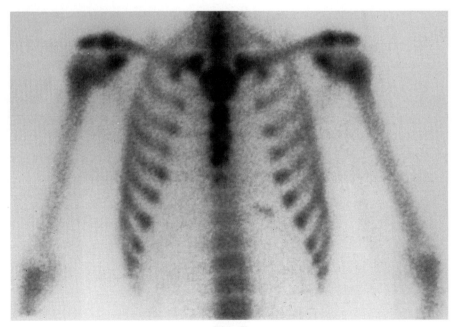

Fig. C

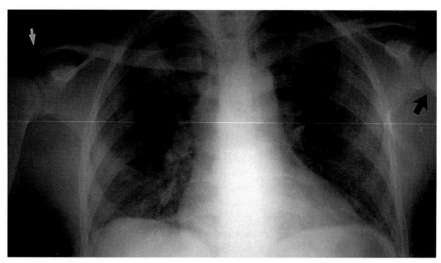

Fig. D

Technique

- 25 mCi technetium-99m–labeled methylene diphosphonate (MDP) administered intravenously.
- Low-energy high-resolution collimator.
- Energy window is 20% centered at 140 keV.
- Static spot views of the head, neck, and trunk (one million counts per view) obtained 3 to 4 hours after radiotracer injection.

Image Interpretation

Spot views of the skeleton (Figs. A through C) show homogeneous tracer uptake throughout the bony structures. The findings are consistent with a superscan appearance with increased uptake in the axial skeleton and high contrast between bone and soft tissue; the kidneys are not visualized (Fig. B). Increased tracer uptake at the costochondral junctions (i.e., beading) and throughout the sternum (so-called "striped tie" sign) are noted on Figure C. A plain radiograph of the chest (Fig. D) shows subperiosteal bone resorption of the distal end of the right clavicle (*white arrow*) with widening of the AC joint. Subperiosteal bony resorption is also seen in the left humeral head inferomedially (*black arrow*).

Differential Diagnosis

- Hyperparathyroidism
- Malignancy

Diagnosis and Clinical Follow-up

Findings are suggestive of hyperparathyroidism in this clinical context. No follow-up was available in this patient.

Discussion

The characteristics of hyperparathyroidism on bone scan images range from normal in the case of primary hyperparathyroidism to severe metabolic changes in hyperparathyroidism secondary to renal osteodystrophy. The latter pattern is seen on bone scan in approximately 50% of patients; radiographic evidence is seen in only 25% of cases.

Suggested Readings

Fogelman I, Carr D. A comparison of bone scanning and radiographs in the evaluation of patients with metabolic bone disease. *Clin Radiol* 31:321–326, 1980.

Taylor A Jr, Datz FL, eds. *Clinical Practice of Nuclear Medicine.* New York:Churchill Livingstone, 1991.

Case 32

Clinical Presentation

37-year-old man presenting with left hip pain. Total left hip replacement using a noncemented prosthesis was performed 1 year ago.

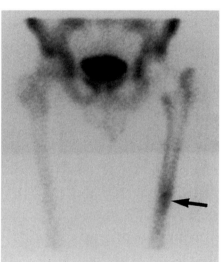
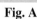

Fig. A

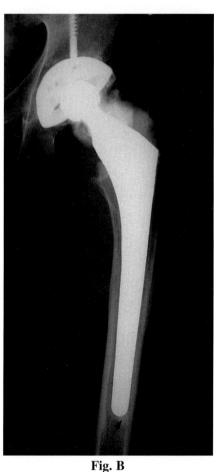

Fig. B

Technique

- 24 mCi technetium-99m–labeled methylene diphosphonate (MDP) administered intravenously.
- Low-energy high-resolution collimator.
- Energy window is 20% centered at 140 keV.
- Spot view of the left hip (0.5 million counts) obtained 3 to 4 hours after tracer injection.

Image Interpretation

The anterior view of the left hip and proximal left femur (Fig. A) shows a focus of increased tracer uptake at the tip of the femoral component of a total hip prosthesis (*arrow*). An arthrogram of the left hip (Fig. B) shows a contiguous collection of contrast over the posterosuperior aspect of the greater trochanter, most

PEARLS/PITFALLS

- Focal uptake at the tip of the femoral component of a cemented prosthesis when accompanied by clinical symptoms is worrisome for loosening.

- Focal tracer uptake at the tip of the femoral component of a noncemented prosthesis could be due to osteoblastic remodeling of the native bone in contact with the prosthesis. It may persist years after surgery and is not always a sign of loosening.

likely indicating pseudocapsule formation. There is a sclerosis at the tip of the prosthesis laterally (*arrow*) that indicates normal pressure response, correlating with the focal tracer uptake in this region. There is no radiographic evidence of loosening of the prosthesis.

Differential Diagnosis

- Loosening
- Infection
- Post-surgical remodeling

Diagnosis and Clinical Follow-up

There is no evidence of loosening of the prosthesis.

Discussion

Differentiation of loosening from postsurgical remodeling of the bone in a surgically implanted prosthesis is often a difficult problem. Persistent tracer uptake on the bone scan may be seen for up to 1 year after surgery and even longer in the region of the greater trochanter when this area has sustained significant trauma.

Suggested Reading

Propst-Proctor SL, Dillingham MF, McDougall IR, Goodwin D. The white blood cell scan in orthopedics. *Clin Orthop* 168:157–165, 1982.

Case 33

Clinical Presentation

43-year-old man, with a history of intravenous drug abuse, presenting with pain and swelling in the anterior tibiae. A bone scan was requested to evaluate the symptoms.

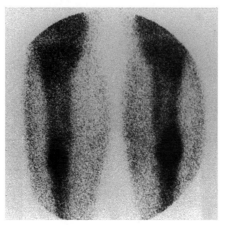

Fig. A

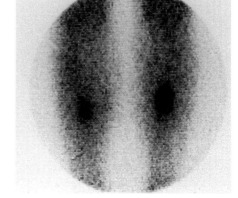

Fig. B

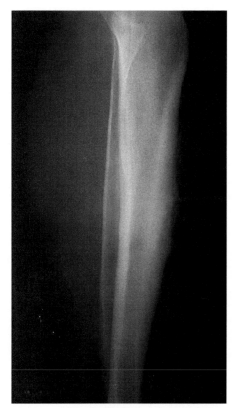

Fig. C

Technique

- 24 mCi technetium-99m–labeled methylene diphosphonate (MDP) administered intravenously.
- Low-energy high-resolution collimator.
- Energy window is 20% centered at 140 keV.
- Planar spot views (0.5 million counts for lower extremities) obtained 3 to 4 hours after tracer injection.

Image Interpretation

Bone scan of the tibiae in the anterior projection (Fig. A) shows focally dense tracer uptake in the midshaft of the tibiae bilaterally. A correlative gallium scan in the same projection (Fig. B) shows very intense tracer uptake in the same anatomic location seen on bone scan. A radiograph of the left tibia in the lateral projection (Fig. C) shows a large cortical erosion involving the anterior cortex. There is solid periosteal reaction and marked soft tissue swelling.

Differential Diagnosis

- Osteomyelitis
- Trauma
- Metastatic/Disease

Diagnosis and Clinical Follow-up

The diagnosis is osteomyelitis. Biopsy of the left tibia showed necrotic bone tissues and *Staphylococcus aureus* coagulase–positive organisms. The patient responded to systemic antibiotic therapy.

Discussion

Bone scintigraphy is almost invariably abnormal by the time symptoms of osteomyelitis are present. Increased tracer uptake is the most common finding. In some children or in cases of increased pressure in the marrow or thrombosis of blood vessels, decreased tracer uptake and a cold photon-deficient lesion may be found.

Suggested Readings

Al-Sheikh W, Sfakianakis GN, Mnaymneh W, et al. Subacute and chronic bone infections: Diagnosis using In-111, Ga-67 and Tc-99m MDP bone scintigraphy and radiography. *Radiology* 155:501–506, 1985.

Schauwecked DS. Osteomyelitis: Diagnosis with In-111 labeled leukocytes. *Radiology* 171:141–146, 1989.

Segal GM, Nino-Murcia M, Jacobs T, Chang K. The role of bone scan and radiography on detection of pedal osteomyelitis in diabetes. *Clin Nucl Med* 14:255–260, 1989.

Case 34

Clinical Presentation

17-year-old male adolescent presenting with a history of low back pain of 5-month duration. A bone scan was requested.

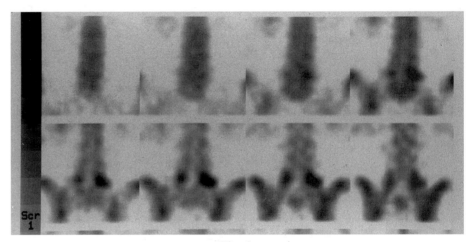

Fig. A

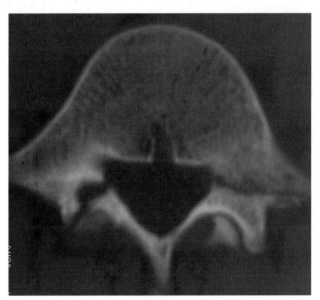

Fig. B

Technique

- 24 mCi technetium-99m–labeled methylene diphosphonate (MDP) administered intravenously.
- Low-energy high-resolution collimator.
- Energy window is 20% centered at 140 keV.
- Single photon emission computed tomography (SPECT) of the lumbar spine obtained 4 hours after tracer injection, using 64 stops at 25 s/stop, and a 360-degree rotation.

Image Interpretation

A coronal SPECT view of the lumbar spine (Fig. A) shows focally increased tracer uptake in the region of the pars interarticularis in L5 (left more than right). Oblique plain film of lumbar spine was unremarkable. Computed tomography of the lumbar spine (Fig. B) shows bilateral pars interarticularis defects at L5. The left pars defect is oriented horizontally and extends into the left transverse process.

Differential Diagnosis

- Spondylolysis
- Trauma
- Osteomyelitis (unlikely to be bilateral)

Diagnosis and Clinical Follow-up

CT scan findings are diagnostic of pars interarticularis defects. No follow-up was obtained.

Discussion

The defect in the pars interarticularis of the spine can often be seen on oblique radiographs of the spine. The bone scan, however, has a higher sensitivity for early diagnosis of spondylolysis, particularly when using SPECT.

Suggested Reading

Calabrese AS, Freiberger RH. Acquired spondylolysis after spinal fusion. *Radiology* 81:492–494, 1963.

Section II

Cardiac Scintigraphy

Case 35

Clinical Presentation

82-year-old female presenting with atypical chest pain. An exercise thallium study was performed to rule out coronary artery disease.

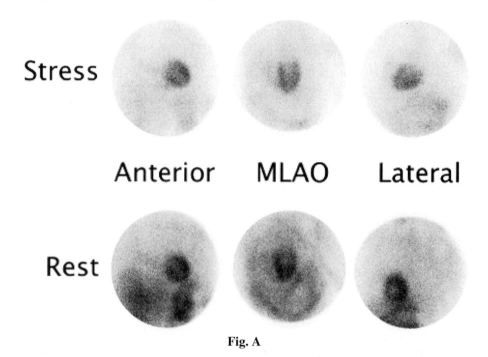

Fig. A

Technique

The following protocol is used in our department and is provided as an example of one possible imaging protocol. For other acceptable protocols, see the Society of Nuclear Medicine Guideline for Myocardial Perfusion Imaging in the Health Care Policy section of the Society of Nuclear Medicine web page (see Suggested Readings, below).

- Patient takes nothing by mouth for 3 hours prior to the test.
- Exercise is performed to increase myocardial perfusion and may be accomplished using a variety of protocols. Consult with your nuclear medicine or cardiology department to familiarize yourself with your institution's protocol.
- 1.6 mCi thallium-201 thallous chloride administered intravenously at peak exercise.
- Imaging begins within 5 minutes of exercise termination.
- Energy window is 20% centered on 70 keV (for Hg X rays), 20% centered on 167 keV (for thallium-201 gamma rays).
- Use slant hole collimator. Supine images are obtained in the anterior, 40-degree modified left anterior oblique (MLAO), and decubitus 70-degree left anterior oblique (LAO).
- Upright images are then obtained in anterior and 70-degree LAO projections to compare with supine images for movement of soft tissue attenuation artifacts.

PEARLS/PITFALLS

- Soft tissue attenuation is an important problem in planar imaging. Repeating views in upright and supine positions may help distinguish soft tissue attenuation from perfusion defects.

- Digital images that allow background subtraction and pixel intensity to be manipulated by the physician reading the study are preferred. Viewing these images on a computer display decreases the reliance on the technologist to film the study at the correct exposure settings.

- Familiarize yourself with the distribution of the major coronary arteries to correlate myocardial defects with the appropriate coronary artery.

- Fixed perfusion defects are not always indicative of previous infarction. More than 20% of fixed defects will demonstrate viability with positron-emission tomography (PET) imaging.

- Images should be obtained as soon as possible after exercise to prevent redistribution from obliterating exercise-induced perfusion defects.

- The influence of the exercise data (symptoms during exercise, electrocardiographic changes, exercise tolerance, etc.) on image interpretation is yet to be determined. Some physicians prefer to read perfusion images with no clinical information available. Others believe the clinical information improves the accuracy of study interpretation.

- Resting images are obtained three to four hours later.
- 2 mCi thallium-201 thallous chloride is injected 15 minutes prior to obtaining resting images.

Image Interpretation

Planar images (Fig. A) demonstrate normal tracer distribution throughout the left ventricular myocardium. Patient exercised for 13 minutes on a modified Bruce protocol, achieving 104% of maximum predicted heart rate. No symptoms were elicited during or after exercise. No electrocardiographic changes were demonstrated. No upright images were obtained.

Differential Diagnosis

- Normal myocardial perfusion
- False negative exercise perfusion studies can occur for many technical and physiological reasons, including lesion too small to be detected, balanced lesions in all coronary arteries, globally diminished perfusion, exercise not maintained long enough after tracer injection, location of lesion (sensitivity for circumflex disease is less than that for other vessels), submaximal stress, patient motion during image acquisition, and camera uniformity maladjustment.

Diagnosis and Clinical Follow-up

Exercise myocardial perfusion study was normal. A second exercise test was also normal 3 months later. Patient is doing well, with mild hypertension 1.5 years after initial exercise test.

Discussion

Although planar images have been replaced in many nuclear medicine facilities by single photon emission computed tomography (SPECT) images, the debate as to the superiority of one technique over the other continues. Many nuclear medicine physicians remain comfortable reading planar studies, and thus planar myocardial perfusion images are still common at many institutions.

Planar images are usually displayed in at least three views: anterior, lateral, and 45-degree LAO. The LAO view can be modified (MLAO) such that there is a cephalad tilt on the camera head (camera tilted slightly to point more inferiorly). This elongates the left ventricle in this view and better visualizes the apex and the posterolateral and septal walls. The three views demonstrate tracer distribution in the myocardium (Fig. B).

Imaging protocols vary considerably. Stress may be accomplished by exercise or pharmacologically. Stress images can be obtained either before or after resting images. Stress and rest images can be done with either one or two radiopharmaceuticals. If resting images are obtained after exercise, they can be done early (approximately 4 hours after stress) or late (approximately 24 hours after stress), or both, either with or without reinjection of the radiotracer.

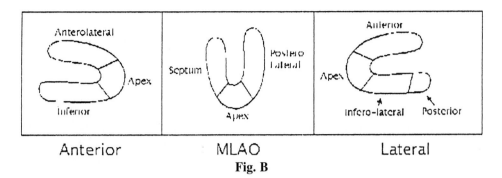

Anterior   MLAO   Lateral

Fig. B

Suggested Readings

Burt RW, Perkins OW, Oppenheim BE, et al. Direct comparison of fluorine-18-FDG SPECT, fluorine-18-FDG PET and rest thallium-201 SPECT for detection of myocardial viability. *J Nucl Med* 36:176–179, 1995.

Cramer MJ, van der Wall EE, Verzijlbergen JF, et al. SPECT versus planar 99mTc-sestamibi myocardial scintigraphy: Comparison of accuracy and impact on patient management in chronic ischemic heart disease. *QJ Nucl Med* 41:1–9, 1997.

Kiat H, Berman DS, Maddahi J. Comparison of planar and tomographic exercise thallium-201 imaging methods for the evaluation of coronary artery disease. *J Am Coll Cardiol* 13:613–616, 1989.

Mahmarian JJ, Verani MS. Exercise thallium-201 perfusion scintigraphy in the assessment of coronary artery disease. *Am J Cardiol* 67:2D–11D, 1991.

Roach PJ, Hansen PS, Scott AM, et al. Comparison of optimised planar scintigraphy with SPECT thallium, exercise ECG and angiography in the detection of coronary artery disease. *Aust N Z J Med* 26:806–812, 1996.

Simons M, Parker JA, Udelson JE, et al. The role of clinical data in interpretation of perfusion images. *J Nucl Med* 35:740–741, 1994.

Society of Nuclear Medicine. *The Society of Nuclear Medicine Guideline for Myocardial Perfusion Imaging, Health Care Policy.* Available: http://www.snm.org/guide.html

Taylor DN, Choraria SK, Maughan J, et al. Diagnosis of coronary artery disease using thallium imaging: tomographic versus planar imaging. *Nucl Med Commun* 10:401–407, 1989.

Case 36

Clinical Presentation

83-year-old man presenting with unstable angina. Four years earlier he had an equivocal coronary artery catheterization.

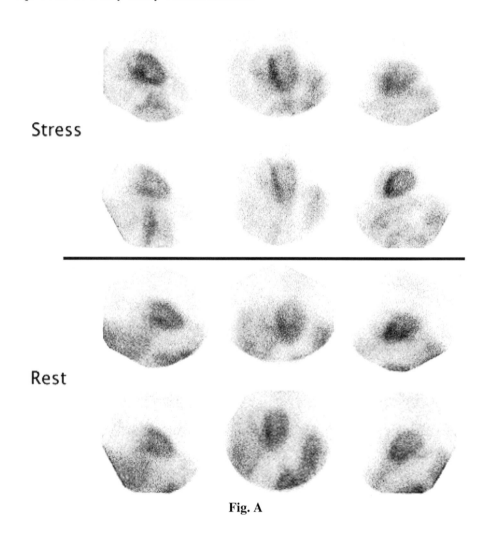

Stress

Rest

Fig. A

Technique

The following protocol is used in our department and is provided as an example of one possible imaging protocol. For other acceptable protocols, see the Society of Nuclear Medicine Guideline for Myocardial Perfusion Imaging in the Health Care Policy section of the Society of Nuclear Medicine web page (see Suggested Readings, below).

- Patient takes nothing by mouth for 3 hours prior to the test.
- Exercise is performed to increase myocardial perfusion and may be accomplished using a variety of protocols. Consult with your nuclear medicine or cardiology department to familiarize yourself with your institution's protocol.

- 1.6 mCi thallium-201 thallous chloride administered intravenously at peak exercise.
- Imaging begins within 5 minutes of exercise termination.
- Energy window is 20% centered on 70 keV (for Hg X rays), 20% centered on 167 keV (for thallium-201 gamma rays).
- Use slant hole collimator. Supine images are obtained in the anterior, 40-degree modified left anterior oblique (MLAO), and decubitus 70-degree left anterior oblique (LAO).
- Upright images are then obtained in anterior and 70-degree LAO projections to compare with supine images for movement of soft tissue attenuation artifacts.

Image Interpretation

Stress images (Fig. A) show diminished tracer uptake in the posterolateral wall on the 40-degree (MLAO) images. The tracer uptake is more uniformly distributed on the rest images.

Differential Diagnosis

- Coronary artery disease
- Soft tissue attenuation
- Idiopathic
- Patient motion
- Camera non-uniformity

Diagnosis and Clinical Follow-up

Diagnosis was exercise-induced ischemia of the posterolateral left ventricular myocardium. Repeat coronary catheterization demonstrated a 90% diagonal, 80% proximal circumflex and lesions in obtuse marginal (OM) branches 1 and 2.

Discussion

The defects demonstrated in this case are moderate defects, typical for what is noted with ischemia in planar perfusion. The persistence of the defects on both upright and supine stress images and the improvement in the defect on rest images make it unlikely to be caused by soft tissue attenuation.

Suggested Readings

Society of Nuclear Medicine. *The Society of Nuclear Medicine Guideline for Myocardial Perfusion Imaging, Health Care Policy.* Available: http://www.snm.org/guide.html 1999.

Wackers FJT. Myocardial perfusion imaging. In: Harbert JC, Eckelman WC, Neumann RD, eds. *Nuclear Medicine Diagnosis and Therapy.* New York: Thieme, 1996, p. 445.

Case 37

Clinical Presentation

75-year-old man with a history of coronary artery disease was sent for evaluation of shortness of breath.

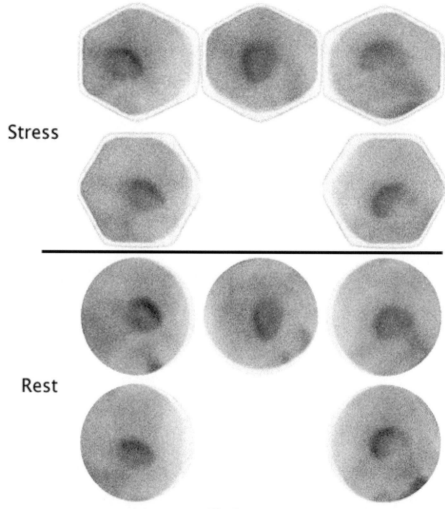

Fig. A

Technique

The following protocol is used in our department and is provided as an example of one possible imaging protocol. For other acceptable protocols, see the Society of Nuclear Medicine Guideline for Myocardial Perfusion Imaging in the Health Care Policy section of the Society of Nuclear Medicine web page (see Suggested Reading, below).

- Patient takes nothing by mouth for 3 hours prior to the test.
- Exercise is performed to increase myocardial perfusion and may be accomplished using a variety of protocols. Consult your nuclear medicine or cardiology department to familiarize yourself with your institution's protocol.

- 1.6 mCi thallium-201 thallous chloride administered intravenously at peak exercise.
- Imaging begins within 5 minutes of exercise termination.
- Energy window is 20% centered on 70 keV (for Hg X rays), 20% centered on 167 keV (for thallium-201 gamma rays).
- Use slant hole collimator. Supine images are obtained in the anterior, 40-degree modified left anterior oblique (MLAO), and decubitus 70-degree left anterior oblique (LAO).
- Upright images are then obtained in anterior and 70-degree LAO projections to compare with supine images for movement of soft tissue attenuation artifacts.

Image Interpretation

Stress and rest images (Fig. A) show poor tracer distribution to the inferior, inferolateral, and adjacent posterolateral walls.

Differential Diagnosis

- Coronary artery disease
- Soft tissue attenuation
- Normal apical thinning
- Idiopathic
- Patient motion
- Camera non-uniformity

Diagnosis and Clinical Follow-up

Inferior, inferolateral, and posterolateral infarcts were diagnosed. Echocardiogram showed fibrosis and akinesis of the inferior, posterior, and apical walls.

Discussion

Fixed tracer defects may not always indicate previous myocardial infarction. As mentioned in Case 35, as many as 20% of fixed defects are shown to contain underlying viable myocardium.

Suggested Reading

Society of Nuclear Medicine. *The Society of Nuclear Medicine Guideline for Myocardial Perfusion Imaging, Health Care Policy.* Available: http://www.snm.org/guide.html 1999.

Case 38

Clinical Presentation

78-year-old woman presenting with a history of aortic stenosis and angina.

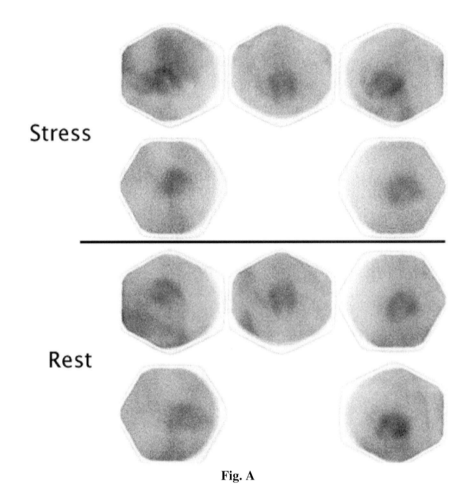

Stress

Rest

Fig. A

Technique

The following protocol is used in our department and is provided as an example of one possible imaging protocol. For other acceptable protocols, see the Society of Nuclear Medicine Guideline for Myocardial Perfusion Imaging in the Health Care Policy section of the Society of Nuclear Medicine web page (see Suggested Readings, below).

- Patient takes nothing by mouth for 3 hours prior to the test.
- Exercise is performed to increase myocardial perfusion and may be accomplished using a variety of protocols. Consult your nuclear medicine or cardiology department to familiarize yourself with your institution's protocol.
- 1.6 mCi thallium-201 thallous chloride administered intravenously at peak exercise.
- Imaging begins within 5 minutes of exercise termination.

PEARLS/PITFALLS

- Always look for lung uptake on planar images. If single photon emission computed tomography (SPECT) imaging is performed, a quick planar image prior to obtaining the SPECT data will allow evaluation of lung uptake.

- To be diagnosed as lung uptake, the extracardiac tracer activity should be seen directly lateral to the myocardium.

- Do not wait for more than 5 minutes to obtain the anterior post-exercise image. This view is best suited for the evaluation of lung uptake.

- Tracer uptake in the pectoral muscles may be mistaken for lung uptake. Pectoral muscle uptake is usually more superior to the myocardium and is not seen lateral to the left ventricular apex.

- Although the SPECT raw data may include the lungs in the field of view, this method of evaluation for lung uptake is not as well-documented in the literature.

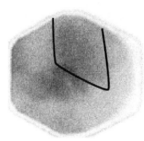

Fig. B

- Energy window is 20% centered on 70 keV (for Hg X rays), 20% centered on 167 keV (for thallium-201 gamma rays).
- Use slant hole collimator. Supine images are obtained in the anterior, 40-degree modified left anterior oblique (MLAO), and decubitus 70-degree left anterior oblique (LAO).
- Upright images are then obtained in anterior and 70-degree LAO projections to compare with supine images for movement of soft tissue attenuation artifacts.

Image Interpretation

Stress images (Fig. A) show a complete (severe) defect in tracer uptake in the apex and adjacent inferior wall. Uptake in the lungs is also noted, particularly in the anterior stress view (outlined in Fig. B). Resting images show resolution of the lung uptake but otherwise no significant change in tracer distribution in the myocardium.

Differential Diagnosis

- Lung uptake secondary to poor left ventricular function
- Thallium uptake in chest wall, particularly pectoral muscle
- Kaposi's sarcoma
- ARDS (however, it is unlikely that a patient with ARDS will be exercising on the treadmill).
- Sarcoidosis

Diagnosis and Clinical Follow-up

Left ventricular decompensation with exercise was the diagnosis. The patient had poor exercise tolerance, exercising to only 60% of maximum predicted heart rate. Exercise was terminated following a sudden drop in systolic pressure (20 mmHg). Echocardiography demonstrated a dyskinetic apex, moderate aortic stenosis and aortic insufficiency, and mitral regurgitation.

Discussion

Thallium uptake in the lungs with stress has been shown to be one of the best indicators of poor prognosis, whether or not the patient has myocardial perfusion defects. The mechanism for the lung uptake is unclear but is associated with elevated left atrial pressure.

Suggested Readings

Gill JB, Ruddy TD, Newell JB, et al. Prognostic importance of thallium uptake by the lungs during exercise in coronary artery disease. *N Engl J Med* 317:1486–1489, 1987.

Jain D, Thompson B, Wackers FJ, et al. Relevance of increased lung thallium uptake on stress imaging in patients with unstable angina and non-Q wave myocardial infarction: Results of the thrombolysis in myocardial infarction (TIMI)-IIIB Study [in process citation]. *J Am Coll Cardiol* 30:421–429, 1997.

Society of Nuclear Medicine. *The Society of Nuclear Medicine Guideline for Myocardial Perfusion Imaging, Health Care Policy*. Available: http://www.snm.org/guide.html 1999.

Case 39

Clinical Presentation

44-year-old obese woman presenting with atypical chest pain.

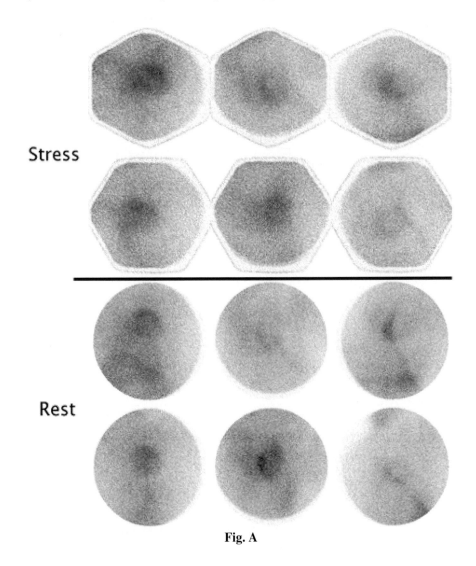

Stress

Rest

Fig. A

Technique

The following protocol is used in our department and is provided as an example of one possible imaging protocol. For other acceptable protocols, see the Society of Nuclear Medicine Guideline for Myocardial Perfusion Imaging in the Health Care Policy section of the Society of Nuclear Medicine web page (see Suggested Reading, below).

- Patient takes nothing by mouth for 3 hours prior to the test.
- Exercise is performed to increase myocardial perfusion and may be accomplished using a variety of protocols. Consult your nuclear medicine or cardiology department to familiarize yourself with your institution's protocol.

- 1.6 mCi thallium-201 thallous chloride administered intravenously at peak exercise.
- Imaging begins within 5 minutes of exercise termination.
- Energy window 20% centered on 70 keV (for Hg X rays), 20% centered on 167 keV (for thallium-201 gamma rays).
- Use slant hole collimator. Supine images are obtained in the anterior, 40-degree modified left anterior oblique (MLAO), and decubitus 70-degree left anterior oblique (LAO).
- Upright images are then obtained in anterior and 70-degree LAO projections to compare with supine images for movement of soft tissue attenuation artifacts.

Image Interpretation

Stress and rest images (Fig. A) show poor definition of the myocardium with several inconsistent defects (defects seen in one view but not where expected in a complimentary view). Note the linear attenuation defect caused by the left arm soft tissues in the 70-degree LAO views.

Differential Diagnosis

- Multiple infarcts
- Global ischemia
- Non-coronary cardiomyopathy
- Tracer infiltration
- Obesity causing severe attenuation
- Metabolic acidosis
- Off-peak energy setting on camera

Diagnosis and Clinical Follow-up

The study was indeterminate secondary to morbid obesity and soft tissue attenuation. The patient weighed more than 300 lb. Cardiac catheterization was not performed.

Discussion

Soft tissue attenuation is one of the most common obstacles to accurate interpretation of planar thallium studies. In obese individuals or in women (or men) with large breasts, the study may be uninterpretable. It is important to communicate the difficulties in scan interpretation to the referring physician. The referring physician should realize that any estimation of perfusion defect does not carry with it the same sensitivity and specificity as an exercise thallium study done on a patient with a normal body habitus.

Other causes of poor visualization of the myocardium include infiltration of the tracer dose, incorrect energy peak of the gamma camera, and injection of the wrong radiopharmaceutical.

Suggested Reading

Society of Nuclear Medicine. *The Society of Nuclear Medicine Guideline for Myocardial Perfusion Imaging, Health Care Policy*. Available: http://www.snm.org/guide.html 1999.

Case 40

Clinical Presentation

39-year-old man presenting with possible cardiomyopathy and atypical chest pain.

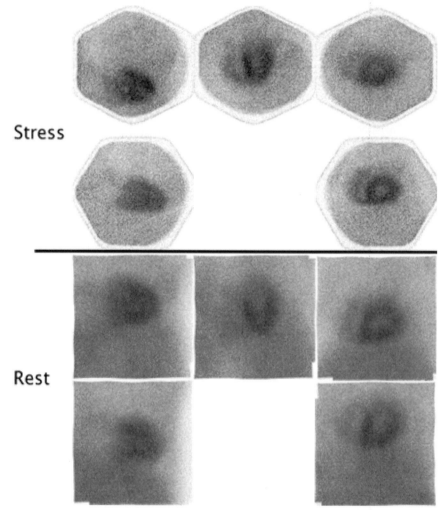

Stress

Rest

Fig. A

Technique

The following protocol is used in our department and is provided as an example of one possible imaging protocol. For other acceptable protocols, see the Society of Nuclear Medicine Guideline for Myocardial Perfusion Imaging in the Health Care Policy section of the Society of Nuclear Medicine web page (see Suggested Readings, below).

- Patient takes nothing by mouth for 3 hours prior to the test.
- Exercise is performed to increase myocardial perfusion and may be accomplished using a variety of protocols. Consult your nuclear medicine or cardiology department to familiarize yourself with your institution's protocol.

- 1.6 mCi thallium-201 thallous chloride administered intravenously at peak exercise.
- Imaging begins within 5 minutes of exercise termination.
- Energy window 20% centered on 70 keV (for Hg X rays), 20% centered on 167 keV (for thallium-201 gamma rays).
- Use slant hole collimator. Supine images are obtained in the anterior, 40-degree modified left anterior oblique (MLAO), and decubitus 70-degree left anterior oblique (LAO).
- Upright images are then obtained in anterior and 70-degree LAO projections to compare with supine images for movement of soft tissue attenuation artifacts.

Image Interpretation

Stress images (Fig. A) show a prominent right ventricle (RV) and no perfusion defects. Rest images show continued visualization of the RV, diminished from the stress images.

Differential Diagnosis

- Right ventricular overload, which may be caused by many factors, including atrial septal defect, congestive cardiomyopathy, chronic obstructive lung disease, myocardial infarction, hypertrophic cardiomyopathy, and incomplete resolution of pulmonary embolism.

Diagnosis and Clinical Follow-up

Right ventricular hypertrophy secondary to pulmonary hypertension was the diagnosis. The echocardiogram showed mild pulmonary hypertension.

Discussion

The RV is most often either not visualized or only minimally seen on exercise images because the blood flow and muscle mass of the RV are so much less than they are for the left. It is unusual to see the RV on planar rest images. Visualization of the RV, therefore, most commonly occurs when there is RV hypertrophy caused by increased demand on the right from elevated pulmonary pressures.

Suggested Readings

Nakajima K, Fotouhi F, Taki J, et al. Estimation of right ventricular pressure by 201TI scintigraphy in paediatric cardiac disease. *Nucl Med Commun* 11:667–684, 1990.

Schulman DS, Lazar JM, Ziady G, et al. Right ventricular thallium-201 kinetics in pulmonary hypertension: Relation to right ventricular size and function. *J Nucl Med* 34:1695–1700, 1993.

Society of Nuclear Medicine. *The Society of Nuclear Medicine Guideline for Myocardial Perfusion Imaging, Health Care Policy*. Available: http://www.snm.org/guide.html 1999.

Case 41

Clinical Presentation

74-year-old woman presenting with mitral valve prosthesis and decreased left ventricle (LV) ejection fraction (EF) on echocardiography.

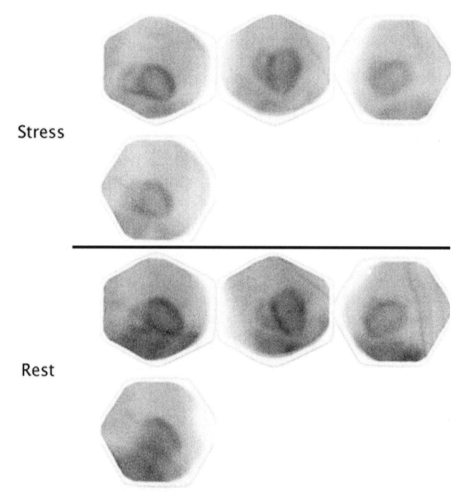

Stress

Rest

Fig. A

Technique

The following protocol is used in our department and is provided as an example of one possible imaging protocol. For other acceptable protocols, see the Society of Nuclear Medicine Guideline for Myocardial Perfusion Imaging in the Health Care Policy section of the Society of Nuclear Medicine web page (see Suggested Readings, below).

- Patient takes nothing by mouth for 3 hours prior to the test.
- Exercise is performed to increase myocardial perfusion and may be accomplished using a variety of protocols. Consult your nuclear medicine or cardiology department to familiarize yourself with your institution's protocol.

PEARLS/PITFALLS

- Transient dilatation of the LV may be seen only on the first planar image obtained. The ventricle size may appear relatively decreased on subsequent views as the hemodynamics return to the resting state.

- Multivessel perfusion defects in patients with ischemic cardiomyopathy may make identification of a single territory of reversibility more difficult. Images should be carefully reviewed for small areas of reversibility that may indicate more extensive regions of viable myocardium.

- When comparing stress and rest images for transient left ventricular dilatation during stress, it is important to make sure the same gamma camera was used for both sets of images.

- Dilatation of the LV with exercise, as compared with rest, suggests a poorer prognosis, but there is little evidence in the literature confirming this hypothesis.

- 1.6 mCi thallium-201 thallous chloride administered intravenously at peak exercise.
- Imaging begins within 5 minutes of exercise termination.
- Energy window 20% centered on 70 keV (for Hg X rays), 20% centered on 167 keV (for thallium-201 gamma rays).
- Use slant hole collimator. Supine images are obtained in the anterior, 40-degree modified left anterior oblique (MLAO), and decubitus 70-degree left anterior oblique (LAO).
- Upright images are then obtained in anterior and 70-degree LAO projections to compare with supine images for movement of soft tissue attenuation artifacts.

Image Interpretation

Stress images (Fig. A) show a moderately enlarged LV with poor apical uptake. No obvious difference in distribution of the tracer is noted in the resting images (no ischemia noted).

Differential Diagnosis

- Triple vessel coronary artery disease
- Viral myocarditis
- Cardiotoxic chemotherapeutic agents such as adriamycin
- Valvular heart disease
- Dominant left anterior descending coronary artery stenosis with hypoxia

Diagnosis and Clinical Follow-up

Severe LV dysfunction was diagnosed. Echocardiography showed a left ventricular EF of 20%. There was severe LV dysfunction, dilated atria, and a mitral valve prosthesis.

Discussion

Assessment of ventricular size is most easily and accurately accomplished with echocardiography. LV enlargement may also be demonstrated with planar thallium imaging, and, when noted, the finding should be included in the study report. Although size markers or region of interest computer analysis may be used, qualitative visual assessment is often adequate to diagnose ventricular dilatation. This is most easily done when there is some familiarity with images obtained from the particular gamma camera being used so that the size of the ventricle may be compared with the camera field of view.

In this case, the chamber size is enlarged out of proportion to the thickness of the myocardial walls. This finding suggests dilatation even without extensive experience with this particular camera field of view.

Suggested Readings

Machac J, Levin H, Balk E, et al. Computer modeling of planar myocardial perfusion imaging: Effect of heart rate and ejection fraction on wall thickness and chamber size. *J Nucl Med* 27:653–659, 1986.

Manno B, Hakki AH, Kane SA, et al. Usefulness of left ventricular wall thickness-to-diameter ratio in thallium-201 scintigraphy. *Cathet Cardiovasc Diagn* 9:483–491, 1983.

Society of Nuclear Medicine. *The Society of Nuclear Medicine Guideline for Myocardial Perfusion Imaging, Health Care Policy.* Available: http://www.snm.org/guide.html 1999.

Case 42

Clinical Presentation

68-year-old man presenting with increasing shortness of breath.

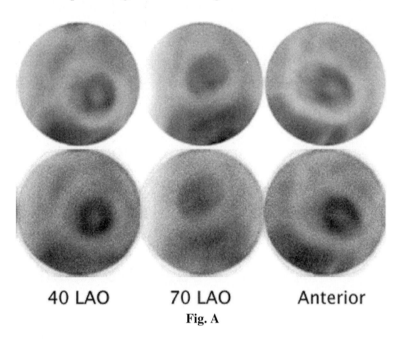

40 LAO   70 LAO   Anterior

Fig. A

Technique

The following protocol is used in our department and is provided as an example of one possible imaging protocol. For other acceptable protocols, see the Society of Nuclear Medicine Guideline for Myocardial Perfusion Imaging in the Health Care Policy section of the Society of Nuclear Medicine web page (see Suggested Readings, below).

- Patient takes nothing by mouth for 3 hours prior to the test.
- Exercise is performed to increase myocardial perfusion and may be accomplished using a variety of protocols. Consult your nuclear medicine or cardiology department to familiarize yourself with your institution's protocol.
- 1.6 mCi thallium-201 thallous chloride administered intravenously at peak exercise.
- Imaging begins within 5 minutes of exercise termination.
- Energy window 20% centered on 70 keV (for Hg X rays), 20% centered on 167 keV (for thallium-201 gamma rays).
- Use slant hole collimator. Supine images are obtained in the anterior, 40-degree modified left anterior oblique (MLAO), and decubitus 70-degree left anterior oblique (LAO).

Image Interpretation

Images in both stress and rest (Fig. A) show a "halo" of decreased tracer activity around the left ventricular myocardium. Cinematic images (not available) show

- Cinematic images are helpful when the pericardial effusion is large. The abnormal myocardial movement within the effusion helps confirm the diagnosis.

- The finding of a "halo" around the left ventricle is very nonspecific and must always be correlated with echocardiography.

the myocardium moving superiorly and inferiorly as it contracts within the confines of the area of decreased tracer activity.

Differential Diagnosis

- Pericardial fluid
- Normal variant (although usually not when the abnormality is this prominent)
- Mediastinal or pericardial fat
- Pericardial cyst or tumor
- Pleural fluid
- Pneumopericardium

Diagnosis and Clinical Follow-up

Echocardiogram showed a large pericardial effusion.

Discussion

Pericardial effusion should be considered when an area of diminished tracer activity is noted around the left ventricular myocardial uptake. Unless rapidly forming at the time of tracer injection, the pericardial effusion will not concentrate the perfusion tracer.

Suggested Readings

Nestico PF, Hakki AH, Iskandrian AS, et al. Thallium-201 imaging in pericardial effusion. *Clin Nucl Med* 11:213, 1986.

Society of Nuclear Medicine. *The Society of Nuclear Medicine Guideline for Myocardial Perfusion Imaging, Health Care Policy*. Available: http://www.snm.org/guide.html 1999.

Vasinrapee P, Cook R, Reese I. Pericardial and mediastinal involvement from bronchogenic carcinoma demonstrated by TI-201 imaging. *Clin Nucl Med* 20:1027, 1995.

Case 43

Clinical Presentation

An elderly woman with no history of coronary artery disease presenting with atypical chest pain.

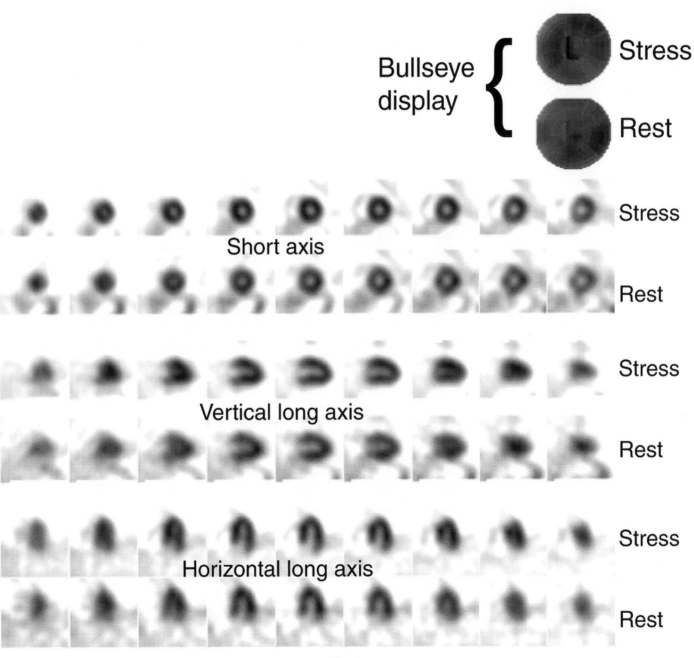

Fig. A

Short axis

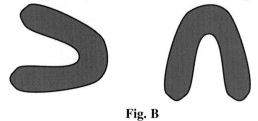

Vertical long axis   Horizontal long axis

Fig. B

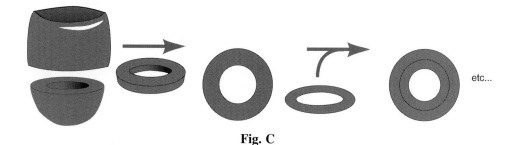

etc...

Fig. C

Technique

- 2 mCi thallium-201 thallous chloride is injected intravenously while the patient is at rest.
- Thallium images are acquired using a dual-headed gamma camera with heads set at 90 degrees from each other.
- Images are acquired for 180 degrees beginning at right anterior oblique and finishing at left posterior oblique projection (each head acquires 90 degrees of data).
- Sixty images are acquired (3 degrees per stop, 30 seconds per stop).
- Patient is placed in the prone position with arms above the head.
- Immediately following rest imaging, the patient is stressed (either with treadmill or pharmacologically).
- At peak stress, 20 mCi Tc-99m-sestamibi (MIBI) is injected intravenously.
- Single photon emission computed tomography (SPECT) images are obtained in the same manner as the rest images just described, except at only 20 seconds per stop.
- Images are processed and displayed in bull's eye format as well as short axis, horizontal long axis, and vertical long axis.

- Always review the rotating images (raw data) to check for patient motion during image acquisition.

- Technetium-labeled perfusion agents such as MIBI and tetrofosmin have higher photon flux and are less subject to attenuation from soft tissue.

- Describe not only the reversibility or fixed nature of defects but also the size, intensity, and degree of reversibility to better assist the referring physician in determining the importance of a finding.

- SPECT images increase contrast. The improved sensitivity is accompanied by a decrease in specificity. Minor irregularities in the image should be interpreted with caution.

- Not all investigators believe that SPECT is more accurate than planar imaging for the diagnosis of coronary artery perfusion abnormalities.

- As with planar images, knowledge of the history, physical exam findings, previous history of coronary artery disease, stress tolerance, symptoms during stress, and electrocardiogram (EKG) findings may influence image interpretation. Some investigators feel the images should be read without this information; some feel it is important for providing an accurate interpretation of images.

- There is some debate as to the optimum patient positioning: prone or supine.

Image Interpretation

SPECT slices and bull's eye display (Fig. A) show normal tracer distribution throughout the left ventricular myocardium.

Diagnosis and Clinical Follow-up

Patient exercised for 9.5 minutes on a Bruce protocol. There was no electrocardiographic evidence of ischemia. Images were interpreted as normal. Catheterization was not performed.

Discussion

Review of a SPECT perfusion study should begin with the cinematic display of the planar images acquired at each projection angle over 180 degrees. This cinematic display will provide information about patient motion during image acquisition. The next step is to review the reconstructed slices. This can be done in a number of ways.

One method is to review the short axis slices first. These slices demonstrate perfusion to all the left ventricular myocardium except the apex. The apical perfusion can then be viewed on either long axis view. Figure B shows a diagrammatic representation of myocardial segments visualized on the reconstructed SPECT slices.

Besides displaying myocardial perfusion of individual slices, the short axis images can be "stacked" together and displayed as a "bull's eye" plot. In this representation, the slices toward the apex are in the center of the disk and the slices toward the base are at the periphery. This display shows all the myocardium in one image and allows a more complete display of the extent of a defect (Fig. C).

SPECT has provided an increase in sensitivity over that of planar images, but this improvement is accompanied by a decrease in specificity. Overall, the accuracy of the SPECT study is probably better than that of the planar study. A more substantial benefit of SPECT may be in the improved ability to map the location and extent of perfusion defects. This allows a closer region-by-region comparison of stress and rest images and may allow a closer correlation with findings on coronary arteriography.

Perfusion defects noted during stress and resolving at rest are the typical findings seen with myocardium at risk for infarction; defects noted on both stress and rest images suggest prior infarction. It has been shown, however, that as many as 20% of perfusion defects seen on both stress and rest images ("fixed" defects) do not reflect infarction. Therefore, these fixed defects reflect areas of viable myocardium that is "hibernating" secondary to chronically diminished blood flow. The viability of the underlying myocardium can be imaged most accurately with ^{18}F-fluorodeoxyglucose (^{18}FDG), described in the section on myocardial viability.

Although the myocardial metabolism of MIBI and thallium-201 is quite different, both tracers are deposited in relation to blood flow and therefore provide important information about myocardial perfusion.

Suggested Readings

Alexander C, Oberhausen E. Myocardial scintigraphy. *Semin Nucl Med* 25:195–201, 1995.

Beller GA. Myocardial perfusion imaging with thallium-201. *J Nucl Med* 35:674–680, 1994.

Gerson MC. *Cardiac Nuclear Medicine*. 3rd ed. New York: McGraw-Hill, 1997.

Merz CN, Berman DS. Imaging techniques for coronary artery disease: Current status and future directions. *Clin Cardiol* 20:526–532, 1997.

Case 44

Clinical Presentation

54-year-old man presenting with chest pain and no prior history of coronary artery disease.

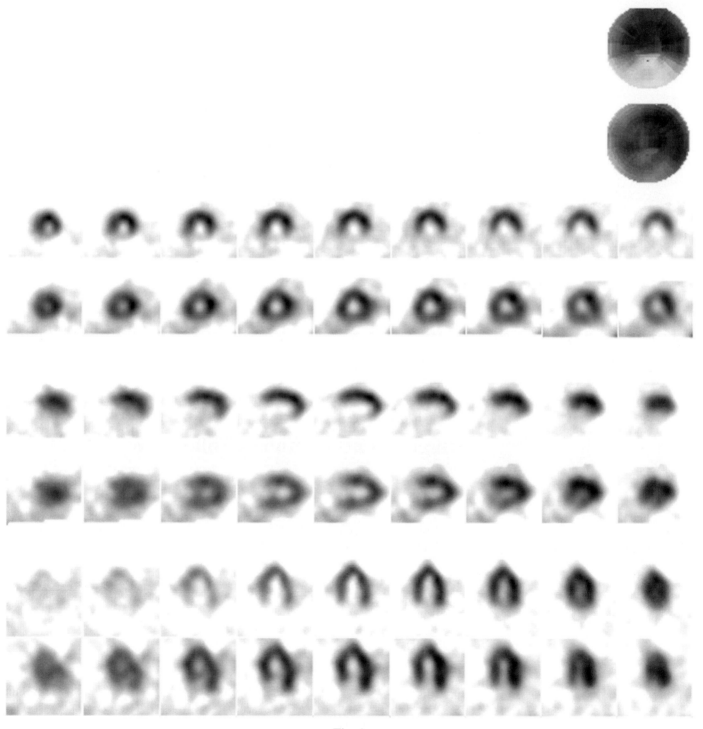

Fig. A

Technique

- 2 mCi thallium-201 thallous chloride is injected intravenously while the patient is at rest.
- Thallium images are acquired using a dual-headed gamma camera with heads set at 90 degrees from each other.
- Images are acquired for 180 degrees beginning at right anterior oblique and finishing at left posterior oblique projection (each head acquires 90 degrees of data).
- Sixty images are acquired (3 degrees per stop, 30 seconds per stop).
- The patient is placed in the prone position with arms above the head.
- Immediately following rest imaging, the patient is stressed (either with treadmill or pharmacologically).
- At peak stress, 20 mCi Tc-99m-sestamibi (MIBI) is injected intravenously.
- Single photon emission computed tomography (SPECT) images are obtained in the same manner as the rest images just described, except at only 20 seconds per stop.
- Images are processed and displayed in bull's eye format as well as short axis, horizontal long axis, and vertical long axis.

Image Interpretation

A severe tracer defect is seen in the inferior wall extending into the posterior wall on exercise images (Fig A). Delayed images show normal tracer distribution throughout the myocardium other than a small amount of mild residual defect in the inferior wall.

Differential Diagnosis

- Coronary artery disease
- Coronary artery spasm
- Diaphragmatic attenuation
- Motion artifact
- Sarcoidosis

Diagnosis and Clinical Follow-up

The patient was sent to the emergency room to be admitted to the coronary care unit. In the emergency room, he experienced a vagal episode during intravenous (IV) placement. He quickly developed chest pain and S-T segment elevations on electrocardiogram (EKG). The pain could not be relieved with initial maneuvers, so the patient was taken immediately to the catheterization suite. Coronary artery catheterization demonstrated a 90% stenotic lesion in the circumflex artery that was stented. Other coronary arteries were normal. The patient recovered uneventfully. Creatine kinase (CK) enzymes remained normal.

Discussion

The severe, reversible defect noted on the SPECT images is consistent with a large area of ischemia in the inferior and posterior portions of the left ventricular myocardium. The inferior wall is often subject to attenuation defects and reconstruction artifacts probably caused by adjacent diaphragmatic attenuation. When

PEARLS/PITFALLS

- Fixed defects should not be called *infarcts*. As many as 20% of fixed defects contain underlying viable myocardium, as demonstrated by positron-emission tomography or revascularization.

- Cinematic display of the raw data should be reviewed for soft tissue attenuation in the region of the inferior wall when the cause of an inferior wall defect is questioned.

- As described previously, diaphragmatic or other soft tissue attenuation can often cause inferior wall defects.

- Prior knowledge of the results of exercise testing (symptoms, EKG findings, work level achieved) may improve the specificity of image readings, although some argue that images should be read without other knowledge of the patient.

defects are as complete and as large as the exercise defect noted in this case, however, and there is such a dramatic improvement in resting images, the defect is almost certainly caused by left ventricular ischemia.

Describing the severity and extent of a perfusion defect provides much more information to the referring physician than merely stating that a defect is present. A qualitative assessment such as mild, moderate, or severe, as well as a description of the size of the defect, will help the referring physician determine the meaning of a defect. A young man with a low pretest likelihood of disease may be more likely to be given a clean bill of health if a perfusion defect is described as "mild, small, fixed" than if it is described as "severe, large, and reversible."

Suggested Readings

Heiba SI, Hayat NJ, Salman HS, et al. Technetium-99m-MIBI myocardial SPECT: Supine versus right lateral imaging and comparison with coronary arteriography. *J Nucl Med* 38:1510–1514, 1997.

Nuyts J, Dupont P, Van den Maegdenbergh V, et al. A study of the liver-heart artifact in emission tomography. *J Nucl Med* 36:133–139, 1995.

Royal HD. How do you differentiate a genuine reversible inferior wall defect on thallium stress tests from an artifact due to respiration during the stress portion of a thallium stress test? *AJR Am J Roentgenol* 165:1004–1005, 1995.

Simons M, Parker JA, Udelson JE, et al. The role of clinical data in interpretation of perfusion images. *J Nucl Med* 35:740–741, 1994.

Van Heertum RL, Nour R. False-positive diagnoses of reversible inferior wall defects on 201TI-SPECT images. *AJR Am J Roentgenol* 163:740–741, 1994.

Case 45

Clinical Presentation

96-year-old man presenting with exertional chest pressure and a history of coronary artery disease.

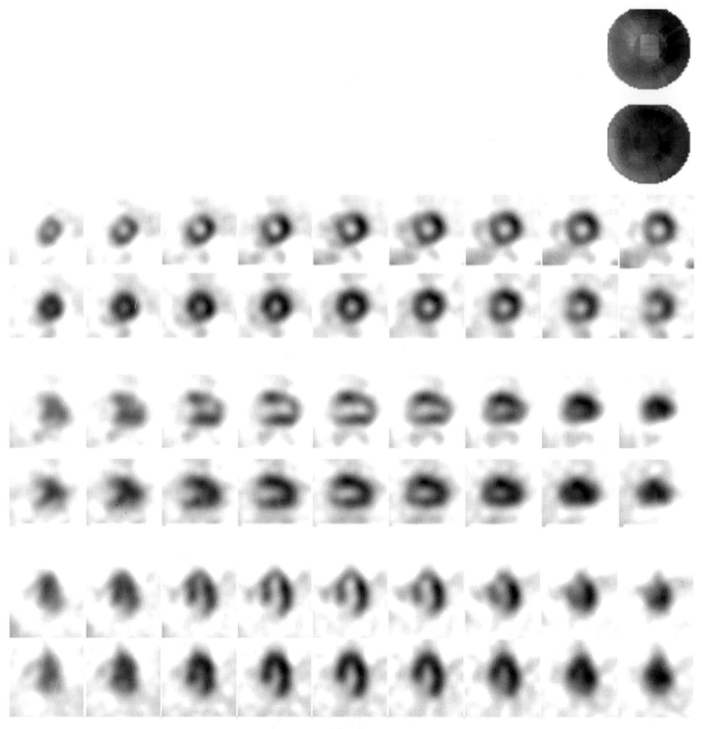

Fig. A

Technique

- 2 mCi thallium-201 thallous chloride is injected intravenously while the patient is at rest.
- Thallium images are acquired using a dual-headed gamma camera with heads set at 90 degrees from each other.
- Images are acquired for 180 degrees beginning at right anterior oblique and finishing at left posterior oblique projection (each head acquires 90 degrees of data).
- Sixty images are acquired (3 degrees per stop, 30 seconds per stop).
- The patient is placed in the prone position with arms above the head.
- Immediately following rest imaging, the patient is stressed (either with treadmill or pharmacologically).
- At peak stress, 20 mCi Tc-99m-sestamibi (MIBI) is injected intravenously.
- Single photon emission computed tomography (SPECT) images are obtained in the same manner as the rest images just described, except at only 20 seconds per stop.
- Images are processed and displayed in bullseye format as well as short axis, horizontal long axis, and vertical long axis.

Image Interpretation

Exercise images show a large, moderate defect of tracer uptake at the distal anterior wall and apex; rest images show normal tracer distribution throughout the myocardium (Fig. A).

Differential Diagnosis

- Coronary artery disease
- Soft tissue attenuation (breast or chest wall)
- Motion artifact
- Coronary artery spasm
- Idiopathic
- Sarcoidosis

Diagnosis and Clinical Follow-up

Catheterization showed a 95% proximal left anterior descending (LAD) stenosis. The lesion was treated with a rotablade, after which minimal (30%) stenosis remained.

Discussion

The exercise perfusion defect here is qualitatively classified as a moderate defect in that it is clearly visible but not characterized by complete absence of tracer uptake seen in the previous case (see Case 44). When a defect of this character resolves completely on resting images, it is less likely secondary to artifact, although shifting soft tissue attenuation, such as breast tissue, can cause reversible mild or moderate defects. Review of the cinematic display of raw data helps to demonstrate focal soft tissue masses that might cause attenuation artifacts.

Suggested Reading

Gerson MC. *Cardiac Nuclear Medicine*. 3rd ed. New York: McGraw-Hill, 1997.

Case 46

Clinical Presentation

55-year-old man presenting with hypertension and poor exercise tolerance.

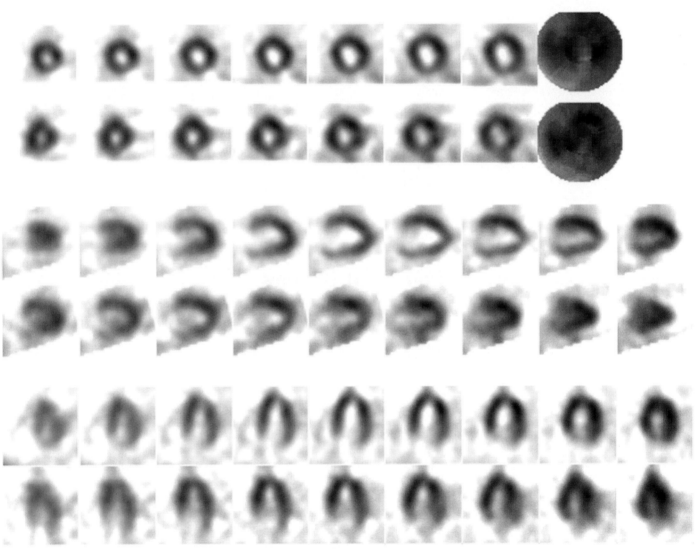

Fig. A

Technique

- 2 mCi thallium-201 thallous chloride is injected intravenously while the patient is at rest.
- Thallium images are acquired using a dual-headed gamma camera with heads set at 90 degrees from each other.
- Images are acquired for 180 degrees beginning at right anterior oblique and finishing at left posterior oblique projection (each head acquires 90 degrees of data).
- Sixty images are acquired (3 degrees per stop, 30 seconds per stop).

- The patient is placed in the prone position with arms above the head.
- Immediately following rest imaging, the patient is stressed (either with treadmill or pharmacologically).
- At peak stress, 20 mCi Tc-99m-sestamibi (MIBI) is injected intravenously.
- Single photon emission computed tomography (SPECT) images are obtained in the same manner as the rest images just described, except at only 20 seconds per stop.
- Images are processed and displayed in bullseye format as well as short axis, horizontal long axis, and vertical long axis.

Image Interpretation

SPECT images (Fig. A) show patchy tracer distribution throughout a dilated left ventricle (LV). No clear areas of improved perfusion are noted at rest.

Differential Diagnosis

- Triple vessel coronary artery disease
- Viral myocarditis
- Cardiotoxic chemotherapeutic agents such as adriamycin
- Valvular heart disease
- Dominant left anterior descending coronary artery stenosis with hypoxia

Diagnosis and Clinical Follow-up

Coronary artery catheterization showed a dilated LV with global hypokinesis and an LV ejection fraction of 41%. Coronary arteries were normal.

Discussion

Idiopathic cardiomyopathy is one of the many causes of perfusion defects seen with myocardial scintigraphy. It should be considered when the LV chamber is dilated and there is irregular tracer distribution throughout the myocardium. When perfusion defects are present, they are most often fixed.

Suggested Reading

Tauberg SG, Orie JE, Bartlett BE, et al. Usefulness of thallium-201 for distinction of ischemic from idiopathic dilated cardiomyopathy. *Am J Cardiol* 71:674–680, 1993.

Case 47

Clinical Presentation

50-year-old woman presenting with shortness of breath.

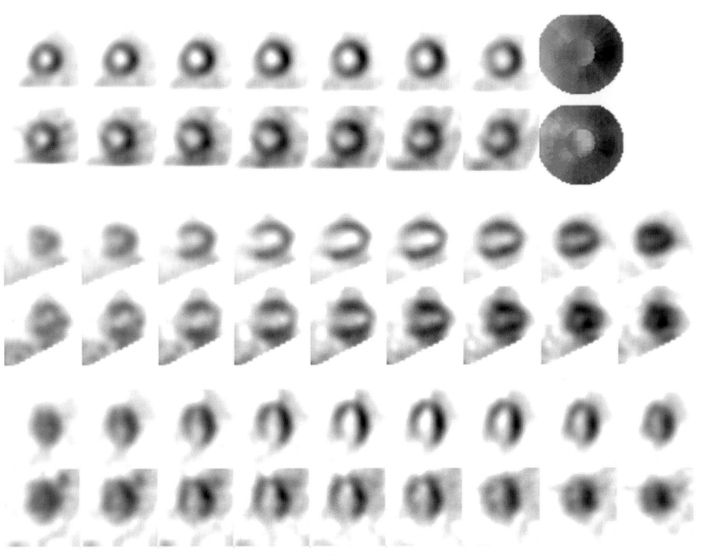

Fig. A

Technique

- 2 mCi thallium-201 thallous chloride is injected intravenously while the patient is at rest.
- Thallium images are acquired using a dual-headed gamma camera with heads set at 90 degrees from each other.
- Images are acquired for 180 degrees beginning at right anterior oblique and finishing at left posterior oblique projection (each head acquires 90 degrees of data).
- Sixty images are acquired (3 degrees per stop, 30 seconds per stop).

- The patient is placed in the prone position with arms above the head.
- Immediately following rest imaging, the patient is stressed (either with treadmill or pharmacologically).
- At peak stress, 20 mCi Tc-99m-sestamibi (MIBI) is injected intravenously.
- Single photon emission computed tomography (SPECT) images are obtained in the same manner as the rest images just described, except at only 20 seconds per stop.
- Images are processed and displayed in bullseye format as well as short axis, horizontal long axis, and vertical long axis.

Image Interpretation

SPECT images (Fig. A) show a dilated left ventricular cavity and decreased tracer activity in the septum, extending into the apex, on both exercise and delayed images.

Differential Diagnosis

For septal defect:

- Coronary artery disease
- Soft tissue attenuation
- Left bundle branch block
- Motion artifact
- Coronary artery spasm
- Alignment artifact

Diagnosis and Clinical Follow-up

Diffuse hypokinesis and normal coronary arteries were noted on cardiac catheterization. The patient had left bundle branch block on EKG.

Discussion

Left bundle branch block (LBBB) is known to cause decreased blood flow, and therefore decreased tracer distribution, in the region of the interventricular septum, especially during exercise. The defect noted on this study is atypical for an exercise-induced LBBB septal perfusion defect in that it extends into the apex and is fixed (i.e., it is unchanged between exercise and rest images). This atypical appearance may be caused by the underlying cardiomyopathy.

The most common LBBB defect is noted during exercise with improvement on resting images. The defect is probably caused by decreased blood flow to the septum during asynchronous systole. The delayed contraction of the septum diminishes blood flow to that area of the myocardium when coronary artery flow to the rest of the myocardium is greatest.

Suggested Reading

Gerson MC. *Cardiac Nuclear Medicine.* 3rd ed. New York: McGraw-Hill, 1997.

Case 48

Clinical Presentation

55-year-old man presenting with a history of hypertension, non–insulin-dependent diabetes, and poor left ventricular wall motion onechocardiogram. A stress Tc-99m-sestamibi (MIBI) study was done to rule out coronary artery disease.

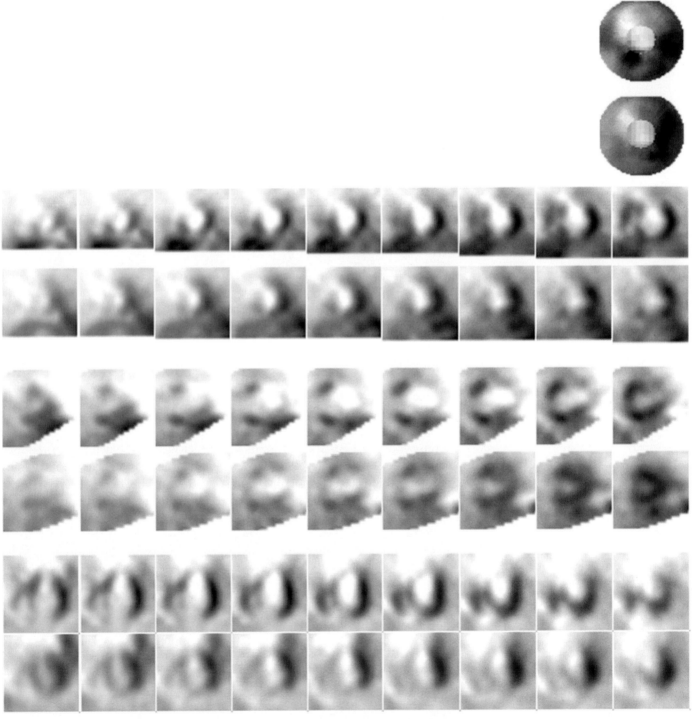

Fig. A

Technique

- 2 mCi thallium-201 thallous chloride is injected intravenously while the patient is at rest.
- Thallium images are acquired using a dual-headed gamma camera with heads set at 90 degrees from each other.
- Images are acquired for 180 degrees beginning at right anterior oblique and finishing at left posterior oblique projection (each head acquires 90 degrees of data).
- Sixty images are acquired (3 degrees per stop, 30 seconds per stop).
- The patient is placed in the prone position with arms above the head.
- Immediately following rest imaging, the patient is stressed (either with treadmill or pharmacologically).
- At peak stress, 20 mCi Tc-99m-sestamibi (MIBI) is injected intravenously.
- Single photon emission computed tomography (SPECT) images are obtained in the same manner as the rest images just described, except at only 20 seconds per stop.
- Images are processed and displayed in bullseye format as well as short axis, horizontal long axis, and vertical long axis.

Image Interpretation

Stress and rest images (Fig. A) show a markedly dilated left ventricle with severe fixed perfusion defects throughout.

Differential Diagnosis

- Triple vessel coronary artery disease
- Viral myocarditis
- Cardiotoxic chemotherapeutic agents such as adriamycin
- Valvular heart disease
- Idiopathic cardiomyopathy

Diagnosis and Clinical Follow-up

The patient went to cardiac catheterization to rule out coronary artery disease. Coronary arteries showed no evidence of disease. The left ventricle was dilated with global hypokinesis. Ejection fraction was calculated to be approximately 30%.

Discussion

Although we tend to think of myocardial perfusion defects as relating to disease in the major coronary arteries, perfusion defects are nonspecific and may relate to microvascular changes or flow changes based on underlying tissue damage that is not related to a primary perfusion abnormality.

Suggested Readings

Li LX, Nohara R, Okuda K, et al. Comparative study of 201 Tl-scintigraphic image and myocardial pathologic findings in patients with dilated cardiomyopathy. *Ann Nucl Med* 10:307–314, 1996.

Tamai J, Nagata S, Nishimura T, et al. Hemodynamic and prognostic value of thallium-201 myocardial imaging in patients with dilated cardiomyopathy. *Int J Cardiol* 24:219–224, 1989.

Case 49

Clinical Presentation

50-year-old woman presenting with hypertension, obesity, and recent onset of chest pain.

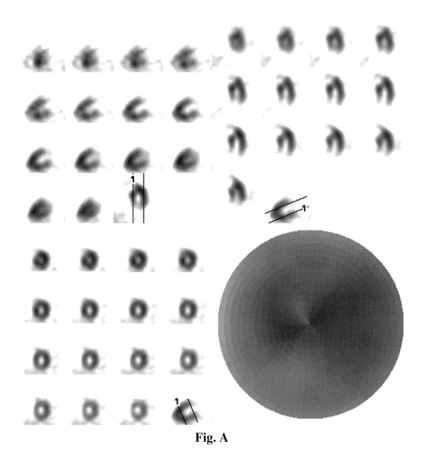

Fig. A

Technique

- While the patient is experiencing chest pain, 20 mCi Tc-99m-sestamibi (MIBI) is injected intravenously.
- The patient is placed in the prone position with arms above the head.
- Images are acquired for 180 degrees beginning at right anterior oblique and finishing at left posterior oblique projection.
- Sixty images are acquired (3 degrees per stop, 20 seconds per stop).
- Images are processed and displayed in bullseye format as well as short axis, horizontal long axis, and vertical long axis.

Image Interpretation

Figure A shows a defect at the apex toward the septum, seen well on the horizontal long axis images. An extension of activity is seen from the lateral wall out past the apex, also noted on the horizontal long axis images.

Differential Diagnosis

- Coronary artery disease
- Physiologic apical thinning
- Motion artifact
- Soft tissue attenuation (chest wall)
- Coronary artery spasm
- Misalignment of camera center of rotation

Diagnosis and Clinical Follow-up

The pattern of tracer activity suggests motion artifact causing the finger-like extension of activity past the apex. Cinematic images (not shown) demonstrate motion during the initial tracer acquisition. A second set of images (Fig. B) was obtained immediately after the first, showing resolution of the apical defect and the abnormal projection of activity beyond the apex.

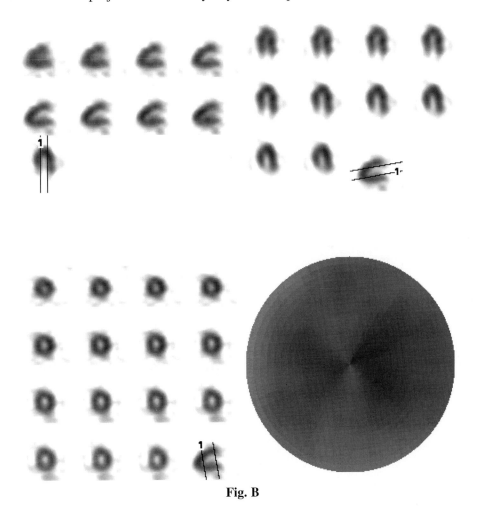

Fig. B

Discussion

Patient motion during image acquisition can introduce a number of artifacts into the image. If the motion occurs during single photon emission computed tomography (SPECT) acquisition, computer processing of the image data can make the motion more difficult to detect, particularly if the only images reviewed are the reconstructed images.

Patient motion during the first acquisition created a defect that may have been mistaken for an apical perfusion abnormality and a nonanatomic extension of the lateral wall past the apex.

Suggested Readings

Cooper JA, Neumann PH, McCandless BK. Effect of patient motion on tomographic myocardial perfusion imaging [see comments]. *J Nucl Med* 33:1566–1571, 1992.

DePuey EGr. How to detect and avoid myocardial perfusion SPECT artifacts. *J Nucl Med* 35:699–702, 1994.

Prigent FM, Hyun M, Berman DS, et al. Effect of motion on thallium-201 SPECT studies: A simulation and clinical study. *J Nucl Med* 34:1845–1850, 1993.

Sorrell V, Figueroa B, Hansen CL. The "hurricane sign": Evidence of patient motion artifact on cardiac single-photon emission computed tomographic imaging. *J Nucl Cardiol* 3:86–88, 1996.

Case 50

Clinical Presentation

64-year-old woman presenting with breast cancer. Radionuclide ventriculography was ordered prior to chemotherapy.

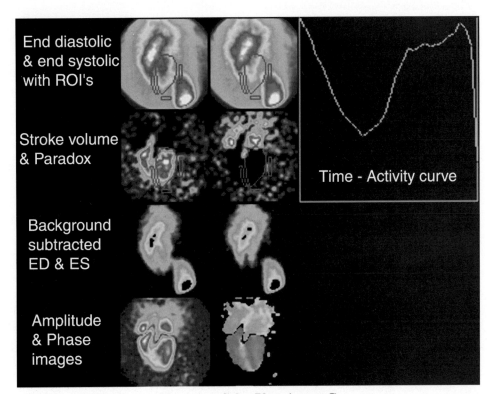

Fig. A (see Color Plate 1, page I)

Technique

- It is important that special precautions be taken to ensure that blood being labeled in the radiopharmacy is injected into the correct patient. In our lab, the technologist that drew the blood must also be the one to inject the blood back into the patient. If that is not possible, two technologists must be involved during the injection, and both must verify that the patient is receiving the appropriate blood.
- As soon as the blood is taken from the patient for labeling, a special wrist band should be attached to the patient for identification.
- The radiopharmacy will label only one blood specimen at a time to avoid confusing two or more samples.
- Three milliliters autologous red blood cells labeled with 20 to 25 mCi technetium-99m in vitro and injected intravenously.
- Images obtained in anterior, 40-degree modified left anterior oblique (MLAO) and left posterior oblique (LPO) views.
- Left ventricular ejection fraction (LVEF) calculated from the 40-degree MLAO view.

Image Interpretation

Cinematic images (Fig. A) demonstrate normal wall motion. All walls visualized move inward toward the center of the left ventricle in a coordinated fashion. Functional images (explained later) show normal stroke volume (SV), paradox, amplitude, and phase. LVEF was calculated to be 64%.

Differential Diagnosis

- Normal study
- False negative in a patient with a depressed ejection fraction and background region of interest (ROI) drawn incorrectly over a region of high activity, such as the right ventricular blood pool.
- A normal ejection fraction does not rule out other cardiac pathology, such as valvular disease or cardiac shunts. Therefore, the ejection fraction should not be reported without knowledge of the patient history and the reason the referring physician ordered the study.

Diagnosis and Clinical Follow-up

The radionuclide ventriculogram was normal. The patient received chemotherapy without incident. Follow-up studies performed 1 and 2 months later showed no change in myocardial function.

Discussion

The radionuclide ventriculogram is the most accurate and reproducible study for determining LVEF. Reproducibility is approximately 5% (in ejection fraction units). In addition, several functional images can be obtained, including SV, paradoxical motion, amplitude, and phase. The values in those images can be displayed as different colors or different shades of gray for a visual display of the data that is easy to understand. Several programs for calculating these data are available, and all may display the data differently. The underlying principle for calculation of these data is the same in most programs, however.

An SV image is obtained by subtracting the end-systolic (ES) image from the end-diastolic (ED) image on a pixel by pixel basis. All negative values (areas with paradoxical motion) are set to zero. Pixels with higher numbers are displayed as white, decreasing to black in areas of zero counts. Therefore, pixels with large changes in counts between ED and ES (large SV) will show brighter color.

The paradox image displays paradoxical changes in activity in the left ventricle ROI. If counts in a particular region of the left ventricle increase during systole rather than decrease as expected, this area of paradoxical ventricular filling is represented by a color whereas other areas demonstrating the normal decrease in counts during systole are represented by black. For example, if there is a dyskinetic region of wall motion causing blood to fill an area of the left ventricle during systole, the ES pixels in the ROI will have more counts than the same ED pixels have. The image therefore displays in color just the pixels with negative values from the result of ED minus ES.

Amplitude images show similar information to SV images; the two values have important differences, however. Amplitude is calculated using the entire cardiac cycle (not just ED and ES frames), resulting in a smoother (less noisy) image.

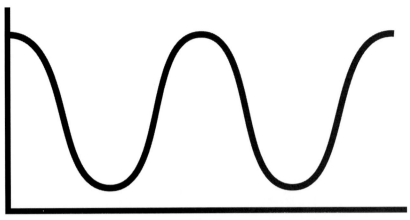

Fig. B

Also, all values are displayed as positive; in other words, in areas of paradoxical motion, the negative difference between ED and ES counts is not changed to zero, as it is in the SV image, but rather the negative value is displayed as a positive value of the same magnitude (the SV plus paradox volume). This means that the amplitude of paradoxically moving areas is displayed with that of the normally contracting ventricle.

The phase images provide information complementary to that of the previously discussed functional images. When observed over time, the tracer activity in the left ventricle (or in each pixel over the cardiac blood pool) increases and decreases throughout the cardiac cycle. This variation in activity can be fit to a sine wave function (Fig. B). The complete cardiac cycle (one cycle of the sine wave) is assigned 360 degrees on the x-axis of the time-activity curve. A color scale can also be assigned to the x-axis. The color corresponding to the location on the color scale of the peak (or trough) of the sine wave can then be assigned to each pixel. A pixel in the left ventricular ROI would show decreasing activity during systole and increasing activity in diastole (Fig. C). A pixel in a heart with a poor ejection fraction would show decreased amplitude over a pixel in a left ventricle with a good ejection fraction (Fig. D).

Not all pixels in the image show the same time-activity curve as those in the left ventricle, however. The atria, for example, are filling with blood as the ventricles are contracting. Filling of the atria is completely opposite the left ventricle; therefore, it is said to be "180 degrees out of phase" with the left ventricle (Fig. E). Similarly, if there is an intraventricular conduction defect and a particular ventricular wall is not contracting until late in the cardiac cycle, it will have a different color than the rest of the ventricle has (Fig. F).

For calculating and displaying the phase image, all pixels representing sine waves in the same phase (peaks all occur at the same place) are assigned the same color. Pixels that peak at a different time in the time-activity curve are assigned another color. This results in a color-coded image demonstrating the coordination of the left ventricular contraction. The amplitude of the sine wave within each pixel is not considered for the phase image. For example, the two pixels demonstrated in Figure D would be assigned the same color.

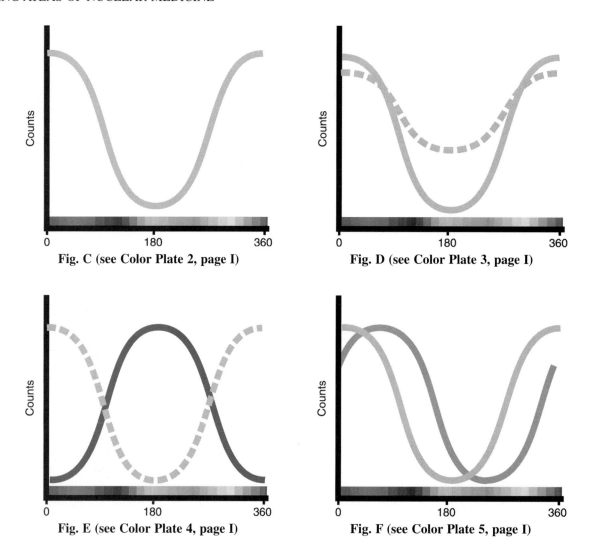

Fig. C (see Color Plate 2, page I)

Fig. D (see Color Plate 3, page I)

Fig. E (see Color Plate 4, page I)

Fig. F (see Color Plate 5, page I)

Suggested Readings

Borges-Neto S, Coleman RE. Radionuclide ventricular function analysis. *Radiol Clin North Am* 31:817–830, 1993.

Botvinick EH, Dae MW, O'Connell JW. Functional imaging and phase analysis of blood-pool scintigrams. In: Gerson MC, ed. *Cardiac Nuclear Medicine*. New York: McGraw-Hill, 1997, pp. 371–386.

Wackers FJT. Equilibrium radionuclide angiocardiography. In: Gerson MC, ed. *Cardiac Nuclear Medicine*. New York: McGraw-Hill, 1997, pp. 315–345.

Watson NE Jr, Cowan RJ, Ball JD. Conventional radionuclide cardiac imaging. *Radiol Clin North Am* 32:477–500, 1994.

Case 51

Clinical Presentation

45-year-old man presenting with shortness of breath, cough, and symptoms of congestive heart failure (CHF).

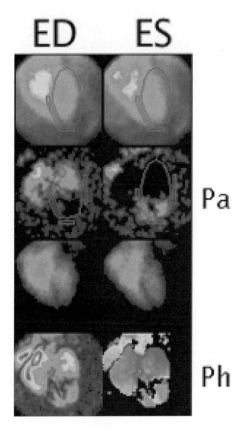

Fig. A (see Color Plate 6, page II)

Technique

- It is important that special precautions be taken to ensure that blood being labeled in the radiopharmacy is injected into the correct patient. In our lab, the technologist that drew the blood must also be the one to inject the blood back into the patient. If that is not possible, two technologists must be involved during the injection, and both must verify that the patient is receiving the appropriate blood.
- As soon as the blood is taken from the patient for labeling, a special wrist band should be attached to the patient for identification.
- The radiopharmacy will label only one blood specimen at a time to avoid confusing two or more samples.
- Three milliliters autologous red blood cells are labeled with 20 to 25 mCi technetium-99m in vitro and injected intravenously.
- Images obtained in anterior, 40-degree modified left anterior oblique (MLAO), and left posterior oblique (LPO) views.
- Left ventricular ejection fraction (LVEF) calculated from the 40-degree MLAO view.

Image Interpretation

Selected views of functional images (Fig. A) (described in Normal Radionuclide Ventriculogram, Case 50) demonstrate a large area of dyskinesis at the apex. Phase images (Ph) show the cardiac apex is filling and emptying in synchrony with the atria. Paradox images (Pa) show a large area of paradoxical filling at the apex consistent with an apical aneurysm.

Differential Diagnosis

- Apical aneurysm
- Pseudoaneurysm (This aneurysm should include a narrow neck attaching the extraventricular blood pool to the ventricular blood pool, but this finding is not always visible on RVG.)

Diagnosis and Clinical Follow-up

The focal abnormality raised the suspicion for coronary artery disease. Cardiac catheterization demonstrated clean coronary arteries. The final diagnosis was idiopathic cardiomyopathy with apical aneurysm.

Discussion

In this case, paradoxical motion is seen on both functional images and the cinematic display (Fig. B). Cinematic display is helpful to confirm abnormal wall motion, but occasionally small areas of dyskinetic motion may be missed without the functional images.

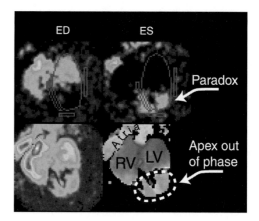

Fig. B (see Color Plate 7, page II)

Suggested Reading

Botvinick EH, Dae MW, O'Connell JW. Functional imaging and phase analysis of blood-pool scintigrams. In: Gerson MC, ed. *Cardiac Nuclear Medicine*. New York: McGraw-Hill, 1997, pp. 371–386.

Case 52

Clinical Presentation

63-year-old man presenting with coronary artery disease and who had suffered a previous myocardial infarction of the anterior wall. Exercise/rest injected technetium-99m–sestamibi (MIBI) myocardial perfusion imaging (not shown here) showed equivocal evidence for a small amount of viable tissue in the left anterior descending (LAD) coronary artery territory.

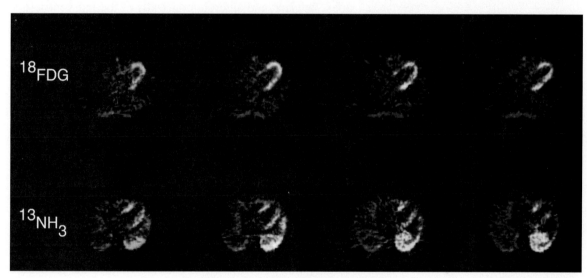

Fig. A (see Color Plate 8, page II)

Technique

- Patient preparation: patient takes nothing by mouth for 12 hours before radiopharmaceutical administration. Switch all glucose-containing intravenous solution to normal saline on the day before imaging. Measure blood glucose concentration before injecting ^{18}FDG.
- 30 mCi of ^{13}NH$_3$ and 10 mCi of ^{18}FDG intravenously at rest, 45 minutes prior to image acquisition.
- Imaging device: whole-body positron emission tomography (PET) camera with in-plane and axial resolutions of 5.0 mm full width half-maximum (FWHM), 9.5-cm field of view, 15 contiguous slices of 6.5-mm separation, and sensitivity of approximately 5000 cps/mCi.
- Perfusion imaging: acquire a transmission image (10 minutes) with a rotating pin source containing germanium-68. Inject ^{13}NH$_3$ over 30 seconds and acquire dynamic images (40 frames of 6 sec duration and 5 frames of 2 min duration).
- Metabolic imaging: if the blood glucose concentration is in the normal range, give glucose (50 g by mouth) and inject ^{18}FDG 45 minutes later. After an additional 45 minutes (uptake period), acquire a single 15-minute emission image followed by a 10-minute transmission image.

- Image reconstruction: use a conventional filtered back projection algorithm to an in-plane resolution of 7 mm FWHM. All projection data are corrected for nonuniformity of detector response, dead time, random coincidences, attenuation, and scattered radiation.
- Image display: sum the images acquired during the final 10 minutes of the perfusion study for comparison with the ^{18}FDG data. Alternatively, the complete set of images can be used to calculate absolute values for regional myocardial perfusion.

Image Interpretation

^{13}NH$_3$ and ^{18}FDG PET images of the myocardium (Fig. A) are displayed in the transaxial projection, and the two studies are independently normalized.

The images show a large area of significantly reduced uptake of ^{13}NH$_3$ in the apex, anterior, and anterolateral walls of the left ventricle. In contrast, the ^{18}FDG images show increased tracer accumulation in all regions of reduced perfusion.

Differential Diagnosis

A defect on ^{13}NH$_3$ images may be caused by any of the typical causes of perfusion defects. The differential diagnosis of discrepant ^{13}NH$_3$ and ^{18}FDG images includes:

1. Hybernating myocardium
2. Image misalignment

Diagnosis and Clinical Follow-up

Based on the results of the ^{13}NH$_3$ and ^{18}FDG PET study, coronary artery bypass surgery was performed. The patient tolerated the procedure well and was free of angina postoperatively.

Discussion

The mismatched pattern of increased glucose metabolism in regions of reduced flow demonstrated by the ^{13}NH$_3$ indicates the presence of a significant amount of viable (hibernating or ischemic) myocardium. Repeat analysis of the exercise/rest technetium-99m-MIBI single photon emission computed tomography (SPECT) images indicated a small increase in perfusion to the apex and anterior walls in the rest study. However, the difference in blood flow to the LAD territory between exercise and rest was less pronounced than the flow-metabolism mismatch.

Suggested Readings

See Case 54.

Case 53

Clinical Presentation

68-year-old man presenting with severe coronary artery disease and had suffered two previous myocardial infarctions. Although hemodynamically stable with a left ventricular ejection fraction of 32%, the patient was severely debilitated by his condition and confined to a "bed-to-chair" lifestyle. Exercise/rest technetium-99m–sestamibi (MIBI) myocardial perfusion imaging revealed equivocal evidence for a small amount of viable muscle in the territory of the left anterior descending (LAD) coronary artery.

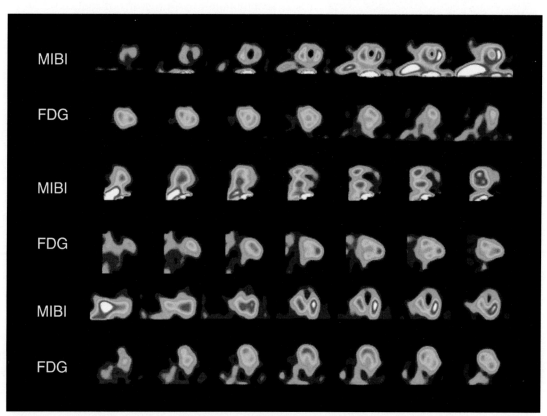

Fig. A (see Color Plate 9, page III)

Technique

- Patient preparation: patient takes nothing by mouth for 12 hours before radiopharmaceutical administration. Switch all glucose-containing intravenous solution to normal saline on the day before imaging. Measure blood glucose concentration before injecting ^{18}F-fluorodeoxyglucose (^{18}FDG).
- 20 mCi technetium-99m–MIBI and 10 mCi ^{18}FDG intravenously at rest, 45 minutes prior to image acquisition.
- Imaging device: dual head gamma camera.
- Collimators: Use ultra high-energy collimator.
- Energy windows: 15%, centered at 140 and 511 keV.

- Measurement of blood glucose concentration is essential, particularly in patients with known or suspected diabetes mellitus.

- In patients with diabetes mellitus, it is useful to acquire a preliminary anterior planar [18]FDG image at 15 minutes after injection. If a considerable amount of radioactivity is present in the blood pool, 2-5 units of regular insulin (depending on the patient's sensitivity) should be administered intravenously before SPECT imaging.

- It is essential to use the same set of axes for constructing horizontal and vertical long axis projections of the [18]FDG and technetium-99m–MIBI data.

- Since [18]FDG may be present only focally in the myocardium, it is helpful to use the technetium-99m–MIBI images for positioning the axes for generating horizontal and vertical long axis projections.

- Image acquisition: 360-degree acquisition (180 degrees per head) with 128 projections. Each projection is acquired for 20 seconds.
- Image reconstruction: order of 7, Butterworth filter with a cutoff of 0.5 times the Nyquist frequency. The same set of axes are used to generate horizontal and vertical long axis projections of the technetium-99m and fluorine-18 data.

Image Interpretation

Simultaneously acquired technetium-99m–MIBI and 18FDG single photon emission computed tomography (SPECT) images are displayed in short, horizontal long, and vertical long axis projections (Fig. A). The technetium-99m–MIBI and [18]FDG images are independently normalized. The images show a large area of markedly reduced uptake of technetium-99m–MIBI involving the apex, anterior, and anterolateral walls of the left ventricle. This defect is clearly demarcated in all three projections. In contrast, the [18]FDG images show intensely increased tracer accumulation in all regions of reduced flow.

Differential Diagnosis

- Hybernating myocardium
- Image misalignment

Diagnosis and Clinical Follow-up

Based on the results of the [18]FDG and technetium-99m–MIBI SPECT studies, coronary artery bypass surgery was performed. The patient tolerated the procedure well, and postoperatively the left ventricular ejection fraction increased to 55% and clinical symptoms were considerably less severe.

Discussion

The pattern of increased glucose metabolism in a region of reduced flow is almost pathognomonic for the presence of viable hibernating myocardium. Retrospective analysis of the exercise/rest technetium-99m–MIBI SPECT images suggested a small increase in perfusion to the apex, and anterior walls in the rest injected study. However, the difference in flow to the left anterior descending LAD territory between exercise and rest, was much less pronounced than the flow-metabolism mismatch.

Suggested Readings

See Case 54.

Case 54

Clinical Presentation

59-year-old man presenting with severe coronary artery disease and had sustained a large myocardial infarction. Although hemodynamically stable, he was severely debilitated and not a candidate for exercise or pharmacological stress myocardial perfusion imaging.

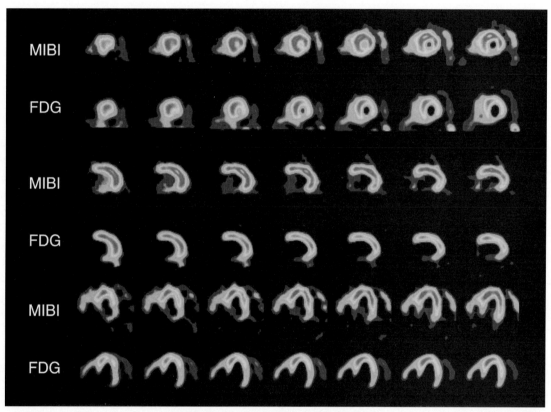

Fig. A (see Color Plate 10, page III)

Technique

- Patient preparation: patient takes nothing by mouth for 12 hours before radiopharmaceutical administration. Switch all glucose-containing intravenous solution to normal saline on the day before imaging. Measure blood glucose concentration before injecting ^{18}FDG.
- 20 mCi of technetium-99m–sestamibi (MIBI) and 10 mCi of ^{18}FDG intravenously at rest, 45 minutes prior to image acquisition.
- Imaging device: dual head gamma camera.
- Collimators: ultra high-energy (UHE) collimator.
- Energy windows: 15%, centered at 140 and 511 keV.
- Image acquisition: 360-degree acquisition (180 degrees per head) with 128 projections. Each projection is acquired for 20 seconds.

- Image reconstruction: order of 7, Butterworth filter with a cutoff of 0.5 times the Nyquist frequency. The same set of axes are used to generate horizontal and vertical long axis projections of the technetium-99m and fluorine-18 data.

Image Interpretation

Simultaneously acquired technetium-99m–MIBI and [18]FDG single photon emission computed tomography (SPECT) images are displayed in short, horizontal long, and vertical long axis projections (Fig. A). The technetium-99m–MIBI and [18]FDG are independently normalized. The images show a large area of absent uptake of technetium-99m–MIBI in the inferior wall of the left ventricle. This defect is clearly visualized in all three projections. The [18]FDG images are remarkably similar, with nearly no tracer accumulation in the inferior wall.

Differential Diagnosis

- Myocardial infarct
- Cardiomyopathy

Diagnosis and Clinical Follow-up

The pattern of matched reductions in myocardial perfusion and glucose metabolism indicates that the area of previous infarction does not contain a significant amount of viable tissue. Based on the results of the [18]FDG and technetium-99m–MIBI SPECT study, coronary artery bypass surgery was not performed and medical management was continued. The patient is currently being evaluated as a candidate for cardiac transplantation.

Discussion

Stress/rest perfusion imaging with thallium-201 thallous chloride or technetium-99m–MIBI currently plays a central role in the noninvasive evaluation of myocardial viability and ischemia. Although SPECT imaging with these agents has provided important clinical information in numerous patients, in many situations (such as Cases 52–54) uncertain or equivocal results have been obtained.

In recent years, positron-emission tomography (PET) has been applied as an alternative to SPECT for evaluating myocardial viability and ischemia (Go et al., 1994; Gould, 1991; Schwaiger and Muzik, 1991). Compared with SPECT, PET has several distinct advantages: (1) PET has considerably higher resolution than SPECT has; (2) because of the fundamental physics of the positron annihilation process, PET images can be accurately corrected for attenuation and scattered radiation, therefore eliminating most artifacts; (3) PET images are intrinsically quantitative; and, (4) most importantly, metabolic imaging can be performed with [18]FDG (Schelbert, 1994; Maddahi et al., 1994; Schwaiger and Hutchins, 1992). When used in conjunction with perfusion imaging, this radiopharmaceutical can provide important additional information about myocardial viability and ischemia. In general, three patterns of perfusion and [18]FDG accumulation can occur. In ischemic or hibernating myocardium, perfusion is reduced whereas [18]FDG accumulation is normal or increased (perfusion-metabolism mismatch). In stunned myocardium, perfusion is normal and [18]FDG accumulation is normal or increased (perfusion-metabolism mismatch) and in regions of infarction, both perfusion and [18]FDG accumulation are reduced (perfusion-metabolism match). These patterns are summarized in Table 1.

PEARLS/PITFALLS

- Oral administration of glucose approximately 45 minutes before injecting ^{18}FDG may be superior to fasting studies for identifying viable myocardium.

Table 1. Patterns of blood flow and FDG metabolism in contractile dysfunction

	Perfusion	^{18}FDG uptake	Clinical state
Acute ischemia	↓	NL or ↑	Acute symptoms
Hibernation	↓	NL or ↑	Chronic, stable
Stunning	NL	NL or ↑	Following an acute event
Repetitive stunning	NL	NL or ↑	
Infarction	↓	↓	Chronic, stable

Over the past decade, ^{18}FDG-PET imaging of the myocardium has been performed in numerous patients and currently is the noninvasive gold standard for detection of ischemic or viable myocardium. Unfortunately, because of the cost and complexity of the instrumentation that is required, use of this procedure has been limited to large academic centers. Very recently, however, three factors have altered this situation: (1) compared with most PET radionuclides, fluorine-18 has a relatively long physical half life (110 minutes), and commercial facilities for distributing ^{18}FDG have been established in several regions of the United States; (2) over the past 2 to 3 years, several instrument manufacturers have introduced UHE collimators that can be used to image 511 keV photons of ^{18}FDG with conventional gamma cameras (Bax et al, 1995; Martin et al., 1995; Burt et al., 1995); and (3) some dual-headed conventional gamma cameras can be upgraded for coincidence detection.

Gamma cameras equipped with UHE collimators yield images with relatively low resolution and count density and therefore cannot be considered general substitutes for PET cameras. Because of resolution limitations, they are unlikely to be very useful for brain imaging, and their low sensitivity will limit oncological applications. These imaging devices are well-suited for cardiac SPECT, however.

Several protocols have been used for ^{18}FDG SPECT imaging of the myocardium. In the simplest procedure, patients fast for at least 12 hours prior to imaging and intravenous infusions containing glucose are discontinued. Approximately 10 mCi of ^{18}FDG plus 20 mCi of technetium-99m–MIBI are coinjected, and after a 45-minute uptake period, the patient is positioned in the gantry. A gamma camera equipped with UHE collimators is used and peaked to 140 and 511 keV photons (15% windows). SPECT acquisition is performed in both windows, and the ^{18}FDG and technetium-99m–MIBI images are reconstructed in identical orientations using a standard filtered back-projection algorithm. In a modification of this procedure, an oral glucose load is administered at 45 minutes before radiopharmaceutical injection.

In most situations, ^{18}FDG SPECT has yielded diagnostic-quality images, with resolutions that are comparable with thallium-201 SPECT. Image interpretation is performed by the same algorithm that is used for analyzing ^{18}FDG PET studies. Although reports of ^{18}FDG SPECT studies are limited, the results have been encouraging. In one small series, ^{18}FDG SPECT was compared with ^{18}FDG PET in nine patients with heart disease, and similar diagnostic information about the amount of viable myocardium present was obtained. In a larger series, 20 patients with proven coronary artery disease and persistent perfusion defects shown by rest reinjection thallium-201 SPECT underwent ^{18}FDG PET and subsequent ^{18}FDG SPECT (Burt et al, 1995). In this study, 13 of 60 fixed segments were shown to be viable by ^{18}FDG SPECT (8 of 20 patients) and 14 of 60 were shown to be viable by ^{18}FDG PET (7 of 20 patients). In 2 patients, fixed thallium defects were found to be viable with ^{18}FDG SPECT alone and 1 by PET alone.

These results indicate that [18]FDG and technetium-99m–MIBI SPECT have several important characteristics: (1) [18]FDG SPECT with 511 keV collimation is less expensive and technically simpler than PET; (2) dual photon acquisition ensures exact registration between perfusion and metabolic images; (3) The short imaging time of the procedure (< 30 minutes for a complete study) is applicable to severely ill unstable patients and could replace rest-redistribution thallium-201 imaging; and, (4) most importantly, [18]FDG SPECT makes metabolic imaging of the heart possible at almost every nuclear medicine facility.

Suggested Readings

Bax JJ, Visser FC, van Lingen A, Visser CA, Teule GJ. Myocardial F-18 fluorodeoxyglucose imaging by SPECT. *Clin Nucl Med* 20:486–490, 1995.

Burt RW, Perkins OW, Oppenheim BE, et al. Direct comparison of fluorine-18-FDG SPECT, fluorine-18-FDG PET and rest thallium-201 SPECT for detection of myocardial viability. *J Nucl Med* 36:176–179, 1995.

Go RT, MacIntyre WJ, Chen EQ, et al. Current status of the clinical applications of cardiac positron emission tomography. *Radiol Clin North Am* 32:501–519, 1994.

Gould KL. Clinical cardiac positron emission tomography: State of the art. *Circulation* 84 (suppl):122–136, 1991.

Maddahi J, Schelbert H, Brunken R, Di Carli M. Role of thallium-201 and PET imaging in evaluation of myocardial viability and management of patients with coronary artery disease and left ventricular dysfunction. *J Nucl Med* 35:707–715, 1994.

Martin WH, Delbeke D, Patton JA, et al. FDG-SPECT: Correlation with FDG-PET. *J Nucl Med* 36:988–995, 1995.

Schelbert HR. Cardiac PET: Microcirculation and substrate transport in normal and diseased human myocardium. *Ann Nucl Med* 8:91–100, 1994.

Schelbert HR. Metabolic imaging to assess myocardial viability. *J Nucl Med* 35(suppl):8S–14S, 1994.

Schwaiger M, Hutchins GD. Evaluation of coronary artery disease with positron emission tomography. *Semin Nucl Med* 22:210–223, 1992.

Schwaiger M, Muzik O. Assessment of myocardial perfusion by positron emission tomography. *Am J Cardiol* 67:35–43, 1991.

Section III

Pulmonary Scintigraphy

Case 55

Clinical Presentation

26-year-old man presenting with shortness of breath and chest discomfort.

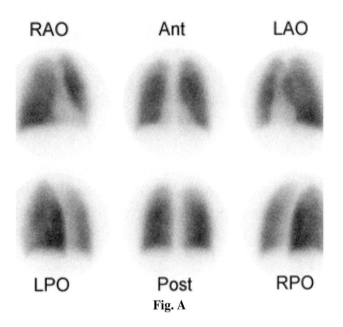

Fig. A

Technique

- 3.0 mCi technetium-99m macroaggregated albumin (MAA) administered intravenously with the patient supine.
- Patient should cough and take several deep breaths prior to administration of the MAA to clear any areas of resting atelectasis.
- Patient should breath normally during tracer injection.
- Use low-energy all-purpose collimator.
- Energy window 20% centered at 140 keV.
- Imaging time is 500,000 counts per view.
- Matrix is 128 × 128.
- Views are anterior, right anterior oblique, left anterior oblique, posterior, right posterior oblique, and left posterior oblique. Lateral views can also be obtained, although the contribution of counts from the contralateral lung tends to compromise the diagnostic value of these views.

Image Interpretation

Homogeneous tracer distribution is seen throughout both lung fields (Fig. A). The lungs are of normal contour. The cardiac sillhouette is noted in the left lung field in the anterior projection.

Differential Diagnosis

- No evidence of pulmonary embolism. There may be many causes of shortness of breath or chest pain that are not caused by pulmonary embolism. A normal lung scan essentially rules out significant perfusion abnormality.

Diagnosis and Clinical Follow-up

The lung perfusion pattern is normal. Shortness of breath and chest discomfort were felt secondary to anxiety and gastritis. No further follow-up was obtained.

Discussion

Lung perfusion scans provide a method for diagnosis of pulmonary embolism that is noninvasive and effective. A normal lung scan essentially rules out pulmonary embolism.

When a perfusion defect is identified, one must first determine the size and anatomic extent of the defect(s). Nonsegmental defects do not occupy known vascular distributions and would therefore be less likely to be caused by a thromboembolus. Nonsegmental defects would include cardiomegaly (Fig. B, *arrow*), pleural effusion (Fig. C, *arrow*), cardiac pacemaker superimposed on the chest wall (Fig. D, *arrow*), and an elevated hemidiaphragm (Fig. E, *arrow*).

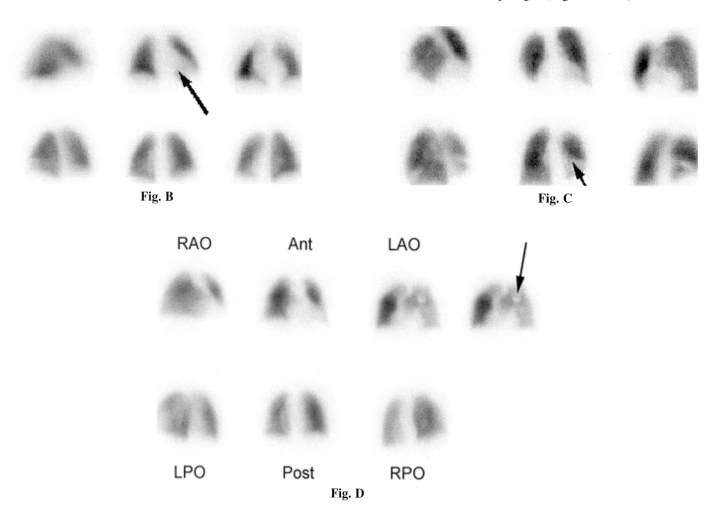

Fig. B

Fig. C

RAO   Ant   LAO

LPO   Post   RPO

Fig. D

PEARLS/PITFALLS

- The likelihood of pulmonary embolism based on the lung scan alone must be combined with the clinical probability of pulmonary embolism to determine the overall probability of pulmonary embolism. Patients with intermediate likelihood scans should often go on to pulmonary arteriography or leg ultrasonography.

- The biological half life of technetium-99m MAA in the lungs is approximately 5 hours. As a result, if a patient becomes acutely short of breath 24 hours after a normal lung scan, the patient can be reinjected for a second lung scan.

- Using the standard 200,000 to 400,000 particle injection of a single dose of technetium-99m MAA, approximately 1 out of 1000 of the pulmonary capillaries are temporarily occluded. Fewer particles (60,000 to 100,000) may be given if there is a history of right to left shunting or pulmonary artery hypertension.

- An oblique band of relative photopenia oriented superomedially to inferolaterally is often seen on the left anterior oblique view (Fig. F, *arrow*). This is a normal variant and corresponds to the aortic arch. This should not be mistaken for a lingula defect. *(continued)*

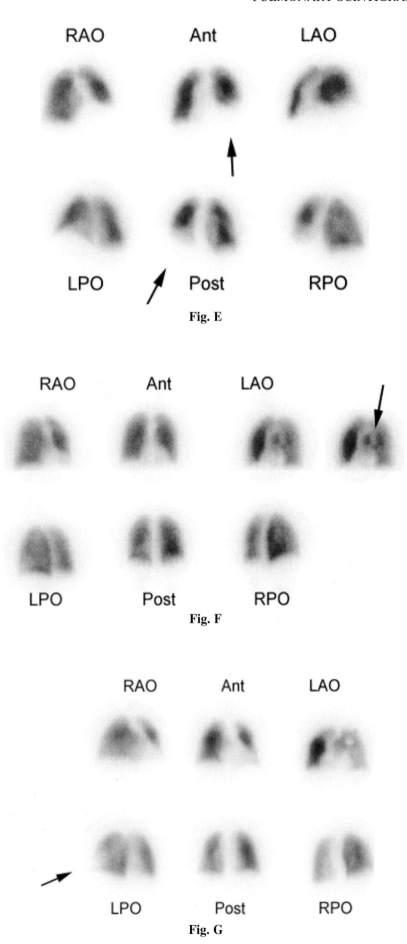

Fig. E

Fig. F

Fig. G

- *(continued)* An area of photopenia is often seen in the region of the junction of the lateral basal segment of the left lower lobe and the inferior lingula segment on the left posterior oblique view (Fig. G, *arrow*). This defect is characteristically of an intensity that gradually fades when compared with the surrounding normally perfused lung. This is a normal variant and corresponds to the cardiac apex.

- Defects due to pulmonary embolism classically extend all the way to the lung periphery. When normally perfused lung surrounds a defect (the stripe sign), the defect is nonsegmental and unlikely to be due to acute pulmonary embolism (Fig. H, *arrow*).

- Pregnancy is not an absolute contraindication to lung scintigraphy. Any theoretical radiation risk to the fetus is minimal in comparison to the risk to the fetus should the mother die of pulmonary embolism.

- When imaging pregnant patients, the dose is often lowered to 1.0 mCi. Although this lowers the fetal dose, the dose to the fetus from the standard 3.0 mCi of technetium-99m MAA is still less than 1/400th the minimal effective dose known to cause an adverse effect on the fetus (approximately 10 rads, see United Nations Scientific Committee, 1977).

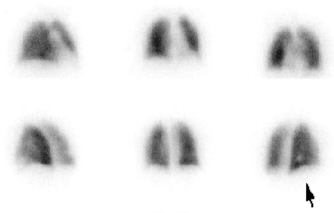

Fig. H

Table 1. Likelihood of Pulmonary Embolism Based on Lung Scan Findings

Lung Scan Findings	Likelihood of Pulmonary Embolism
Clear chest x-ray in same location as perfusion defect	
Nonsegmental perfusion defect	Low
Segmental perfusion defect	
Small	Low
Moderate–Large	
Matched by ventilation abnormality	
Matched ventilation and perfusion defects compose $\leq$ 50% of both lung fields	Low
Matched ventilation and perfusion defects compose > 50% of both lung fields	Intermediate
Not matched by ventilation abnormality	
< 2 large segmental mismatch equivalents	Intermediate
$\geq$ 2 large segmental mismatch equivalents	High
Opacity on chest x-ray in same location as perfusion defect	
Nonsegmental perfusion defects	Low
Segmental perfusion defects	
Small	
Smaller than chest x-ray abnormality	Low
Matched by chest x-ray abnormality	Low/Intermediate
Larger than chest x-ray abnormality	Low
Moderate–Large	
Smaller than chest x-ray abnormality	Low
Matched by chest x-ray abnormality	Intermediate
Greater than chest x-ray abnormality	
Matched by ventilation abnormality	
Matched ventilation and perfusion defects compose $\leq$ 50% of both lung fields	Low
Matched ventilation and perfusion defects compose > 50% of both lung fields	Intermediate
Not matched by ventilation abnormality	
< 2 large segmental mismatch equivalents	Intermediate
$\geq$ 2 large segmental mismatch equivalents	High

Low likelihood corresponds to a < 20% chance of pulmonary embolism.

Intermediate likelihood corresponds to a 20 to 80% chance of pulmonary embolism.

High likelihood corresponds to a > 80% chance of pulmonary embolism.

The above probabilities are based on a pulmonary embolism prevalence of approximately 33%.

Once it has been determined that the defect corresponds to a lung segment, the size of the defect must be determined. A small defect composes less than 25% of a lung segment, a moderate defect composes 25 to 75% of a lung segment, and a large defect composes greater than 75% of a lung segment. Two moderate defects are equivalent to one large defect. Multiple small defects are not equivalent to moderate or large defects, however.

The best way to assess any lung scan for likelihood of pulmonary embolism is to combine the results of the revised (Gottschalk et al, 1993) and modified (Freitas et al, 1995) Prospective Investigation of Pulmonary Embolic Disease (PIOPED) criteria with one's overall "gestalt" of the lung perfusion pattern. This is summarized in Table 1.

Suggested Readings

Freitas JE, Sarosi MG, Nagle CC, et al. Modified PIOPED criteria used in clinical practice. *J Nucl Med* 36:1573–1578, 1995.

Gottschalk A, Sostman HD, Coleman RE, et al. Ventilation-perfusion scintigraphy in the PIOPED Study. Part II. Evaluation of the scintigraphic criteria and interpretation. *J Nucl Med* 34:1119–1126, 1993.

Pulmolite packet insert. Du Pont Merck Pharmaceutical Co., June 1994.

United Nations Scientific Committee on the Effects of Atomic Radiation. *Sources and Effects of Ionizing Radiation.* New York: United Nations, 1977.

Case 56

Clinical Presentation

54-year-old man presenting with acute shortness of breath and chest pain.

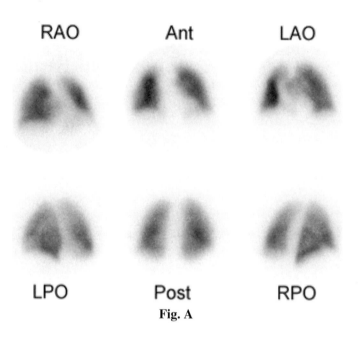

Fig. A

Technique

- 3.0 mCi technetium-99m macroaggregated albumin (MAA) administered intravenously with the patient supine.
- Patient should cough and take several deep breaths prior to administration of the MAA to clear any areas of resting atelectasis.
- Patient should breath normally during tracer injection.
- Use low-energy all-purpose collimator.
- Energy window 20% centered at 140 keV.
- Imaging time is 500,000 counts per view.
- Matrix is 128 × 128.
- The views are anterior, right anterior oblique, left anterior oblique, posterior, right posterior oblique, and left posterior oblique. Lateral views can also be obtained, although the contribution of counts from the contralateral lung tends to compromise the diagnostic value of these views.

Image Interpretation

There is a small defect involving the anterior basal segment of the right lower lobe, best seen abutting the expected location of the right major fissure on the right posterior oblique view (Fig. A). No other segmental defects are identified. The chest X-ray was clear.

Differential Diagnosis

A small perfusion defect is non-specific, and can be secondary to many causes, including:

- Atelectasis
- Bronchitis
- Asthma, COPD
- Pleural effusion
- Pneumonia
- Unresolved previous pulmonary embolism
- Previous surgery
- Attenuation artifact

Diagnosis and Clinical Follow-up

Given the small size of this defect, the scan was read as being low likelihood of pulmonary embolism. Chest pain was due to bronchitis.

Discussion

If only small subsegmental defects are noted on a lung perfusion scan the study is read as a low likelihood of pulmonary embolism (Gottschalk et al, 1993), given a clear chest X-ray. Any ventilation findings will not alter this diagnosis.

Suggested Reading

Gottschalk A, Sostman HD, Coleman RE, et al. Ventilation-perfusion scintigraphy in the PIOPED Study. Part II. Evaluation of the scintigraphic criteria and interpretation. *J Nucl Med* 34:1119–1126, 1993.

Case 57

Clinical Presentation

70-year-old woman, status post–total hip replacement, presenting with chest pain.

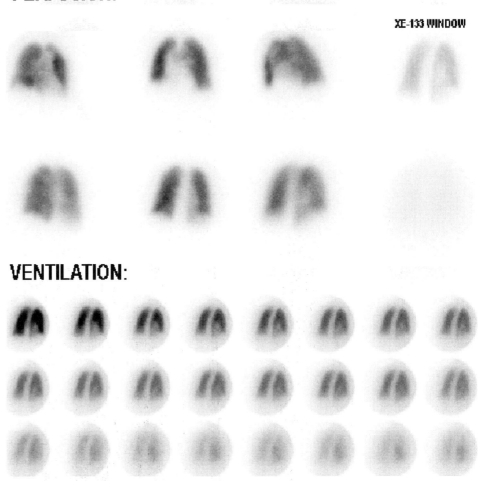

PERFUSION:

XE-133 WINDOW

VENTILATION:

Fig. A

Technique

Lung Perfusion Scan

- 3.0 mCi technetium-99m macroaggregated albumin (MAA) administered intravenously with the patient supine.
- Patient should cough and take several deep breaths prior to administration of the MAA to clear any areas of resting atelectasis.
- Patient should breath normally during tracer injection.
- Use low-energy all-purpose collimator.
- Energy window 20% centered at 140 keV.
- Imaging time is 500,000 counts per view.

- A ventilation equilibrium phase of at least 4 minutes is helpful to allow the xenon to penetrate obstructed airways.

- Visualization of small areas of washout abnormality are better seen if the ventilation portion of the study is done prior to the perfusion imaging.

- The cardiac silhouette on chest X-ray is often less prominent than that on perfusion images because the former is obtained during maximal inspiration and the latter during tidal breathing. A left lingular defect on perfusion images is often caused by the normal position of the cardiac apex, even though it may not appear to extend that far laterally on the chest X-ray.

- Some imaging centers perform the ventilation scan after the perfusion scan. The advantage of this method allows one to select the optimal view in which to perform the ventilation scan and to avoid the ventilation study completely when perfusion images are normal. The disadvantage is that the 140 keV photons from the technetium-99m MAA perfusion scan will be "down scattering" into the 80-keV window of the xenon-133 image, making interpretation of the ventilation study slightly more difficult. It is important to acquire an MAA downscatter image with the 80-keV window before performing the ventilation scan. This helps to distinguish tracer activity caused by trapping from that caused by downscatter. Trapping, a sign of airway obstruction, is generally considered to be present if tracer activity persists in the lungs during washout.

- Matrix is 128 × 128.
- Views are anterior, right anterior oblique, left anterior oblique, posterior, right posterior oblique, and left posterior oblique. Lateral views can also be obtained, although the contribution of counts from the contralateral lung tends to compromise the diagnostic value of these views.

Lung Ventilation Scan

- The view that best demonstrates the significant perfusion defects is chosen.
- 20.0 mCi xenon-133 breathed in via mask with the patient sitting up.
- Use low-energy all-purpose collimator.
- Energy window 20% centered at 80 keV.
- Matrix is 128 × 128.
- Imaging sequence: initial breath image: one 15-second image; equilibrium phase, 15 images, 15 seconds per image; washout phase, 15 images, 15 seconds per image; trapping image: one 60-second image.

Image Interpretation

The lung perfusion images demonstrate large defects involving the posterior basal, lateral basal, and superior segments of the right lower lobe (Fig. A). No other segmental defects are identified. On the ventilation images, these defects are completely matched by defects on the initial breath and equilibrium phase images. The chest X-ray was clear.

Differential Diagnosis

(large, matching defects):

- COPD
- Acute asthma exacerbation
- Pneumonia
- Congestive heart failure (defects usually smaller in size)
- Adult respiratory distress syndrome
- Mucous plugging of the airways
- Foreign body aspiration
- Pneumonectomy

Diagnosis and Clinical Follow-up

The scan was read as being low likelihood of pulmonary embolism. Chest pain was caused by gastroesophageal reflux.

Discussion

If the segmental defects on a lung perfusion scan are completely matched by ventilation abnormalities, the likelihood of pulmonary embolism is low, unless the abnormalities involve more than 50% of both lung fields (in which case the scan is intermediate likelihood), or if the chest X-ray is abnormal at the site of the perfusion defects (Freitas et al, 1995). If the chest X-ray has a corresponding opacity that is significantly larger than the perfusion defect, the final diagnosis is low likelihood. If the chest X ray has a corresponding opacity that is the same size as the perfusion defect, the final diagnosis is intermediate likelihood of pulmonary embolism.

Suggested Reading

Freitas JE, Sarosi MG, Nagle CC, et al. Modified PIOPED criteria used in clinical practice. *J Nucl Med* 36:1573–1578, 1995.

Case 58

Clinical Presentation

31-year-old man presenting with increasing oxygen requirements. The chest X-ray was clear.

PERFUSION:

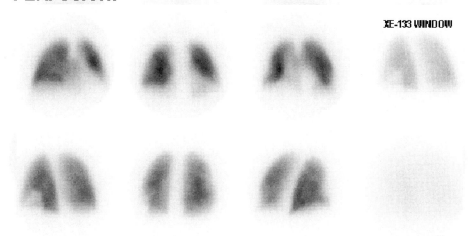

XE-133 WINDOW

VENTILATION:

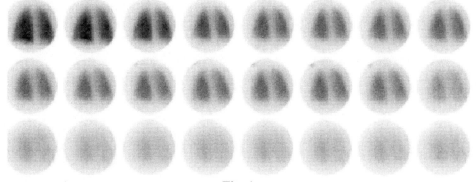

Fig. A

Technique

Lung Perfusion Scan

- 3.0 mCi technetium-99m macroaggregated albumin (MAA), administered intravenously with the patient supine.
- Patient should cough and take several deep breaths prior to administration of the MAA to clear any areas of resting atelectasis.
- Patient should breath normally during tracer injection.
- Use low-energy all-purpose collimator.
- Energy window 20% centered at 140 keV.
- Imaging time: 500,000 counts per view.
- Matrix is 128 × 128.

• Views are anterior, right anterior oblique, left anterior oblique, posterior, right posterior oblique, and left posterior oblique. Lateral views can also be obtained, although the contribution of counts from the contralateral lung tends to compromise the diagnostic value of these views.

Lung Ventilation Scan

• The view that best demonstrates the significant perfusion defects is chosen.
• Radiopharmaceutical is 20.0 mCi xenon-133 breathed in via mask with the patient sitting up.
• Use low-energy all-purpose collimator.
• Energy window 20% centered at 80 keV.
• Matrix is 128 × 128.
• Imaging time: initial breath image is obtained for approximately 15 seconds; equilibrium phase, 15 images, 15 seconds per image; washout phase, 15 images, 15 seconds per image; trapping image, one 60-second image.

Image Interpretation

The lung perfusion images demonstrate a large defect involving the anteromedial basal segment of the left lower lobe and a moderate defect involving the lateral basal segment of the left lower lobe (Fig. A). No other segmental defects are identified. The ventilation images are normal.

Differential Diagnosis

• Pulmonary embolism (acute)
• Pulmonary embolism (previous)
• Lung cancer (primary or metastatic)
• Histoplasmosis
• Pneumonia
• Sarcoidosis

Diagnosis and Clinical Follow-up

The scan was read as indicating intermediate likelihood of pulmonary embolism. The patient was treated with anticoagulants for presumed pulmonary embolism.

Discussion

If the segmental defects on a lung perfusion scan are moderate or large, or both, in size; sum to fewer than two large segment equivalents; and are not matched by a ventilation abnormality, the final interpretation is intermediate likelihood.

Suggested Reading

Freitas JE, Sarosi MG, Nagle CC, et al. Modified PIOPED criteria used in clinical practice. *J Nucl Med* 36:1573–1578, 1995.

Case 59

Clinical Presentation

74-year-old woman presenting with acute onset chest pain and shortness of breath after a 2-day car ride. The chest X-ray was clear.

PERFUSION:

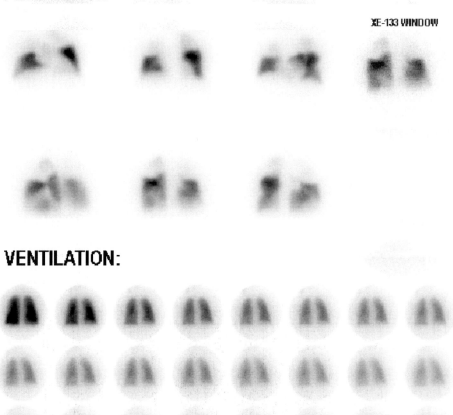

XE-133 WINDOW

VENTILATION:

Fig. A

Technique

Lung Perfusion Scan

- 3.0 mCi technetium-99m macroaggregated albumin (MAA), administered intravenously with the patient supine.
- Patient should cough and take several deep breaths prior to administration of the MAA to clear any areas of resting atelectasis.
- Patient should breath normally during tracer injection.
- Use low-energy all-purpose collimator.
- Energy window 20% centered at 140 keV.
- Imaging time: 500,000 counts per view.
- Matrix is 128×128.

• Views are anterior, right anterior oblique, left anterior oblique, posterior, right posterior oblique, and left posterior oblique. Lateral views can also be obtained, although the contribution of counts from the contralateral lung tends to compromise the diagnostic value of these views.

Lung Ventilation Scan

• 20.0 mCi xenon-133 breathed in via mask with the patient sitting up.
• Use low-energy all-purpose collimator.
• Energy window 20% centered at 80 keV.
• Matrix is 128 × 128.
• Imaging time: initial breath image: one 15-second image; equilibrium phase, 15 images, 15 seconds per image; washout phase, 15 images, 15 seconds per image; trapping image: one 60-second image.
• The view that best demonstrates the significant perfusion defects is chosen.

Image Interpretation

The lung perfusion images demonstrate large defects involving all three segments of the right upper lobe, the superior segment of the right lower lobe, the anterior and apicoposterior segments of the left upper lobe, and the posterior basal and anteromedial basal segments of the left lower lobe (Fig. A). The ventilation images are normal.

Differential Diagnosis

• Acute pulmonary thromboembolism
• Previous pulmonary thromboembolism
• Lung cancer (primary or metastatic to lung)
• Radiation therapy
• Other embolic disease (fat embolism, air embolism)
• Sickle cell disease (not in a patient this age, however)

Diagnosis and Clinical Follow-up

The scan was read as indicating high likelihood of pulmonary embolism. Patient was treated for pulmonary embolism with thrombolysis and anticoagulation.

Discussion

If the segmental defects on a lung perfusion scan are moderate or large, or both, in size; sum to at least two large defect equivalents; and are not matched by a ventilation abnormality, the final interpretation is high likelihood of pulmonary embolism (Freitas et al, 1995). The reading will only change if a corresponding chest X-ray opacity is noted in a distribution similar to that of the perfusion defects, in which case the reading becomes indeterminate likelihood.

Suggested Readings

Freitas JE, Sarosi MG, Nagle CC, et al. Modified PIOPED criteria used in clinical practice. *J Nucl Med* 36:1573–1578, 1995.

The PIOPED Investigators. Value of the ventilation perfusion scan in acute pulmonary embolism. *JAMA* 263:2753–2759, 1990.

Case 60

Clinical Presentation

61-year-old woman presenting with acute shortness of breath.

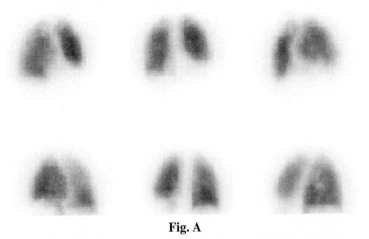

Fig. A

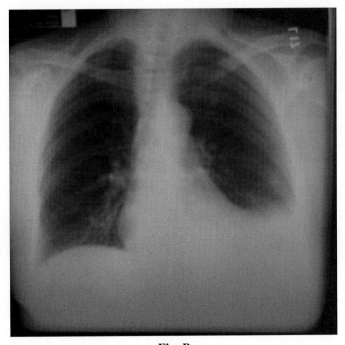

Fig. B

Technique

- 3.0 mCi technetium-99m macroaggregated albumin (MAA), administered intravenously with the patient supine.
- Patient should cough and take several deep breaths prior to administration of the MAA to clear any areas of resting atelectasis.
- Patient should breath normally during tracer injection.
- Use low-energy all-purpose collimator.

- Energy window 20% centered at 140 keV.
- Imaging time: 500,000 counts per view.
- Matrix is 128 × 128.
- Views are anterior, right anterior oblique, left anterior oblique, posterior, right posterior oblique, and left posterior oblique. Lateral views can also be obtained, although the contribution of counts from the contralateral lung tends to compromise the diagnostic value of these views.

Image Interpretation

The lung perfusion scan (Fig. A) demonstrates subsegmental defects in the left lower lobe that are matched by the opacity on chest X-ray (Fig. B).

Differential Diagnosis

- Pulmonary embolism (acute)
- Pulmonary embolism (previous)
- Lung cancer (primary or metastatic)
- Histoplasmosis
- Pneumonia
- Sarcoidosis

Diagnosis and Clinical Follow-up

This is consistent with intermediate likelihood for pulmonary embolism. Pulmonary arteriogram (Fig. C) demonstrates filling defects consistent with emboli in left lower lobe vessels as well as the inferior lingula segment (arrow).

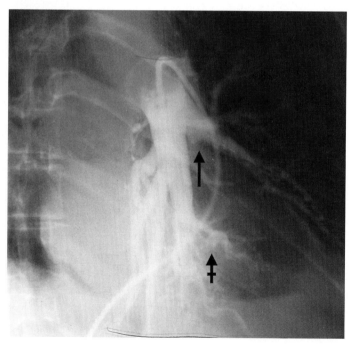

Fig. C

Discussion

When the perfusion defect on lung scan matches the opacity on chest X ray, the scan is intermediate likelihood of pulmonary embolism (Freitas et al, 1995). A ventilation scan is not needed. If the clinical suspicion of pulmonary embolism is not high enough to warrant treatment, these cases usually are further evaluated by pulmonary arteriography.

Suggested Readings

Freitas JE, Sarosi MG, Nagle CC, et al. Modified PIOPED criteria used in clinical practice. *J Nucl Med* 36:1573–1578, 1995.

Gottschalk A, Sostman HD, Coleman RE, et al. Ventilation-perfusion scintigraphy in the PIOPED study. Part II. Evaluation of the scintigraphic criteria and interpretation. *J Nucl Med* 34:1119–1126, 1993.

Case 61

Clinical Presentation

43-year-old woman presenting with acute shortness of breath.

PERFUSION:

XE-133 WINDOW

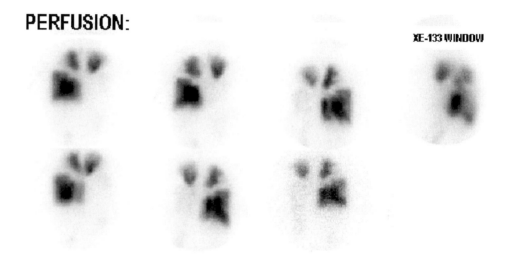

VENTILATION:

Fig. A

Technique

Lung Perfusion Scan

- 3.0 mCi technetium-99m macroaggregated albumin (MAA), administered intravenously with the patient supine.
- Patient should cough and take several deep breaths prior to administration of the MAA to clear any areas of resting atelectasis.
- Patient should breath normally during tracer injection.
- Use low-energy all-purpose collimator.
- Energy window 20% centered at 140 keV.
- Imaging time: 500,000 counts per view.

- Matrix is 128 × 128.
- Views are anterior, right anterior oblique, left anterior oblique, posterior, right posterior oblique, and left posterior oblique. Lateral views can also be obtained, although the contribution of counts from the contralateral lung tends to compromise the diagnostic value of these views.

Lung Ventilation Scan

- 20.0 mCi xenon-133 breathed in via mask with the patient sitting up.
- Use low-energy all-purpose collimator.
- Energy window 20% centered at 80 keV.
- Matrix is 128 × 128.
- Imaging time: initial breath image, one 15 second image; equilibrium phase, 15 images, 15 seconds per image; washout phase, 15 images, 15 seconds per image; trapping image, one 60-second image.
- The view that best demonstrates the significant perfusion defects is chosen.

Image Interpretation

The lung perfusion scan (Fig. A) demonstrates widespread segmental and subsegmental defects throughout both lungs. Among the large defects are the entire left lower lobe, the inferior and superior segments of the lingula, and the superior segment of the right lower lobe. The chest X-ray was clear, and the ventilation images were normal.

Differential Diagnosis

- Acute pulmonary thromboembolism
- Previous pulmonary thromboembolism
- Lung cancer (primary or metastatic to lung)
- Radiation therapy
- Other embolic disease (fat embolism, air embolism)
- Sickle cell disease

Diagnosis and Clinical Follow-up

This is consistent with a high likelihood for pulmonary embolism. Patient was treated for pulmonary embolism with anticoagulation and thrombolysis.

Discussion

If the segmental defects on a lung perfusion scan are moderate or large, or both, in size, sum to at least two large defect equivalents; and are not matched by a ventilation abnormality, the final interpretation is high likelihood of pulmonary embolism (Freitas et al, 1995). The reading will only change if a corresponding chest X-ray opacity is noted in a distribution similar to that of the perfusion defects.

In cases with widespread bilateral defects, such as this, it is important to communicate to the referring clinician not only the likelihood of pulmonary embolism but also the size of the clot burden. Patients with a large amount of pulmonary embolism may need aggressive treatment, such as thrombolysis.

Suggested Reading

Freitas JE, Sarosi MG, Nagle CC, et al. Modified PIOPED criteria used in clinical practice. *J Nucl Med* 36:1573–1578, 1995.

Case 62

Clinical Presentation

63-year-old woman presenting with shortness of breath, swollen left calf, and normal chest X-ray.

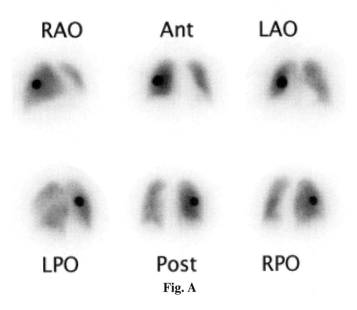

Fig. A

Technique

Lung Perfusion Scan

- 3.0 mCi technetium-99m macroaggregated albumin (MAA), administered intravenously with the patient supine.
- Patient should cough and take several deep breaths prior to administration of the MAA to clear any areas of resting atelectasis.
- Patient should breath normally during tracer injection.
- Use low-energy all-purpose collimator.
- Energy window 20% centered at 140 keV.
- Imaging time: 500,000 counts per view.
- Matrix is 128 × 128.
- Views are anterior, right anterior oblique, left anterior oblique, posterior, right posterior oblique, and left posterior oblique. Lateral views can also be obtained, although the contribution of counts from the contralateral lung tends to compromise the diagnostic value of these views.

Image Interpretation

Images in multiple projections (Fig. A) show a focus of intensely increased tracer activity in the midright lung field. The finding is characteristic of clumping of injected tracer.

Differential Diagnosis

• Clumping of tracer
• Small focus of normally perfused lung in a patient with massive pulmonary embolism
• Atelectasis

Diagnosis and Clinical Follow-up

No evidence of pulmonary embolism. Shortness of breath was thought to be secondary to exacerbation of congestive heart failure.

Discussion

Clumping of MAA at the time of injection is not an uncommon problem. It may be associated with labeling of microthrombi, either on a catheter tip or because a small amount of blood was aspirated into the syringe containing the MAA just before it was injected into the patient.

Suggested Reading

Preston DF, Greenlaw RH. "Hot spots" in lung scans. *J Nucl Med* 11:422–425, 1970.

Case 63

Clinical Presentation

83-year-old woman presenting with shortness of breath following an airplane ride.

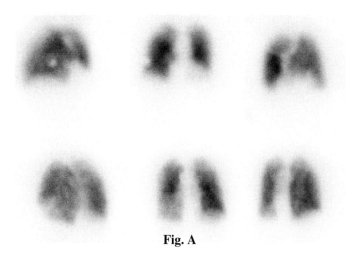

Fig. A

Technique

- 3.0 mCi technetium-99m macroaggregated albumin (MAA), administered intravenously with the patient supine.
- Patient should cough and take several deep breaths prior to administration of the MAA to clear any areas of resting atelectasis.
- Patient should breath normally during tracer injection.
- Use low-energy all-purpose collimator.
- Energy window 20% centered at 140 keV.
- Imaging time: 500,000 counts per view.
- Matrix is 128 × 128.
- Views are anterior, right anterior oblique, left anterior oblique, posterior, right posterior oblique, and left posterior oblique. Lateral views can also be obtained, although the contribution of counts from the contralateral lung tends to compromise the diagnostic value of these views.

Image Interpretation

A focal defect is noted over the right lung field on the right anterior oblique view (Fig. A). It is also noted laterally on the anterior view. Patchy perfusion is noted in both lung fields.

Differential Diagnosis

- Attenuation artifact
- Gamma camera defect (cracked crystal, photomultiplier tube malfunction, collimator abnormality)

Diagnosis and Clinical Follow-up

Chest X-ray demonstrates a pacemaker over the right hemithorax.

Discussion

Pacemakers can be placed in any location in the chest, causing an attenuation artifact that may resemble a pulmonary perfusion defect. Careful analysis of the different projections of the perfusion images will demonstrate that the defect moves separately from the lung parenchyma. Of course, review of the chest X-ray will easily demonstrate the nature of the defect.

Case 64

Clinical Presentation

67-year-old woman presenting with worsening shortness of breath.

PERFUSION:

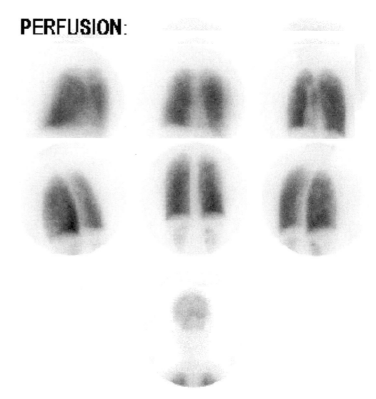

Fig. A

Technique

- 3.0 mCi technetium-99m macroaggregated albumin (MAA), administered intravenously with the patient supine.
- Patient should cough and take several deep breaths prior to administration of the MAA to clear any areas of resting atelectasis.
- Patient should breath normally during tracer injection.
- Use low-energy all-purpose collimator.
- Energy window 20% centered at 140 keV.
- Imaging time: 500,000 counts per view.
- Matrix is 128 × 128.
- Views are anterior, right anterior oblique, left anterior oblique, posterior, right posterior oblique, and left posterior oblique. Lateral views can also be obtained, although the contribution of counts from the contralateral lung tends to compromise the diagnostic value of these views.

Image Interpretation

The lung perfusion images demonstrate overall heterogeneous tracer localization, without segmental defects (Fig. A). The chest X-ray was clear. The scan was read as being low likelihood of pulmonary embolism (Freitas et al, 1995). There is tracer uptake seen in the kidneys on the posterior views. Images of the head demonstrate tracer uptake in the brain, confirming a right-to-left shunt.

Differential Diagnosis

(for tracer uptake outside the lungs):

• Right-to-left shunt
• Particle dissolution (images done several hours after tracer injection)
• Radiopharmaceutical preparation problems
• Pulmonary AVM

Diagnosis and Clinical Follow-up

The patient had an atrial septal defect diagnosed by echocardiography.

Discussion

Tracer uptake outside the pulmonary capillary bed can be seen in a number of organs from a variety of causes. Uptake in the liver can be seen secondary to superior vena cava obstruction or from normal breakdown and passage of particles through the lung. Thyroid uptake is often thought to be caused by free pertcchnctate. The blood flow to the thyroid is quite high, however, and right-to-left shunting may also result in visualization of the thyroid. Kidney uptake can be seen with right-to-left shunts and with free pertechnetate. The most reliable way to confirm a right-to-left shunt, therefore, is to image the brain.

The right-to-left shunt is often caused by an atrial septal defect, although other etiologies include ventriculoseptal defects or intrapulmonic shunts.

Suggested Reading

Freitas JE, Sarosi MG, Nagle CC, et al. Modified PIOPED criteria used in clinical practice. *J Nucl Med* 36:1573–1578, 1995.

Case 65

Clinical Presentation

54-year-old woman presenting with hemoptysis, shortness of breath, and previous pulmonary embolism.

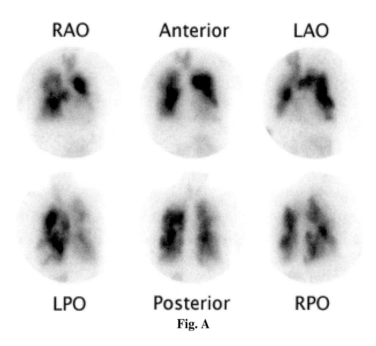

RAO   Anterior   LAO

LPO   Posterior   RPO

Fig. A

Technique

- 3.0 mCi technetium-99m macroaggregated albumin (MAA), administered intravenously with the patient supine.
- Patient should cough and take several deep breaths prior to administration of the MAA to clear any areas of resting atelectasis.
- Patient should breath normally during tracer injection.
- Use low-energy all-purpose collimator.
- Energy window 20% centered at 140 keV.
- Imaging time: 500,000 counts per view.
- Matrix is 128 × 128.
- Views are anterior, right anterior oblique, left anterior oblique, posterior, right posterior oblique, and left posterior oblique. Lateral views can also be obtained, although the contribution of counts from the contralateral lung tends to compromise the diagnostic value of these views.

Image Interpretation

The lung perfusion images (Fig. A) demonstrate irregular perfusion throughout both lung fields, including multiple segmental and subsegmental defects that have not changed since the previous study (not shown). Anterior images (top row) show tracer uptake in the thyroid gland. A subsequent view of the head also shows tracer uptake in the brain (Fig. B). The chest X-ray was clear.

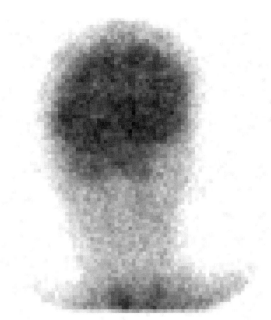

Fig. B

Differential Diagnosis

(for tracer uptake outside the lungs):

- Right-to-left shunt
- Particle dissolution (images done several hours after tracer injection)
- Radiopharmaceutical preparation problems
- Pulmonary AVM

Diagnosis and Clinical Follow-up

Ventilation images on the previous study show relatively normal ventilation throughout both lung fields. Patient was thought to have a right-to-left shunt secondary to pulmonary embolism.

Discussion

Tracer uptake in the thyroid is often thought to be secondary to free pertechnetate. The thyroid is a very vascular organ, however. Visualization of the thyroid should always raise the suspicion of right-to-left shunting. A view of the head is important to distinguish between poor labeling of the MAA and right-to-left shunt.

Suggested Readings

Gale B, Chen C, Chun KJ, et al. Systemic to pulmonary venous shunting in superior vena cava obstruction. Unusual myocardial and thyroid visualization. *Clin Nucl Med* 15:246–250, 1990.

Weissmann HS, Steingart RM, Kiely TM, et al. Myocardial visualization on a perfusion lung scan. *J Nucl Med* 21:745–746, 1980.

Section IV

Endocrine Scintigraphy

Case 66

Clinical Presentation

34-year-old woman presenting with possible right lobe nodule palpated by the referring physician. Thyroid function tests were normal.

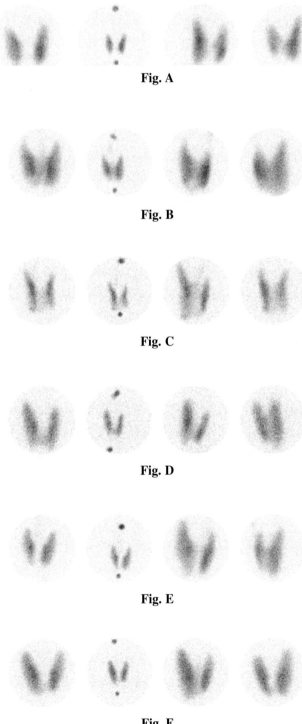

Fig. A

Fig. B

Fig. C

Fig. D

Fig. E

Fig. F

PEARLS/PITFALLS

- Oblique views of the thyroid should always be obtained to look for unusual contours of the posterior portions of the right and left lobes.

- A marker view should always be obtained so that some anatomical landmark can be correlated with the location of the gland (e.g., a marker on the suprasternal notch).

- Including a size marker in one image is helpful to document the size of the gland.

- Size markers should not be included in an image obtained with a pinhole collimator because of the distortion of objects in different planes (see Case 71).

- Similarly, the size of the thyroid gland should not be estimated from the images when a pinhole collimator is used.

- The value of single photon emission computed tomography (SPECT) imaging has not been proved. Because of the shoulders, it is difficult to get close enough to the thyroid to obtain clear images.

- Both technetium-99m and iodine-123 have advantages and disadvantages for thyroid imaging (Table 1). The physician reading the study should be familiar with the properties of the tracer being used.

Technique

- 300 μCi iodine-123 orally 24 hours prior to uptake and scan.
- Pinhole collimator images obtained for 5 minutes in anterior, right anterior oblique (RAO), and left anterior oblique (LAO) projections.
- Marker views also obtained.

Image Interpretation

Images in several views (Fig. A) demonstrate homogeneous tracer distribution throughout the thyroid gland. The gland is normal in contour.

Diagnosis and Clinical Follow-up

On physical exam, the gland was normal in size, configuration, and consistency. No module was palpated. The thyroid scan was normal. Patient was diagnosed as having a normal thyroid. No further follow-up was obtained.

Discussion

Normal iodine-123 thyroid scans (Figs. B through F) show variable appearance of the thyroid gland. It is important to be familiar with the variations of normal. Some glands normally demonstrate the isthmus; others do not. A few normal glands will contain enough functioning tissue in the pyramidal lobe to visualize this structure as well. It is not uncommon for the right and left lobes to be slightly asymmetrical.

Thyroid scans with technetium-99m look quite different from those obtained with iodine-123. There is often more background soft tissue activity and occasional blood pool activity, and, if the field of view is large enough, the salivary glands should be seen. Because technetium-99m is secreted by the salivary glands, salivary activity in the esophagus can also be seen. On oblique images, this salivary activity moves with posterior structures and can therefore be distinguished from a pyramidal lobe that lies anterior to the trachea. Another method to distinguish salivary activity in the esophagus from that in the pyramidal lobe is to have the patient flush the esophageal activity away by drinking water.

Table 1. Comparison of Advantages and Disadvantages of the Two Most Popular Tracers for Thyroid Scintigraphy

Tracer	Advantages	Disadvantages
Technetium-99m	Study started and finished in 1 day Tracer inexpensive and readily available	Not all nodules that do not organify iodine ("cold" nodules) are cold with technetium-99m (discordant nodules) Uptake value is difficult to obtain and subject to more rapid variability over time Blood pool structures and salivary glands may interfere with scan interpretation Requires injection
Iodine-123	The gold standard for documentation of nodule functional status (organification) Uptake can be readily obtained and is not subject to minute to minute variability Good target to background images of the thyroid Oral administration	Usually must be ordered at least 24 hours before the study is begun Requires 2 visits to nuclear medicine facility: first visit to administer isotope, and second visit 24 hours later to perform uptake and/or imaging.

Suggested Readings

Falk S. *Thyroid Disease: Endocrinology, Surgery, Nuclear Medicine, and Radiotherapy.* 2nd ed. New York: Lippincott-Raven, 1997.

Harbert J. The thyroid. In: Harbert J, Eckelman W, Neumann R, eds. *Nuclear Medicine Diagnosis and Therapy.* New York: Thieme, 1996, pp. 407–427.

Ryo UY, Alavi A, Collier DB, et al. *Atlas of Nuclear Medicine Artifacts and Variants.* 2nd ed. Chicago: Year Book Medical Publishers, Inc., 1990.

Case 67

Clinical Presentation

82-year-old woman referred from her primary care physician for a right thyroid mass.

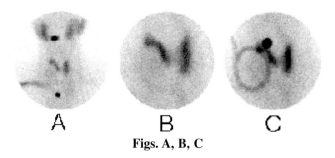

Figs. A, B, C

Technique

- 11 mCi technetium-99m sodium pertechnetate intravenously.
- Pinhole images obtained 20 minutes after tracer injection (anterior, right anterior oblique [RAO], left anterior oblique [LAO], and marker views), 128 × 128 matrix for 5 minutes.
- Marker views obtained with cobalt-57 string and spot markers.

Image Interpretation

Pinhole views demonstrate a large hypofunctioning area in the right lobe of the gland. The anterior view (Fig. A) demonstrates the location of the gland in the neck. Two cobalt-57 markers at the sternal notch and 10 cm above the notch provide some anatomical landmarks. The anterior spot view (Fig. B) demonstrates distortion of the right lobe of the gland. Marker views (Fig. C) with a cobalt-57 string marker show that the palpated right thyroid nodule corresponds to the location of the hypofunctioning area. A cobalt-57 spot marker was also placed on top of what was thought to be a dermal structure between the right and left lobes of the thyroid gland. Salivary glands are also noted, as expected with technetium-99m sodium pertechnetate imaging.

Differential Diagnosis

- Adenoma
- Adenomatous hyperplasia
- Cyst
- Thyroid malignancy
- Hematoma
- Fibrosis following I-131 therapy of hyperfunctioning nodule
- Early lymphocytic thyroiditis
- Metastatic disease to thyroid gland
- Parathyroid mass

(continued) Technetium-99m thyroid images demonstrate ion trapping but not organification. Some thyroid cancers have lost the ability to organify iodine but have not lost the ability for ion trapping. Therefore, if technetium-99m is used for thyroid imaging and a palpated nodule is seen to concentrate the tracer, imaging should be repeated with iodine-123 to ensure that the nodule has retained organification function.

- Cold nodules can occur in the isthmus or at the periphery of the gland, causing little distortion of the normal gland contour. A nodule is a physical exam finding, not a scan finding. All thyroid glands should be palpated. If a palpatory abnormality exists, it should be marked and correlated with scan findings.

- The value of thyroid imaging in patients with nodules is the subject of debate. The reliance on scintigraphy varies according to individual preferences of referring physicians. In many cases, the most cost-effective evaluation of solitary thyroid nodules is by fine needle aspiration. Scintigraphy is most helpful when the biopsy is equivocal.

Diagnosis and Clinical Follow-up

Fine needle aspiration demonstrated thyroid cancer, confirmed at thyroidectomy as papillary carcinoma. Following therapy with 150 mCi iodine-131 on two separate occasions, whole-body views demonstrated no evidence of distant metastases. There is no evidence of recurrence to date.

Discussion

Hypofunctioning, or "cold," nodules noted on thyroid scan are caused by thyroid cancer in 10 to 20% of patients, depending on such factors as patient age and gender, size of nodule, and history of neck irradiation. A solitary hypofunctioning nodule larger than 2 cm in a young man would be more worrisome than a 1-cm nodule in a 40-year-old woman with a multinodular gland. Ultrasound may provide information about internal architecture of the nodule, but anatomical findings are nonspecific and less definitive than histological examination is. On the other hand, ultrasound is helpful for guiding fine needle aspiration if the nodule is difficult to palpate.

Some investigators question the need for thyroid scans in patients with solitary nodules. Because fine needle aspiration provides histological information, the nonspecific findings on the thyroid scan are thought to be of questionable value. Autonomous hyperfunctioning nodules can show atypical cellular changes on fine needle aspiration but are almost never malignant. The thyroid scan is very useful, therefore, if the nodule is noted to be functioning autonomously when there are equivocal results from the fine needle biopsy.

Suggested Readings

Mazzaferri EL. Management of a solitary thyroid nodule. *N Engl J Med* 328:553–559, 1993.

Price DC. Radioisotopic evaluation of the thyroid and the parathyroids. *Radiol Clin North Am* 31:991–1015, 1993.

Case 68

Clinical Presentation

42-year-old woman presenting with symptoms of hyperthyroidism and right thyroid nodule. There was a long history of thyroid enlargement.

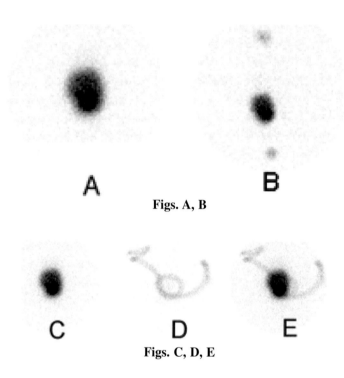

Figs. A, B

Figs. C, D, E

Technique

- 300 μCi iodine-123 orally 24 hours prior to uptake and scan.
- Pinhole collimator images obtained for 5 minutes in anterior, right anterior oblique (RAO), and left anterior oblique (LAO) projections.
- Marker views also obtained.

Images Interpretation

Figures A and B show two pinhole images of the thyroid bed. Figure A is a close up view; Figure B is a view with the pinhole further away from the patient to allow cobalt-57 spot markers to be placed on the supersternal notch and chin. Figures A and B show a focal area of intense tracer localization and no other uptake in the thyroid gland. Figures C through E show three marker views. These images demonstrate that the palpated nodule corresponds to the area of tracer uptake. After a string marker was placed around the palpated nodule, the initial image with the energy window set to iodine-123 showed the tracer uptake in the thyroid nodule (Fig. C). Without moving the patient, the energy window was then set to 122 keV (cobalt-57) to image the string marker (Fig. D). Figures C and D are added to create the final image (Fig. E). Uptake was measured to be 42%.

Differential Diagnosis

- Autonomous hyperfunctioning nodule
- Post-ablative (surgical or iodine-131) remnant
- Hemiagenesis (more often seen as tracer uptake in the shape of a single thyroid lobe).

Diagnosis and Clinical Follow-up

Hyperfunctioning autonomous nodule was the diagnosis. The patient elected to be treated surgically for removal of the nodule.

Discussion

Hyperfunctioning nodules may suppress surrounding thyroid function by inhibiting thyroid-stimulating hormone (TSH) secretion. The suppression of normally functioning thyroid tissue allows a therapeutic dose of iodine-131 to be selectively taken up by the nodule, therefore treating only the hyperfunctioning tissue. This study demonstrates the marked suppression of the normally functioning thyroid tissue, ensuring that there would be minimal injury to the remainder of the gland had therapy with iodine-131 been chosen.

Later scans, after recovery of normal function by the rest of the thyroid gland, can show a cold area at the site of the previously treated hyperfunctioning nodule. This cold area may be mistaken for a potential malignancy if the history is not obtained. Because she was leaving the country soon, this patient elected to have surgical removal of the nodule rather than remain available for monitoring of radioiodine effectiveness.

Suggested Readings

Giuffrida D, Gharib H. Controversies in the management of cold, hot, and occult thyroid nodules. *Am J Med* 99:642–650, 1995.

Hamburger JI. The autonomously functioning thyroid nodule: Goetsch's disease. *Endocr Rev* 8:439–447, 1987.

Case 69

Clinical Presentation

80-year-old woman presenting with new onset atrial fibrillation and hyperthyroidism.

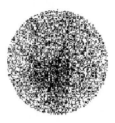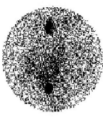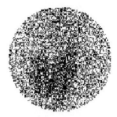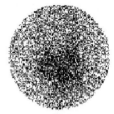

Fig. A

Technique

- 300 μCi iodine-123 orally 24 hours prior to imaging and uptake measurements.
- Images acquired with a pinhole collimator for 5 minutes in a 128 × 128 matrix.

Image Interpretation

Minimal tracer uptake is noted in the region of the thyroid bed (Fig. A). Iodine uptake was measured to be 5%.

Differential Diagnosis

- Subacute thyroiditis
- Previous surgical or iodine-131 ablation of thyroid
- Iatrogenic, such as administration of antithyroid drugs, suppression with exogenous thyroid hormone, recent administration of radiographic contrast material or iodine as expectorant.
- Primary hypothyroidism
- Struma ovarii (more often seen on board exams than in life)

Diagnosis and Clinical Follow-up

The thyroid was palpated to have an irregular surface and was approximately five times normal size. Patient was questioned about medications and recent contrast administration. History revealed recent ingestion of amiodarone. The poor uptake was attributed to iodine excess from amiodarone. The cause of the hyperthyroidism could not be determined in light of the iodine excess.

Discussion

This is a difficult case that can be interpreted only in light of findings on physical exam and medical history. There are many reasons for diminished uptake of io-

PEARLS/PITFALLS

- Careful questioning about medications is important. Do not rely entirely on the medical record. Talk to the patient yourself and be aware of factors that may suppress iodine uptake.

- Make certain the gamma camera and thyroid probe are set at the correct energy window.

- Nodular thyroid disease is common. Two diseases, such as a multinodular gland and subacute thyroiditis, may be superimposed, making the findings on scan, uptake, and physical exam confusing.

dine on thyroid scan. Subacute thyroiditis, previous iodine load, and medications such as antithyroid agents and synthroid may all cause depressed uptake of iodine by the thyroid gland. With the recent history of amiodarone ingestion in this patient, there may be suppression of iodine organification by the thyroid, although some studies have shown amiodarone to suppress radioiodine uptake more commonly in hypothyroid patients and less commonly in hyperthyroid patients.

Suggested Readings

Falk S. *Thyroid Disease: Endocrinology, Surgery, Nuclear Medicine, and Radiotherapy.* 2nd ed. New York: Lippincott-Raven, 1997.

Harbert J. The thyroid. In: Harbert J, Eckelman W, Neumann R, eds. *Nuclear Medicine Diagnosis and Therapy*. New York: Thieme, pp. 407–427, 1996.

Ross DS. Syndromes of thyrotoxicosis with low radioactive iodine uptake. *Endocrinol Metab Clin North Am* 27;169–185, 1998.

Case 70

Clinical Presentation

48-year-old woman presenting with history of recent thyroidectomy for thyroid cancer. Images were obtained following an iodine-131 dose that was given to ablate a postsurgical thyroid remnant.

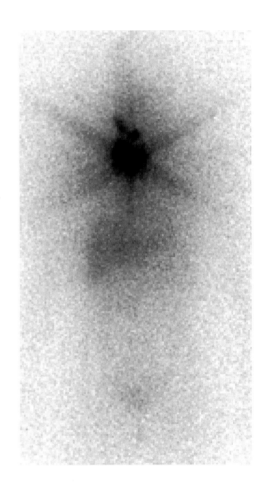

Fig. A

Technique

- 29 mCi iodine-131 3 days prior to imaging.
- Medium-energy collimator images obtained for 5 minutes per view.
- Whole-body image was constructed with adjacent spot views.

Image Interpretation

Six regularly spaced linear streaks can be seen emanating radially from an intense area of uptake in the region of the thyroid bed (Fig. A). Tracer uptake is also noted in the liver.

Differential Diagnosis

- Penetration of collimator septa
- Faulty collimator
- Patient motion (although usually not as symmetric as artifact seen in this case)

Diagnosis and Clinical Follow-up

Images show a star artifact. Patient had an uneventful ablation of thyroid remnant. No distant metastases were noted. The activity in the liver was secondary to metabolism of T3 and T4 labeled with radioiodine.

Discussion

The principle energy photon emitted from iodine-131 is at 364 keV, which is too high to adequately collimate with a medium-energy collimator. If the collimator holes are arranged in a hexagonal pattern (as in this case), the high-energy photons penetrate in the direction of the least amount of lead (Fig. B).

Gamma camera images may be subject to several artifacts that can degrade the images and make accurate interpretation of images difficult. The artifacts may be caused by many factors, including the gamma camera, radiopharmaceutical, technologist, filming process or patient. Physicians aware of the appearance of artifacts are more likely to avoid misreading images containing them.

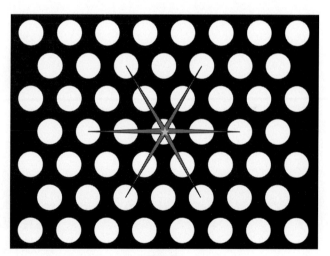

Fig. B

Suggested Readings

Ryo UY, Alavi A, Collier BD, Bekerman C, Pinsky SM. Atlas of Nuclear Medicine Artifacts and Variants. Chicago: Yearbook Medical Publishers, Inc., 1990.

Gentili A, Miron SD, Adler LP. Review of some common artifacts in nuclear medicine. *Clin Nucl Med* 1994; 19:138–43.

Case 71

Clinical Presentation

35-year-old man with no medical history presenting with an asymptomatic thyroid nodule noted on routine physical exam.

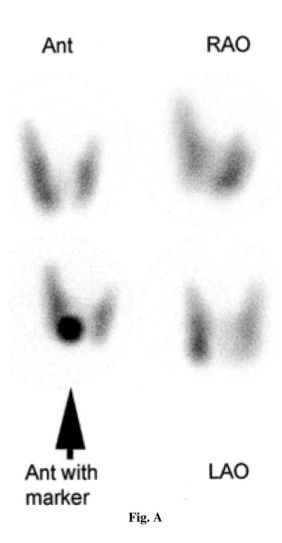

Fig. A

Technique

- 300 µCi iodine-123 orally 24 hours prior to uptake and scan.
- Pinhole collimator images obtained for 5 minutes in anterior, right anterior oblique (RAO), and left anterior oblique (LAO) projections.
- A marker view obtained with the marker placed over the palpated nodule.

Image Interpretation

Figure A shows a thyroid gland that looks normal other than some minimal asymmetry in tracer uptake. The right lobe appears to be larger than the left. The hot spot noted on the marker view (image at lower left of Fig. A) is a cobalt marker placed on the palpated nodule. Figure B demonstrates the same patient imaged after a suppressive dose of thyroid hormone. The nodule is shown to continue functioning despite the suppressed thyroid-stimulating hormone (TSH). It is very unlikely that an autonomous functioning nodule such as this would be cancerous.

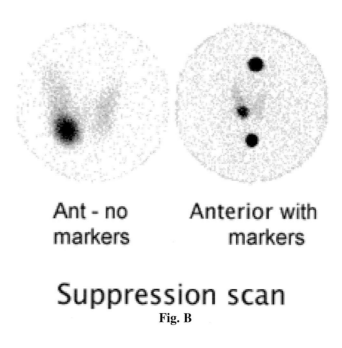

Ant - no markers   Anterior with markers

Suppression scan
Fig. B

Differential Diagnosis

- Autonomous nodule
- Primary thyroid cancer (extremely rare)

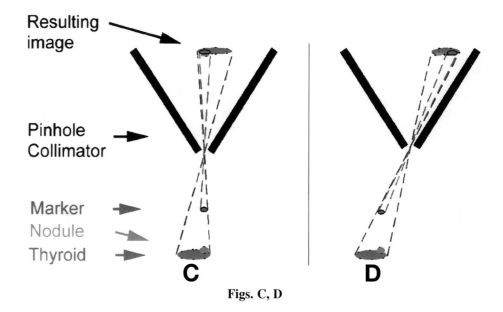

Resulting image

Pinhole Collimator

Marker
Nodule
Thyroid

C   D

Figs. C, D

Diagnosis and Clinical Follow-up

Autonomous nodule without hyperfunction. The nodule was followed clinically and showed no signs of enlargement. Thyroid function tests remained normal.

Discussion

When a nodule is palpated but not clearly seen to correspond to any area of decreased tracer uptake on the scan, the nodule may have a number of causes, including a cold nodule surrounded by functioning tissue, a functioning nodule, or an extrathyroidal mass such as a lymph node or lipoma. If the nodule is functioning, it may be autonomously functioning but not hyperfunctioning to the extent that it suppresses the surrounding normal thyroid tissue. This is an important distinction because if the nodule is functioning and autonomous, it is very unlikely that it is a carcinoma.

To distinguish an autonomous functioning nodule from a cold nodule, a suppression scan may be done. A suppression scan is obtained in a manner similar to the technique described previously, except that images are obtained after the patient is put on a suppressive dose of thyroid hormone (Fig. B). The thyroid hormone should suppress iodine uptake in all tissue normally responsive to TSH but not in the autonomous nodule.

Suggested Reading

Cavalieri RR, McDougall IR. In Vivo Isotopic Tests and Imaging. In: Braverman LE, Utiger RD, eds. Werner and Ingbar's The Thyroid. Philadelphia: Lippincott-Raven, 1996:352–376.

Case 72

Clinical Presentation

36-year-old man with no previous medical history presenting with a thyroid nodule that was removed and found to be papillary follicular cancer. Images with iodine-123 after withdrawal from thyroid hormone were obtained.

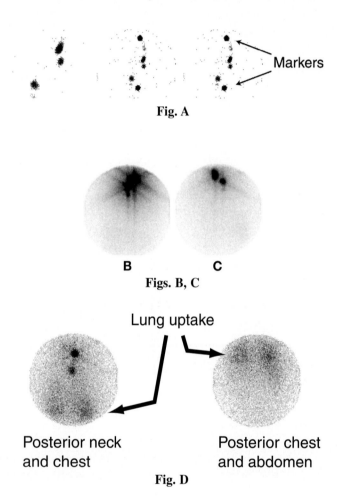

Fig. A

Figs. B, C

Fig. D

Technique

- For thyroid hormone withdrawal, stop T4 and start the patient on T3 (shorter half-life) 6 weeks prior to testing. Two weeks prior to planned imaging, T3 should be stopped. One to two weeks later, the thyroid-stimulating hormone (TSH) level is drawn and the imaging is done. TSH should be at least five times the upper limit of normal. Making patients hypothyroid is not a trivial matter. Patients should be closely followed by an experienced physician during this time. Patients can also be put on a low-iodine diet to maximize tracer uptake.
- 300 μCi iodine-123 orally 24 hours prior to imaging.
- Pinhole views of tracer uptake in the neck at 24 hours obtained in a 128 × 128 matrix.
- 5 mCi iodine-131 orally following the iodine-123 images.

- Pinhole views of the neck and parallel hole collimator images with a medium-energy collimator obtained of the torso and proximal extremities (anterior and posterior) at 3 days.

Image Interpretation

Figure A shows iodine-123 uptake in residual functioning thyroid tissue in the neck. The focal uptake may be either surgical remnants of normal thyroid tissue or local metastases.

Following the iodine-123 images, the patient was given 5 mCi iodine-131 for whole-body search images.

Anterior (Fig. B) and posterior (Fig. C) views of the neck (residual functioning thyroid tissue at the top of the image) and chest show no evidence of distant metastases. A later scan done after an iodine-131 therapy dose of 100 mCi administered to eliminate the residual tissue in the neck demonstrates tracer uptake in the base of both lungs (Fig. D).

Differential Diagnosis

- Metastatic thyroid cancer
- Gastric uptake (base of left lung)
- Liver uptake (base of right lung)
- Breast uptake (should be seen best in anterior view)
- Chronic inflammatory lung disease
- Stomach uptake with hiatal hernia
- Aspirated saliva

Diagnosis and Clinical Follow-up

Tracer uptake at the base of both lungs in Figure D is consistent with distant metastatic disease. Patient moved away for employment reasons and was lost to follow-up.

Discussion

Iodine-131 imaging of patients with a history of thyroid cancer is an important tool in the management of thyroid cancer. Iodine uptake in metastases with follicular elements is often seen before the metastases can be detected with other imaging modalities. The withdrawal of thyroid hormone replacement causes TSH to rise, which in turn stimulates any follicular tissue to concentrate iodine. The high iodine uptake allows treatment of metastatic sites with high doses of locally delivered radiation following the administration of iodine-131. Despite being able to administer localized radiotherapy to metastatic sites, distant metastases carry a poorer prognosis than disease confined to the thyroid bed. Iodine-131 therapy, however, remains the most effective treatment option for these functioning metastases.

Additional sites of metastasis not seen with the earlier iodine-131 total-body search dose of 5 mCi can be seen on post-therapy images for several possible reasons. On the post-therapy images, the iodine-131 dose is higher. Delayed imaging at 8 days may allow more thorough clearance of background activity, and the additional few days of hypothyroidism between the whole-body search dose and the treatment dose mean additional days of TSH stimulation of metastatic tissue.

- *(continued)* Iodine-131 is best imaged with a high-energy or ultra high (511 keV photon) collimator. If high energy collimators are not available, medium-energy collimation can be used.

- Diagnostic imaging doses of iodine-131 following thyroidectomy can "stun" thyrocytes and diminish uptake of subsequent therapeutic doses of iodine. The lower the diagnostic dose, however, the less sensitive the study is for the detection of distant metastases. The optimal diagnostic dose is therefore the subject of debate.

Suggested Readings

Cavalieri RR. Nuclear imaging in the management of thyroid carcinoma. *Thyroid* 6:485–492, 1996.

Huic D, Medvedec M, Dodig D, et al. Radioiodine uptake in thyroid cancer patients after diagnostic application of low-dose 131I. *Nucl Med Commun* 17:839–842, 1996.

Nemec J, Rohling S, Zamrazil V, et al. Comparison of the distribution of diagnostic and thyroablative I-131 in the evaluation of differentiated thyroid cancers. *J Nucl Med* 20:92–97, 1979.

Preisman RA, Halpern S. Detection of metastatic thyroid carcinoma after the administration of a therapeutic dose of 131-iodine. *Eur J Nucl Med* 3:69–70, 1978.

Case 73

Clinical Presentation

48-year-old woman presenting with a history of thyroid cancer. Patient is post-thyroidectomy.

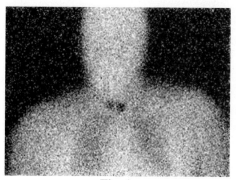

Fig. A

Technique

- 5 mCi iodine-131 orally 72 hours prior to imaging.
- Cobalt-57 flood source placed behind patient, and the camera set to cobalt-57 photopeak (122 keV).
- Following acquisition of image for 45 seconds, camera peak is switched to iodine-131 photopeak (364 keV) and imaging resumes for 5 minutes.
- Two images (cobalt-57 and iodine-131) superimposed.

Image Interpretation

Figure A shows a silhouette of a head, torso, and lungs, with focal tracer uptake in the region of the thyroid bed.

Differential Diagnosis

The cause for the transmission scan should be self-evident. However, increased background activity can also be seen with:

- Someone walking by the camera during imaging, either with a source of radio-activity in hand (dose to be injected in another patient), or a patient walking by that has recently been injected with a radiotracer.
- Contamination in the room on the floor, imaging table or walls
- Flood source mistakenly left in the room.

Diagnosis and Clinical Follow-up

Patient had no distant metastases and did well in follow-up.

PEARLS/PITFALLS

- Any flood source may be used. Merely set the camera for the flood photopeak, then for the iodine 131 photopeak.

- Make sure the patient does not move between the two image acquisitions.

- A point source may also be used by drawing it around the periphery of the body during acquisition.

- Make certain you first review any sites of uptake in the iodine 131 image by itself. If there is faint tracer concentration in the lungs from metastatic disease, a flood source might mask this site of abnormality.

- Although a flood source may increase radiation exposure to the patient, the additional exposure is minimal, and the benefits far outweigh the theoretical risks.

Discussion

Localization of the foci of iodine-131 concentration in the body can be difficult without normal anatomical landmarks. If there are no landmarks to identify the location of the thyroid or metastatic uptake, some method of providing landmarks is needed. A cobalt-57 (or any other) flood source behind the patient outlines lungs and body, allowing improved localization of iodine-131 uptake. The lungs are visualized with cobalt-57 because the air in the lungs attenuates the cobalt-57 photons less than surrounding tissues do. Figure B demonstrates how the iodine-131 and cobalt-57 images look before they are combined to form the final image.

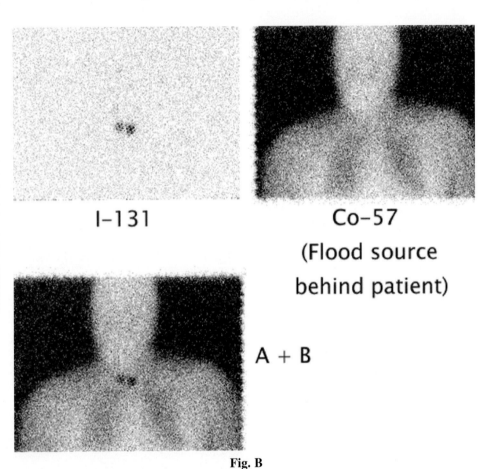

I-131

Co-57
(Flood source behind patient)

A + B

Fig. B

Case 74

Clinical Presentation

37-year-old woman presents with a 10-year history of follicular carcinoma. Total-body iodine-131 diagnostic images were obtained for follow-up (A, B, C). At the time of her follow-up images, the level of thyroid-stimulating hormone (TSH) was elevated at 105 μU/mL. After the diagnostic images, a 150-mCi therapy dose was administered. Seven days later, repeat imaging was obtained (D, E, F).

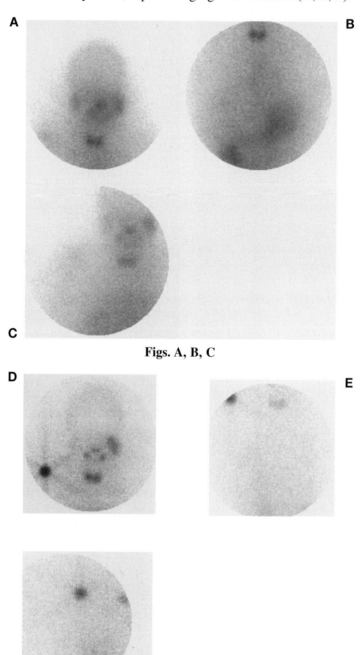

Figs. A, B, C

Figs. D, E, F

Technique

- 2 to 5 mCi iodine-131 for diagnostic imaging (Figs. A–C).
- 150 to 200 mCi sodium iodine-131 for treatment dose (Figs. D–F).
- Medium-, high-, or ultra high-energy collimator.
- Energy window is 20% centered on 364 keV.
- Imaging time is 10 minutes per view.
- Images obtained 48 to 72 hours after administration of diagnostic dose.
- Images obtained 7 to 10 days after administration of therapeutic dose.

Image Interpretation

Anterior views of the head (Fig. A), chest (Fig. B), and right shoulder (Fig. C) taken 24 hours after the ingestion of 5 mCi iodine-131 demonstrate residual thyroidal uptake (24-hour iodine uptake was measured to be 0.5%). Uptake in the right shoulder is unremarkable.

Although there was no evidence of metastatic disease on the iodine-131 diagnostic scan, the patient was scheduled for radioiodine therapy because of the aggressive nature of her tumor and her elevated serum thyroglobulin. A second set of images was obtained 7 days after the ingestion of a 150 mCi therapeutic dose (Figs. D, E, and F).

Repeat images of the head (Fig. D), chest (Fig. E), and right shoulder (Fig. F) after the higher dose of iodine-131 demonstrate intensely increased uptake in a metastatic focus in the right shoulder.

Differential Diagnosis

- Metastatic thyroid carcinoma
- Fungal infection
- Salivary or urinary contamination

Diagnosis and Clinical Follow-up

The patient was restarted on levothyroxine sodium (Synthroid). The right shoulder metastasis was known from earlier images following the initial therapeutic dose of iodine-131.

Discussion

Radioactive iodine therapy is indicated for the treatment of differentiated thyroid carcinomas (papillary and follicular). One criteria for treatment with radioactive iodine is tumor avidity on a low-dose scan using 2 to 5 mCi of iodine-131. Because of a relatively low tumor avidity for iodine-131 (compared with normal thyroid tissue) and relatively higher background counts, metastases may not be visualized 1 to 2 days after administration of diagnostic doses (2 to 5 mCi) of the tracer. After administration of a therapeutic dose of iodine-131 (150 to 200 mCi), it is not uncommon to visualize additional sites of metastatic disease.

Suggested Readings

Mazzaferri EL. Radioiodine and other treatment and outcomes. In: Braverman LE, Utiger RD, eds. *Werner and Ingbar's The Thyroid: A Fundamental and Clinical Text.* Philadelphia: J.B. Lippincott, 1991.

Mazzaferri EL, Jhiang SM. Long-term impact of initial surgical and medical therapy on papillary and follicular thyroid cancer. *Am J Med* 97:418–428, 1994.

Ozata M, Suzuki S, Miyamoto T, et al. Serum thyroglobulin in the follow-up of patients with treated differentiated thyroid cancer. *J Clin Endocrinol Metab* 79;98–105, 1994.

Pacini R, Lippi F, Formica N, et al. Therapeutic doses of iodine-131 reveal undiagnosed metastases in thyroid cancer patients with detectable serum thyroglobulin levels. *J Nucl Med* 28:1888–1891, 1987.

Samaan NA, Schultz PN, Hickey RC, et al. The results of various modalities of treatment of well differentiated thyroid carcinoma: A retrospective review of 1599 patients. *J Clin Endocrinol Metab* 75:714–719, 1992.

Case 75

Clinical Presentation

43-year-old woman presenting with recent diagnosis of renal stones. Elevated calcium and parathyroid hormone noted on blood testing.

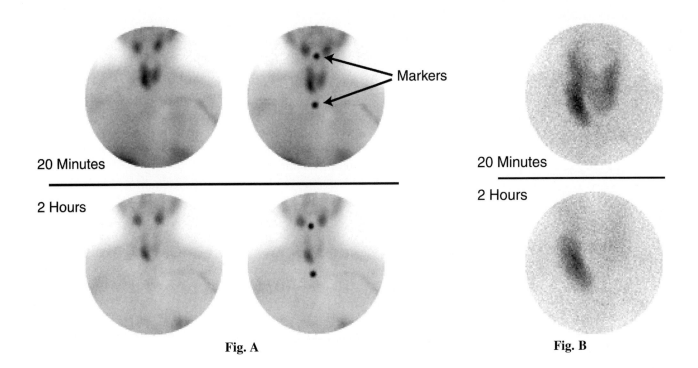

20 Minutes

2 Hours

Markers

20 Minutes

2 Hours

Fig. A

Fig. B

Technique

- 20 mCi technetium-99m–labeled sestamibi intravenously approximately 20 minutes prior to initial set of images.
- High-resolution collimator.
- Anterior view of the neck and chest done at 20 minutes and 2 hours.
- Pinhole view of the thyroid bed done at 20 minutes and 2 hours.

Image Interpretation

Initial images (Figs. A and B, top) show relatively diffuse uptake in the thyroid and a focus of increased tracer uptake in the right lower pole. Two hour–delayed images (Figs. A and B, bottom) show washout of tracer from the thyroid and residual tracer concentration in the region of the right lower pole (Figure B-pinhole image).

Differential Diagnosis

- Parathyroid adenoma
- Parathyroid hyperplasia
- Thyroid adenoma (more commonly not seen)

- Thyroid carcinoma
- Parathyroid carcinoma

Diagnosis and Clinical Follow-up

Ultrasound demonstrated a possible nodule on the left side, but no right side abnormality. Surgical exploration revealed a 3 cm by 2 cm right inferior parathyroid adenoma. Parathyroid hormone levels returned to normal after resection of the adenoma.

Discussion

Parathyroid imaging with sestamibi provides important information about the location of parathyroid adenomas and parathyroid hyperplasia. Its use in the initial management of hyperparathyroidism is questioned, however, because many head and neck surgeons feel it does not alter the initial management. Even though the scan may localize a specific site of uptake, many surgeons believe all parathyroid glands should be palpated and, occasionally, biopsied. When the initial surgical procedure fails to cure the hyperparathyroidism, however, the scan is thought to offer help in localizing the abnormality.

The scan is most accurate for the diagnosis of abnormal parathyroid glands when a focal abnormality is noted on the initial images and better seen on delayed images after the initial thyroid uptake washes out. Some abnormal parathyroid glands can also show tracer washout, however, and some thyroid nodules show persistently increased tracer concentration. These factors must be taken into consideration when the scan is interpreted. Additional imaging studies, such as ultrasound and computed tomography, may be correlated with the finding of the parathyroid study for optimal patient management.

Suggested Readings

Chen CC. Parathyroid scintigraphy. In: Harbert JC, Eckelman WC, Neumann RD, eds. *Nuclear Medicine Diagnosis and Therapy*. New York: Thieme, pp. 429–438, 1996.

Kipper MS, LaBarbera JJ, Krohn LD, et al. Localization of a parathyroid adenoma by the addition of pinhole imaging to Tc-99m sestamibi dual-phase scintigraphy. Report of a case and review of experience. *Clin Nucl Med* 22:73–75, 1997.

Shaha AR, Sarkar S, Strashun A, et al. Sestamibi scan for preoperative localization in primary hyperparathyroidism. *Head Neck* 19:87–91, 1997.

Shen W, Duren M, Morita E, et al. Reoperation for persistent or recurrent primary hyperparathyroidism. *Arch Surg* 131:861–867, 867–869 (discussion), 1996.

Shen W, Sabanci U, Morita ET, et al. Sestamibi scanning is inadequate for directing unilateral neck exploration for first-time parathyroidectomy. *Arch Surg* 132:969–974, 974–966 (discussion), 1997.

Summers GW. Parathyroid update: A review of 220 cases. *Ear Nose Throat J* 75:434–439, 1996.

Case 76

Clinical Presentation

42-year-old woman with a history of hypothyroidism and multinodular goiter presenting with elevated calcium and parathyroid hormone on routine blood testing.

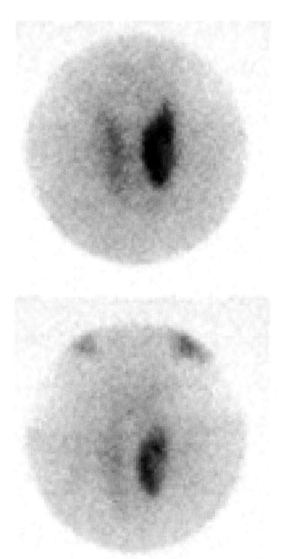

Fig. A

Technique

- 20 mCi technetium-99m–labeled sestamibi intravenously approximately 20 minutes prior to initial set of images.
- High-resolution collimator.
- Anterior view of the neck/chest done at 20 minutes and 2 hours.
- Pinhole view of the thyroid bed done at 20 minutes and 2 hours.

Image Interpretation

Pinhole images (Fig. A) show a large area of relatively increased tracer uptake in the left lobe of the thyroid that does not wash out on delayed image (Fig A, bottom).

Differential Diagnosis

- Parathyroid adenoma
- Parathyroid hyperplasia
- Thyroid adenoma (more commonly not seen)
- Thyroid carcinoma
- Parathyroid carcinoma

Diagnosis and Clinical Follow-up

Exploration of the neck revealed a 3 cm × 2 cm parathyroid adenoma in the upper portion of the left lobe of the thyroid. A second "possibly enlarged" right upper parathyroid gland was also identified and removed.

Discussion

The size and contour of the abnormality noted on the scan suggest thyroid uptake of tracer, possibly in a thyroid nodule in this patient with known multinodular goiter. The size of the removed adenoma, however, suggests that the uptake may have been caused by the adenoma, which was found to weigh more than 4 g. The scan did not show any evidence of a right-sided adenoma, which was suggested at pathology.

Suggested Readings

Caixas A, Berna L, Hernandez A, et al. Efficacy of preoperative diagnostic imaging localization of technetium 99m-sestamibi scintigraphy in hyperparathyroidism. *Surgery* 121:535–541, 1997.

Taillefer R, Boucher Y, Potvin C, et al. Detection and localization of parathyroid adenomas in patients with hyperparathyroidism using a single redionuclide imaging procedure with technetium-99m-sestamibi (double-phase study). *J Nucl Med* 33:1801–1807, 1992.

Zuback J, Patel KA, Guzman R, et al. Preoperative localization of a parathyroid adenoma with Tc-99m sestamibi imaging in a patient with concomitant nontoxic multinodular goiter. *Clin Nucl Med* 20:27–30, 1995.

Case 77

Clinical Presentation

34-year-old woman presenting with a ureteral stone. Subsequent workup revealed an elevated calcium and parathyroid hormone.

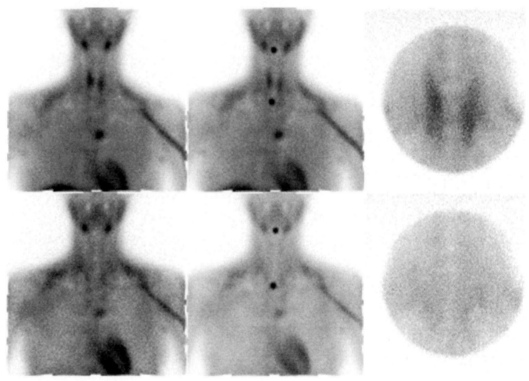

Fig. A

Technique

- 20 mCi technetium-99m–labeled sestamibi intravenously approximately 20 minutes prior to initial set of images.
- High-resolution collimator.
- Anterior view of the neck/chest done at 20 minutes and 2 hours.
- Pinhole view of the thyroid bed done at 20 minutes and 2 hours.

Image Interpretation

Normal uptake and washout is noted in the region of the thyroid bed (Fig. A). A focus of tracer concentration is noted just to the left of midline in the mediastinum, just superior to the heart.

Differential Diagnosis

• Parathyroid adenoma
• Other malignancy that can be seen in mediastinum or lung.

Diagnosis and Clinical Follow-up

Computed tomography scan demonstrated a nodule in the aorto-pulmonic window. Resection resulted in normalization of parathyroid hormone levels. Histological examination revealed a parathyroid adenoma. The patient recovered uneventfully.

Discussion

Parathyroid adenomas are usually found in the region of the thyroid bed but can be seen in the anterior mediastinum in approximately 5% of patients. Nuclear medicine parathyroid scintigraphy is particularly helpful in these patients because many have had an earlier surgical procedure in the region of the thyroid bed that failed to identify the abnormality. This study demonstrates the importance of using a large field of view camera.

Suggested Reading

Taillefer R, Boucher Y, Potvin C, et al. Detection and localization of parathyroid adenomas in patients with hyperparathyroidism using a single radionuclide imaging procedure with technetium-99m-sestamibi (double-phase study). *J Nucl Med* 33:1801–1807, 1992.

Case 78

Clinical Presentation

34-year-old man presenting with a long history of hyperparathyroidism. A sestamibi study is obtained for parathyroid localization.

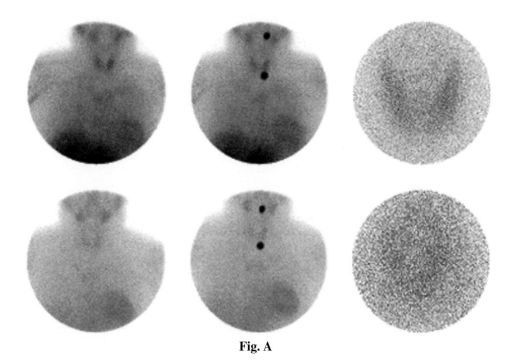

Fig. A

Technique

- 20 mCi technetium-99m–labeled sestamibi intravenously approximately 20 minutes prior to initial set of images.
- High-resolution collimator.
- Anterior view of the neck and chest done at 20 minutes and 2 hours.
- Pinhole view of the thyroid bed done at 20 minutes and 2 hours.

Image Interpretation

Normal uptake is seen in the region of the thyroid bed (Fig. A). A vague blush in the region of the mediastinum is also noted but not seen clearly enough to be diagnostic.

Differential Diagnosis

(for mediastinal uptake):

- Normal blood pool structure
- Parathyroid adenoma
- Other malignancy

Diagnosis and Clinical Follow-up

Angiography showed a blush of vascularity in the mediastinum at the site of the blush noted on sestamibi images. Magnetic resonance imaging and computed tomography showed equivocal soft tissue density in that region. Thoracoscopy revealed the parathyroid adenoma at that location. Thoracoscopic resection of mediastinal parathyroid adenoma was performed, after which the patient became hypoparathyroid.

Discussion

The tracer uptake in the neck is normal. The mediastinal scintigraphic findings were reported as questionable and nondiagnostic. This patient demonstrated equivocal findings in the same location on several studies, providing enough suspicion to warrant thoracoscopy.

Suggested Reading

Berna L, Caixas A, Piera J, et al. Technetium-99m-methoxyisobutylisonitrile in localization of ectopic parathyroid adenoma. *J Nucl Med* 1996; 37:631–633.

Section V

Scintigraphy of Neoplastic Disease

Case 79

Clinical Presentation

A 32-year-old man presenting with biopsy-proven nodular sclerosis Hodgkin's disease (Figs. A–C), and a 34-year-old man presenting with biopsy-proven mixed cellularity Hodgkin's disease (Figs. D–F). Gallium scan was requested for staging in both patients.

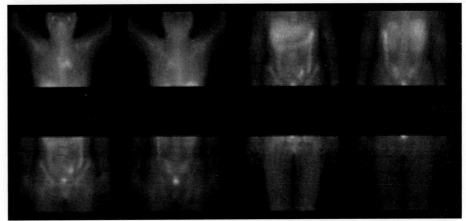

Fig. A

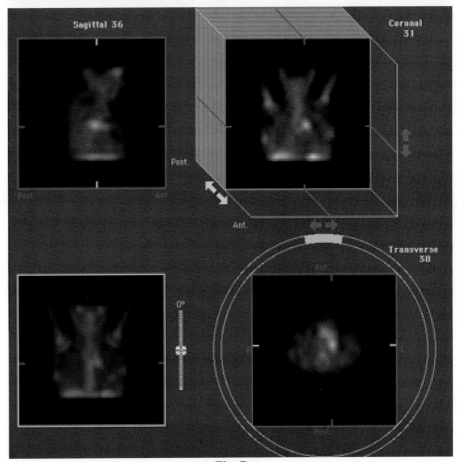

Fig. B

PEARLS/PITFALLS

- Gallium-67 citrate should always be injected first, even if it is only a few hours prior to the start of steroid therapy, chemotherapy, or radiation therapy. Injecting gallium after the start of any therapy, can lead to a false-negative study. For evaluation of response at midtreatment, imaging should be performed just before the next cycle of chemotherapy. This usually represents a 4-week delay between the delivery of the last chemotherapy and the time of the gallium scan.

- Counts are the key when performing gallium scintigraphy. The 10 mCi dose decreases the number of false-negatives and allows appropriate counting statistics for SPECT imaging.

- SPECT increases sensitivity and specificity. A negative SPECT rules out disease with a confidence interval of 81 to 96%. It also increases the certainty of a positive or negative reading and decreases the need for extra views of the abdomen by > 90%.

- "Triangulation," in other words, the capability offered by many SPECT softwares to focus the cursor on a particular finding and display it in three different planes, is extremely helpful in evaluating its significance. For example, a gallium-avid focus in one plane may appear tubular in the others and be consistent with physiological bowel activity, as demonstrated in the first patient. Such a tool significantly decreases the need for delayed views. *(continued)*

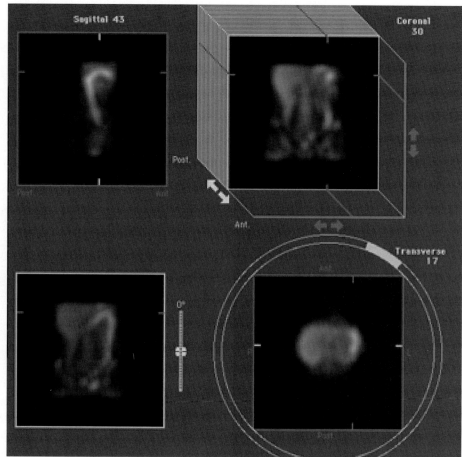

Fig. C

Technique

- 10 mCi (370 MBq) of gallium-67 citrate ($T\frac{1}{2}$ = 78 hours) injected intravenously prior to any therapy or 4 weeks after the end of therapy.
- Imaging at 72 hours, up to 14 days if necessary.
- Bowel preparation is optional.
- Use three photopeaks: 93.3 (37%), 184.6 (20.4%), and 300 (16.6%) keV; 15 to 20% window; medium-energy collimator, large field of view (LFOV).
- Planar study: anterior and posterior spot views of the chest (2 M counts) with the arms up, abdomen (1.5 M), pelvis (1.5 M), femora (for the time of the pelvis), and lateral skull (600 K); 256 × 256 matrix.
- Single photon emission computed tomography (SPECT) study: dual head system, tailored to each patient based on the results of the planar study and includes the neck/chest and abdomen/pelvis; 360 degrees, 64 images; 50 sec/image; 64 × 64 matrix; and reconstruction in three dimensions and coronal, sagittal, and axial planes.

Image Interpretation

Figure A shows anterior and posterior spot views of the head/chest, abdomen, pelvis and femora in the first patient. There is abnormal focal gallium avidity in the chest. The activity in the abdomen appears mostly tubular, suggestive of physiological bowel excretion.

- *(continued)* All studies should be correlated with clinical information and morphological imaging modalities, such as computed tomography (CT) or magnetic resonance imaging (MRI), and follow-up studies should be compared with the baseline study and prior studies.

- It is essential to read the SPECT studies from the computer terminal. If these studies are only read on film, there is a risk to underread or overread the significance of a particular finding. It may also add a degree of uncertainty that frequently leads to unnecessary delays because the patient is often brought back for delayed views to finalize the reading.

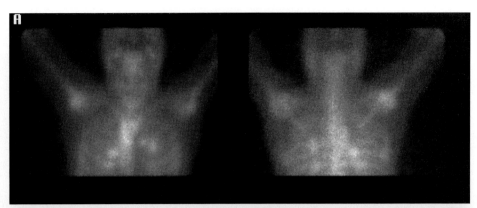

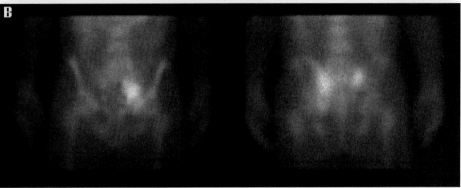

Fig. D

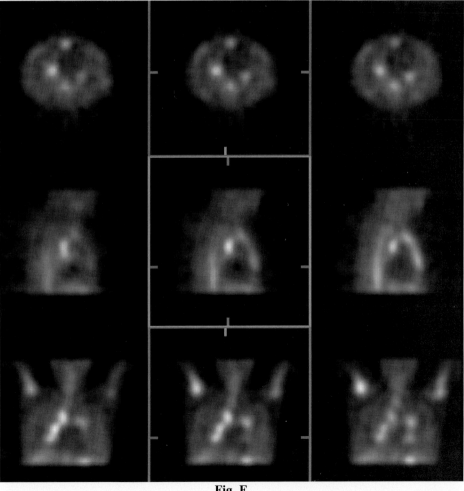

Fig. E

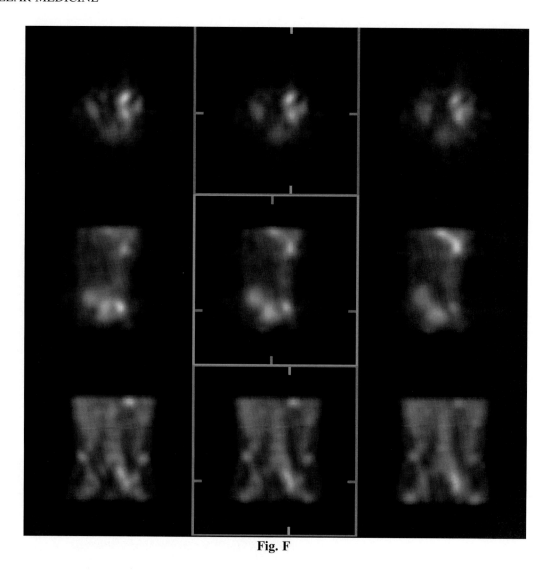

Fig. F

Figure B is a SPECT of the head and chest of the same patient performed with the arms above the head displayed in a clockwise fashion in the sagittal, coronal, and axial planes and in the volume-rendered format. The planes are centered over the gallium-avid mediastinal mass. The focal areas seen on the coronal views in the lateral aspects of the chest are the tips of the scapulae.

Figure C is the SPECT of the abdomen displayed in the same format as the SPECT of the chest and centered over the left upper quadrant (LUQ). The focal area seen in the LUQ on the coronal view appears as a tubular structure on the other views, confirming physiological excretion in the bowel. No delayed views were needed.

Figure D shows anterior and posterior planar views of the chest (A) and the pelvis (B) in the patient with biopsy-proven mixed cellularity Hodgkin's disease. Several areas of gallium avidity are demonstrated above and below the diaphragm, in the mediastinum and hilar regions, as well as in the iliac regions (left more than right).

Figure E is the chest SPECT demonstrating gallium-avid disease extending from the paratracheal region down to the infrahilar regions bilaterally.

Figure F is the abdominal and pelvic SPECT demonstrating gallium-avid disease in the left iliac nodes extending to the level of the bifurcation. The less gallium-avid foci seen on the planar study in the right iliac fossa were consistent with physiological bowel activity.

Differential Diagnosis

- Hodgkin's disease
- Non-Hodgkin's lymphoma (intermediate and high grade)
- Sarcoma
- Lung carcinoma
- Testicular tumors
- Head and neck tumors
- Neuroblastoma and adrenal cortical cancer
- Renal cell carcinoma
- Melanoma
- Multiple myeloma

Gallium-67 citrate is not tumor specific and can also be taken in a variety of inflammatory and infectious disorders. These include

- Sarcoidosis
- Sjögren's syndrome
- Soft-tissue infections
- Pneumocystis carinii pneumonia (PCP), cytomegalovirus (CMV), mycobacterium avium intracellulare (MAI), tuberculosis, and bacterial pneumonias
- Osteomyelitis
- Skeletal trauma or repair
- Radiation therapy sites (early on, later these areas will appear photon deficient)
- Cardiac amyloidosis

Diagnosis and Clinical Follow-up

The findings in the first patient were consistent with nodular sclerosis Hodgkin's disease limited to the mediastinum. The patient was then treated with chemotherapy and had a complete response.

The findings in the second patient were consistent with mixed cellularity Hodgkin's disease above and below the diaphragm. This patient also responded to chemotherapy and had a complete response.

Discussion

Hodgkin's disease is a lymphoproliferative disorder with a bimodal distribution with one peak between ages 15 and 34 and a second peak above 50 years of age. The disease generally involves lymph nodes and tends to progress in an orderly fashion from one nodal site to the next. It consists of four histological subtypes. Nodular sclerosis is the most common, followed by mixed cellularity. The lymphocyte-depleted and lymphocyte-predominant subtypes are the rarest. Both nodular sclerosis and mixed cellularity are gallium-avid, as demonstrated in these two patients. Gallium imaging is a standard imaging study for most patients with Hodgkin's disease and is used at staging as well as to assess response to therapy. Persistent gallium uptake during and after treatment is a poor prognostic sign and suggests a high risk for relapse.

Normal gallium distribution includes bone and bone marrow, liver and spleen (less than liver), bowel, kidneys (faint at 72 hours, more prominent with earlier imaging), lacrimal and salivary glands, nasopharynx, breasts, external genitalia, thymus (in children), and soft tissues. Gallium-67 citrate is taken up by live cells. Gallium-67 citrate scintigraphy therefore allows determination of whether persistent morphological abnormalities seen on chest X ray, CT, or MRI represent viable tumor or scar or edema.

The value of gallium scanning at baseline cannot be overemphasized, especially if gallium scanning is to be used in the follow-up of patients with lymphoma to assess therapeutic response. It provides whole body imaging that cannot always be obtained with conventional imaging modalities and therefore contributes to the staging. It also defines the location and avidity of the primary disease, which helps assess the significance of any new finding in the follow-up of these patients since Hodgkin's disease has a tendency to progress from one nodal site to the next.

In Hodgkin's disease, all disease sites usually have similar gallium avidity at staging. The size of the lesions and the resolution of the camera are the limiting factors. However, even normal-size lymph nodes may be visualized if they are involved with disease. Diffuse bone marrow uptake is commonly seen at presentation and during chemotherapy. This bone marrow expansion or reaction is thought to be related to the presence of growth factors secreted by the tumor at presentation, and secondary to post-therapeutic changes during and shortly after treatment. Heterogeneous bone marrow uptake with focal areas of gallium avidity is suspicious for bone marrow or skeletal involvement, or both.

Liver uptake commonly increases after chemotherapy in a diffuse fashion. Any focal area of gallium avidity should be correlated with conventional imaging modalities to rule out extranodal hepatic involvement. Focal splenic uptake is also worrisome for splenic involvement, particularly if the intensity of uptake is similar to that seen in the primary disease. Normal splenic uptake by gallium limits the sensitivity of detecting occult splenic involvement. Preliminary reports have shown that positron-emission tomography (PET) imaging using F-18 fluorodeoxyglucose (^{18}FDG) may be useful in detecting disease in the spleen.

Gallium-67 citrate is not tumor specific. Because it is an iron analogue, it binds to various iron-binding proteins such as transferrin, ferritin, and lactoferrin. The latter explains the intense breast uptake seen in postpartum women. The tracer is also secreted into the breast milk, which would require the mother to stop breast feeding. However, women who wish to continue breast feeding can undergo ^{18}FDG PET scanning as an alternative to gallium scanning and can be followed with that modality. Gallium-67 citrate also binds to bacterial siderophores and accumulates in neutrophils, lymphocytes, and monocytes, which explains its accumulation in inflammatory and infectious sites.

Suggested Readings

Anderson KC, Leonard RC, Canellos GP, Skarin AT, Kaplan WD. High-dose gallium imaging in lymphoma. *Am J Med* 75:327–331, 1983.

Front D, Bar-Shalom R, Mor M, et al. Hodgkin disease: Prediction of outcome with ^{67}Ga scintigraphy after one cycle of chemotherapy. *Radiology* 210:487–491, 1999.

Hagemeister FB, Purugganan R, Podoloff DA, et al. The gallium scan predicts relapse in patients with Hodgkin's disease treated with combined modality therapy. *Ann Oncol* 5(suppl 2):59–63, 1994.

Henkin PE, Polcyn PE, Quinn JL III. Scanning treated Hodgkin's disease with Ga-67 citrate. *Radiology* 110:151–154, 1974.

Hoekstra OS, Ossenkoppele GJ, Golding R, et al. Early treatment response in malignant lymphoma, as determined by planar fluorine-18-fluorodeoxyglucose scintigraphy. *J Nucl Med* 34:1706–1710, 1993.

Jochelson M, Mauch P, Balikian J, Rosenthal D, Canellos G. The significance of the residual mediastinal mass in treated Hodgkin's disease. *J Clin Oncol* 3:637–640, 1985.

Jochelson MS, Herman TS, Stomper PC, Mauch PM, Kaplan WD. Planning mantle radiation therapy in patients with Hodgkin's disease: Role of gallium-67 scintigraphy. *AJR Am J Roentgenol* 151:1229–1231, 1988.

Kostakoglu L, Yeh SDJ, Portlock C, et al. Validation of gallium-67-citrate single-photon emission computed tomography in biopsy-confirmed residual Hodgkin's disease in the mediastinum. *J Nucl Med* 33:345–350, 1992.

Tumeh ST, Rosenthal DS, Kaplan WD, et al. Lymphoma: Evaluation with Ga-67 SPECT. *Radiology* 164:111–114, 1987.

Wylie BR, Southee AE, Joshua DE, et al. Gallium scanning in the management of mediastinal Hodgkin's disease. *Eur J Haematol* 42:334–347, 1989.

Case 80

Clinical Presentation

55-year-old man presenting with a history of low-grade lymphoma that had waxed and waned over the last 2 years. The patient remains untreated. He now reports a recent increase in nodal size in the neck and axillae and is being restaged by thallium and gallium scintigraphy.

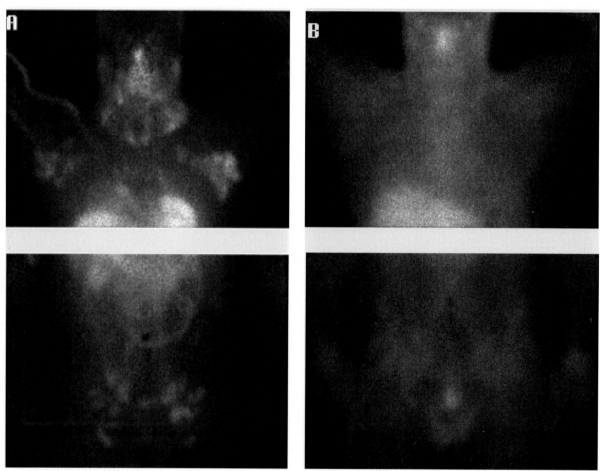

Figs. A, B

Technique

Thallium-201 Thallous Chloride Scintigraphy

- Patient should take nothing by mouth to try to minimize abdominal excretion of the tracer.
- Intravenous injection of 3 mCi (185 MBq) of thallium-201 thallous chloride (group IIIA metallic element, T½ = 73 hours) followed by a 10- to 20-mL saline flush.

- Large field of view (LFOV) camera equipped with low-energy, high-resolution collimator(s); energy window is 25% centered at 75 keV and 167 keV.
- Imaging starts 20 minutes after injection. Planar acquisition includes anterior and posterior views of the chest (1.5 M counts), abdomen/pelvis (1 M counts), femora, and both lateral skulls (600 K counts), 256 × 256 matrix. Single photon emission computed tomography (SPECT) studies are tailored to each patient based on the planar study and include neck/chest and abdomen/pelvis; 360 degrees; 64 projections, 60 sec/step; 64 × 64 matrix; reconstruction in three dimensions and coronal, sagittal, and axial planes.
- At end of thallium acquisition, patient is injected with gallium-67 citrate.

Gallium-67 Citrate Scintigraphy

- See Case 79.
- 10 mCi (370 MBq) of gallium-67 citrate (group IIIA metal, ferric ion analogue, half life is 77.9 hours) injected intravenously.
- Imaging at 72 hours, up to 14 days if necessary.
- Bowel preparation is optional.
- Use the three photopeaks: 93.3 (37%), 184.6 (20.4%), and 300 (16.6%) keV; an energy window at 15 to 20%; medium-energy collimators, and a LFOV camera.
- Planar study consists of anterior and posterior spot views of the chest with the arms up (2 M counts), abdomen (1.5 M), pelvis (1.5 M), femora (for the time of the pelvis), and lateral skull (600 K); matrix is 256 × 256.
- SPECT study is tailored to each patient based on the results of the planar study and includes the neck/chest and abdomen/pelvis. Use a dual head system, 360 degrees, 64 images, 50 sec/image, a 64 × 64 matrix, and reconstruct in three dimensions and coronal, sagittal, and axial planes.

Image Interpretation

Figure A shows anterior views of the chest and pelvis obtained after the injection of thallium-201 thallous chloride. Multiple focal areas of intense thallium uptake are seen bilaterally in the neck, supraclavicular regions, axillae, and inguinal nodal regions extending into the iliac and para-aortic lymph nodes, as was confirmed by SPECT (not shown). Also note the physiological uptake along the vessels in the right upper arm following injection in the right antecubital fossa and in the myocardium, thyroid, bowel, and liver.

Figure B shows anterior views of the chest and pelvis obtained 3 days later in the same patient following the injection of gallium-67 citrate. Only faint gallium uptake can be seen in the neck, axillary, and inguinal and pelvic regions. Note the marked difference between the two studies.

Differential Diagnosis

- Low-grade non-Hodgkin's lymphomas: categories A (small lymphocytic), B (follicular, predominantly small cleaved cell), and C (follicular, mixed small cleaved cell) of the National Cancer Institute Working formulation.
- Many other types of viable tumors
- In skeletal tumors, thallium is useful in assessing soft tissue and skeletal involvement at staging and in evaluating residual skeletal tumor and therapeutic response because reparative changes may remain gallium positive.

- *(continued)* Evaluation of abdominal tumors with thallium-201 thallous chloride or Tc-99m-MIBI is limited because of the unpredictable excretion of the tracer into the small and large portion of the bowel. In addition, biliary and renal excretion of MIBI leads to intense renal and bladder urinary activity that frequently induces artifacts during SPECT reconstruction.

- Thallium uptake is frequently seen (especially on SPECT) in the posterior chest in the region of the scapula ipsilateral to the injection site. This may be related to muscular activity and differential perfusion to this area during the injection process.

- Any skeletal muscular activity can be seen on thallium study such as uptake in the facial muscles if the patient is chewing gum or sartorius muscle if the patient is twitching a leg.

- Another focal area of physiological uptake is commonly seen in the lower chest in the midline in the region of the atria that most likely represents a cardiac structure.

- The combination of thallium and gallium scintigraphy may be helpful in monitoring the biology and natural course of low-grade lymphomas and may be used as a noninvasive functional tool to evaluate changes in the biology of the tumor and possible transformation to a more aggressive lymphoma.

Diagnosis and Clinical Follow-up

Low-grade lymphoma was the diagnosis. Findings were consistent with low-grade non-Hodgkin's lymphoma without scintigraphic evidence of transformation to a higher grade. A watch-and-wait strategy was adopted, and the patient remained untreated. The size of the nodes gradually decreased clinically over time, and the thallium avidity in these nodes decreased significantly on a follow-up scan. The gallium scan at follow-up remained similar to the one presented here. The patient continued to be followed in a similar fashion and remained untreated for 2.5 years.

Discussion

In a prospective study including all grades of non-Hodgkin's lymphomas, Kaplan et al (1990) showed that 26% of disease sites were negative on gallium scan and only seen on thallium scintigraphy. All these sites were low-grade lymphomas. Waxman et al (1996) showed marked differences in sensitivity between thallium and gallium scintigraphy for low-grade lymphomas as well: 100% sensitivity for thallium (per patient and site) versus 56% (per patient) and 32% (per site) for gallium.

Low-grade lymphomas typically wax and wane and remain relatively indolent for several years. In our experience, during that indolent phase of the disease, the thallium scan findings match the waxing and waning clinical phases of the disease, but the gallium scan remains relatively negative, as shown in this patient. If some of the nodal sites defined on the thallium study become positive on the gallium study, it may indicate a change in the biology of the tumor. The patient is then followed more closely to assess if transformation to a higher grade is occurring. In our experience, when the patient has transformed to a higher grade lymphoma, the gallium scan becomes equally or more positive than the thallium scan in both intensity and extent of the disease.

Uptake of thallium by tumor is most likely multifactorial based on flow, leaky capillaries, cell viability, increased permeability, Na/K adenosine triphosphatase pump, calcium ion channel system, and cotransport mechanism.

Technetium-99m-sestamibi (MIBI) has also demonstrated uptake in low-grade lymphomas, and, in our experience, images obtained with either agent compare well. In addition to flow, leaky capillaries, and increased permeability, uptake of MIBI is based on negative membrane potential. MIBI is also a substrate for efflux pumps located on the cell membrane such as p-glycoprotein and MRP, which are encoded for by the MDR-1 gene. Its use as a potential noninvasive functional tool to assess multidrug resistance expression in tumor cells is under study. The biggest advantage for Tc-99m-MIBI is the high photon flux that results in better images and a shorter acquisition time; the disadvantage is the high biliary and renal excretion that can compromise the evaluation of the abdomen and pelvis and lead to artifacts during SPECT reconstruction.

Suggested Readings

Arthur JE, Kehoe K, Van den Abbeele AD. Thallium-201 scintigraphy in low grade non-Hodgkin's lymphoma. *J Nucl Med* 37:258P, 1996.

Kaplan WD, Southee AE, Annese ML, Jochelson MS, Nadler LM. Evaluating low and intermediate grade non-Hodgkin's lymphoma (NHL) with gallium-67 (Ga) and Thallium-201 (TI) imaging. *J Nucl Med* 31:793, 1990. Abstract.

Nejmeddine F, Raphael M, Martin A, et al. [67]Ga scintigraphy in B-cell non-Hodgkin's lymphoma: Correlation of ^{67}Ga uptake with histology and transferrin receptor expression. *J Nucl Med* 40:40–45, 1999.

Waxman AD, Eller D, Ashook G, et al. Comparison of gallium-67-citrate and thallium-201 scintigraphy in peripheral and intrathoracic lymphoma. *J Nucl Med* 37:46–50, 1996.

PEARLS/PITFALLS

• A baseline study is essential because it will demonstrate the baseline tumor avidity for gallium. This is of critical importance in the follow-up of these patients in order to assess response to therapy and recurrence of disease.

• When the scintigraphy is performed at 72 hours, the intensity of gallium uptake in the spleen should be lower than that seen in the liver in normal circumstances. When it equals or surpasses the liver avidity, disease involvement cannot be ruled out, especially if there is associated splenomegaly. Benign increased splenic uptake can, however, be seen if the spleen is used as an extramedullary hematopoietic site. If images are performed later than 72 hours, there is normal physiological increased splenic uptake that may be equal to the avidity seen in the liver.

• Gallium scanning allows determination of whether persistent morphological abnormalities seen on chest X ray, CT, or magnetic resonance imaging (MRI) represent viable tumor or scar or edema. Although changes in tumor size on CT are indicative of response to therapy, there will frequently be a residual mass on CT that does not necessarily represent viable tumor. Therefore, functional assessment by gallium scintigraphy is a very useful adjunct to the morphological information provided by CT. Several groups have demonstrated the prognostic value of a positive or negative gallium scan at midtreatment or even after one *(continued)*

Case 81

Clinical Presentation

56-year-old patient was diagnosed with large cell lymphoma. A gallium scan was requested at baseline for staging (Fig. A, B). A correlative computed tomography (CT) was requested as well (Fig. C). The patient then received cyclophosphamide, hydroxydaunorubicin, Oncovin, and prednisone (CHOP) chemotherapy, and a gallium scan was requested at midtreatment to assess therapeutic response (Fig. D, E). The mid-treatment CT scan is shown in Fig. F.

65-year-old man (Fig. G) and a 28-year-old woman (Fig. H) were diagnosed with Burkitt's lymphoma. Gallium scans were requested at baseline for staging.

62-year-old man was diagnosed with mantle cell lymphoma. A gallium scan was requested for staging (Fig. I) and at midtreatment (Fig. J) to evaluate therapeutic response.

Technique

• 10 mCi (370 MBq) of gallium-67 citrate (group IIIA metal, ferric ion analogue, half life is 78 hours) injected intravenously prior to any therapy or 4 weeks after the end of therapy to prevent the risk of false-negative studies.
• Imaging at 72 hours, up to 14 days if necessary.
• Bowel preparation is optional.
• Three photopeaks: 93.3 (37%), 184.6 (20.4%), and 300 (16.6%) keV; energy window is 15 to 20%; a medium-energy collimator, and a large field of view (LFOV) camera.
• Planar study is anterior and posterior spot views of the chest with the arms up (2 M counts), abdomen (1.5 M), pelvis (1.5 M), femora (for the time of the pelvis), and lateral skull (600 K); matrix is 256×256.
• Single photon emission computed tomography (SPECT) study is performed with a dual head system, tailored to each patient based on the results of the planar study and includes the neck and chest and abdomen and pelvis; 360 degrees, 64 images; 50 s/image; 64×64 matrix; and reconstruction in three dimensions and coronal, sagittal, and axial planes.

(continued) cycle of chemotherapy. Failure-free survival or overall survival was not significantly different between patients with negative or positive CT scans at midtreatment.

- Increase in salivary gland uptake can be seen after radiation or chemotherapy.

- Bihilar uptake is commonly seen after chemotherapy and radiation therapy and may persist for several years. This uptake is usually symmetrical and decreases with time. Unilateral hilar uptake or increase in the intensity of uptake over time should raise the possibility of recurrent disease.

- A negative gallium-67 citrate scan with a positive chest X ray often indicates Kaposi's sarcoma. In these cases, thallium-201 thallous chloride scanning will frequently be positive. A positive Ga-67 scan in a patient with known Kaposi's sarcoma suggests infection or inflammation or lymphoma. *(continued)*

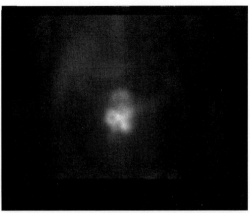

Fig. A

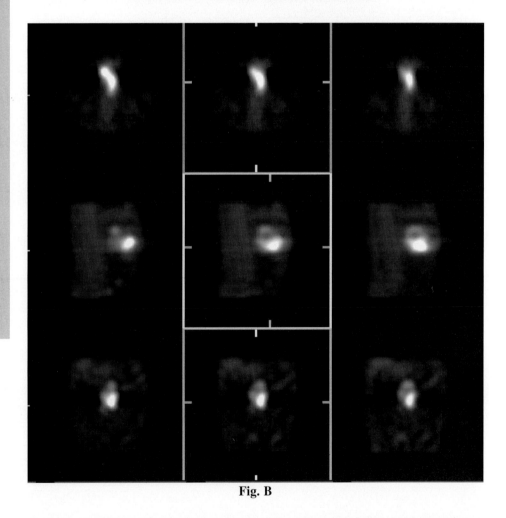

Fig. B

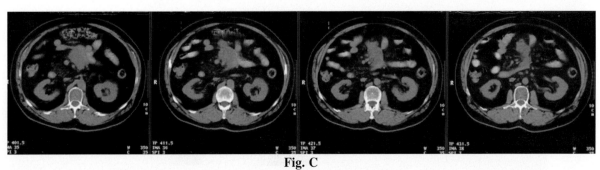

Fig. C

- *(continued)* Gallium-67 citrate is not tumor-specific and can also be taken in a variety of inflammatory and infectious disorders.

- A negative gallium scan in the follow-up of a patient or in the evaluation of a persistent mass on X ray or CT is of little value without knowledge of the avidity of the tumor at baseline and may lead to misinterpretation.

- Diffuse increased bone marrow uptake is often seen at presentation, during chemotherapy, and in the context of increased iron uptake such as in anemia. Conversely, decreased bone marrow uptake can be seen with iron overload such as after a transfusion. *(continued)*

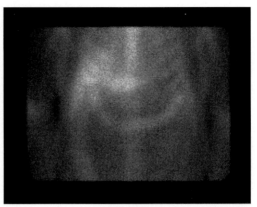

Fig. D

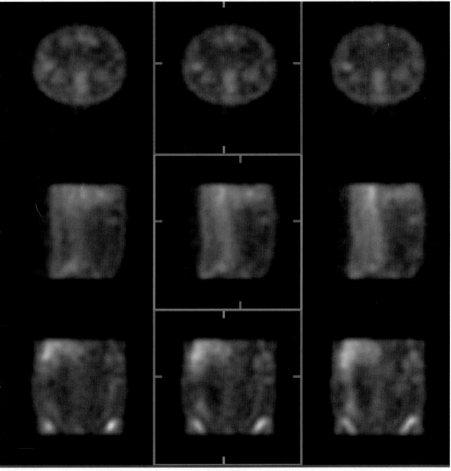

Fig. E

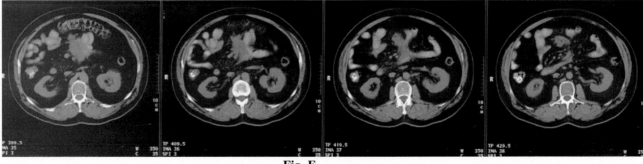

Fig. F

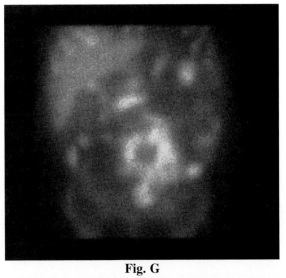

Fig. G

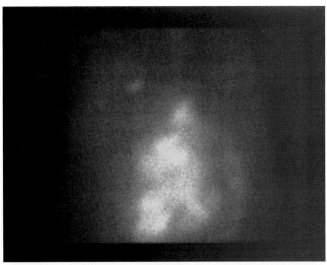

Fig. H

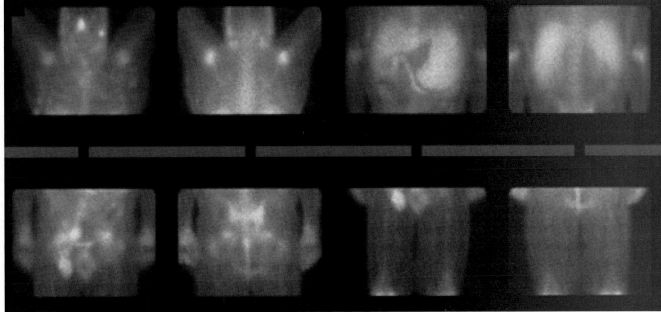

Fig. I

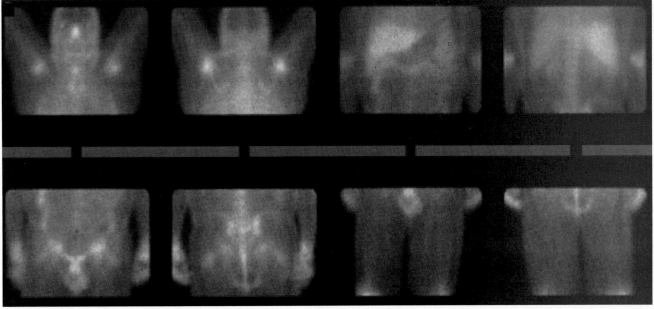

Fig. J

- *(continued)* Focal increased bone marrow uptake at presentation should raise the suspicion of bone marrow or skeletal involvement. Focal decreased bone marrow uptake is often seen after radiation therapy in the region of the radiation port. In that case, normal bone marrow uptake at the edge of the radiation port may appear quite intense in contrast with the depressed bone marrow uptake within the radiation port and should not be confused with bone marrow or skeletal involvement.

- Gallium-67 citrate is contraindicated in postpartum patients who wish to breastfeed because the radiopharmaceutical is excreted in the milk. In those circumstances, positron-emission tomography (PET) with F18-fluorodeoxyglucose (^{18}FDG) may be a useful alternative.

- False-negative studies can be seen if suboptimal techniques are being applied, if the patient has indolent low-grade lymphoma (for which thallium-201 thallous chloride or technetium-99m sestamibi [MIBI] would be indicated), and if the patient has received recent chemotherapy, radiation or steroid therapy (always inject gallium *prior* to the start of any therapy, even if it is only a few hours), a recent barium contrast study, iron supplements or chelators, or a transfusion (which will compete for the receptor sites). *(continued)*

Image Interpretation

Figures A (planar) and B (SPECT) obtained from the patient with large cell lymphoma demonstrate intense gallium uptake in the abdominal mass seen on CT (Fig. C). There was no other scintigraphic evidence of gallium-avid disease. Following three cycles of CHOP chemotherapy, the patient shows no evidence of gallium uptake at the site of the original disease (Figs. D, planar, and E, SPECT). The concomitant CT, however, still demonstrates a residual mass (Fig. F).

Figures G and H obtained in two patients with Burkitt's disease show multiple areas of high gallium avidity within the abdomen. The patient in Figure G had retroperitoneal and mesenteric disease as well as intestinal and hepatic involvement. The patient in Figure H had retroperitoneal, mesenteric, and hepatic involvement.

Figure I shows anterior and posterior spot views of the chest, abdomen, pelvis, and femora in a patient with mantle cell lymphoma. Gallium-avid disease is seen above and below the diaphragm in the left parotid, bilateral neck and axillae, pelvis, and right inguinal region. Also note the splenomegaly and the diffuse increased gallium uptake seen throughout the spleen, which appears more intense than the liver. After three cycles of treatment, there is resolution of the gallium-avid foci (Fig. J). Also note that the spleen has decreased in size and that the gallium intensity within the spleen is now less than that seen in the liver.

Differential Diagnosis

- Intermediate-grade malignant lymphomas (National Cancer Institute Working formulation):
  D. Follicular, predominantly large cell
  E. Diffuse small cleaved cell
  F. Diffuse mixed, small and large cell
  G. Diffuse large cell, cleaved/noncleaved
- High-grade malignant lymphomas (National Cancer Institute Working formulation):
  H. Diffuse large cell, immunoblastic
  I. Lymphoblastic (convoluted/nonconvoluted)
  J. Small noncleaved cell (Burkitt's/non-Burkitt's types)
- Mantle cell lymphoma
- Other gallium-avid tumors (See Case 79) including hepatocellular carcinoma
- Inflammatory and infectious disorders (See Case 79)

Diagnosis and Clinical Follow-up

The gallium avidity seen in the abdominal mass in the patient shown in Figures A through F is typical of that seen in an aggressive lymphoma such as large cell lymphoma, an intermediate-grade lymphoma. The findings after three cycles of CHOP are consistent with therapeutic response. A follow-up study done at the end of chemotherapy showed no evidence gallium-avid disease above or below the diaphragm.

• *(continued)* There is great interest in using ^{18}FDG-PET in lymphoma given the recent Health Care Financing Administration approval for reimbursement and the superior technical characteristics of dedicated PET. PET, may be superior to gallium scintigraphy in evaluating splenic involvement. However, the mechanisms of ^{18}FDG and Ga-67 uptake are based on two different biological processes, one being glucose metabolism and the other the expression of transferrin receptors. This may explain some of the discrepant results reported between the two studies. It is, therefore, premature to assume that ^{18}FDG-PET will replace gallium scintigraphy at this time, until prospective comparative studies can be performed.

Figures G and H illustrate the high gallium avidity seen in two patients with Burkitt's lymphoma, a high-grade lymphoma. Also note the extranodular involvement frequently seen with high-grade lymphomas. The patient shown in Figure G had a partial response to high-dose chemotherapy and went on to salvage chemotherapy and bone marrow transplant, but unfortunately the lymphoma recurred and the patient died of his disease. The patient in Figure H responded to the first line of chemotherapy and had no scintigraphic evidence of disease at the end of chemotherapy.

Figure I demonstrates the gallium avidity seen in mantle cell lymphoma. The midtreatment scan (Fig. J) shows good therapeutic response, and the patient is completing his chemotherapy regimen and will be reassessed at the end of the treatment.

Discussion

Intermediate and high grade non-Hodgkin's lymphomas are very gallium-avid, and gallium-67 citrate is the radiopharmaceutical of choice in those patients, not only for staging but also in the monitoring of therapeutic response and as a predictor of failure-free survival as well as overall survival. We currently routinely use gallium-67 citrate scintigraphy at baseline and midtreatment, at the end of chemotherapy, and in the follow-up of patients with intermediate and high grade lymphomas. Ga-67 scintigraphy is also used to plan radiation therapy and to detect relapse.

The use of Ga-67 scintigraphy has also been proposed after one cycle of chemotherapy as a predictor of outcome and is under study to evaluate whether the dose of chemotherapy could be decreased in patients in whom a good outcome can be predicted. This would be particularly useful in the pediatric population.

Mantle cell lymphoma is a lymphoma that used to be considered low grade. However, it behaved aggressively biologically, and these patients required chemotherapy. It is now considered to be one of the aggressive lymphomas by the REAL (Revised European American Lymphoma) classification. Interestingly, the gallium avidity seen in these tumors is similar to that seen in intermediate and high grade lymphomas as opposed to the low gallium avidity noted in indolent low grade lymphomas, as shown in Case 80.

Suggested Readings

Anderson KC, Leonard RC, Canellos GP, Skarin AT, Kaplan WD. High-dose gallium imaging in lymphoma. *Am J Med* 75:327–331, 1983.

Front D, Bar-Shalom R, Mor M, et al. Hodgkin disease: Prediction of outcome with Ga-67 scintigraphy after one cycle of chemotherapy. *Radiology* 210:487–491, 1999.

Front D, Ben-Haim S, Israel O, et al. Lymphoma: Predictive value of Ga-67 scintigraphy after treatment. *Radiology* 182:359–363, 1992.

Front D, Israel O. The role of Ga-67 scintigraphy in evaluating the results of therapy of lymphoma patients. *Semin Nucl Med* 1:60–71, 1995.

Israel O, Front D, Lam M, et al. Gallium-67 imaging in monitoring lymphoma response to treatment. *Cancer* 61:2439–2443, 1988.

Israel O, Front D, Epelbaum R, et al. Residual mass and negative gallium scintigraphy in treated lymphoma. *J Nucl Med* 31:365–368, 1990.

Janicek M, Kaplan W, Neuberg D, et al. Early restaging gallium scans predict outcome in poor-prognosis patients with aggressive non-Hodgkin's lymphoma treated with high-dose CHOP chemotherapy. *J Clin Oncol* 15:1631–1637, 1997.

Jochelson MS, Herman TS, Stomper PC, Mauch PM, Kaplan WD. Planning mantle radiation therapy in patients with Hodgkin's disease: role of gallium-67 scintigraphy. *AJR Am J Roentgenol* 151:1229–1231, 1988.

Kaplan WD. Residual mass and negative gallium scintigraphy in treated lymphoma: When is the gallium scan really negative? *J Nucl Med* 31:369–371, 1990. Editorial.

Kaplan WD, Jochelson MS, Herman TS, et al. Gallium-67 imaging: a predictor of residual tumor viability and clinical outcome in patients with diffuse large-cell lymphoma. *J Clin Oncol* 8:1966–1970, 1990.

Nejmeddine F, Raphael M, Martin A, et al. [67]Ga scintigraphy in B-cell non-Hodgkin's lymphoma: Correlation of ^{67}Ga uptake with histology and transferrin receptor expression. *J Nucl Med* 40:40–45, 1999.

Tumeh ST, Rosenthal DS, Kaplan WD, et al. Lymphoma: Evaluation with Ga-67 SPECT. *Radiology* 164:111–114, 1987.

Case 82

Clinical Presentation

70-year-old woman presenting with insulin-dependent diabetes, a left breast mass, and difficult-to-interpret mammograms.

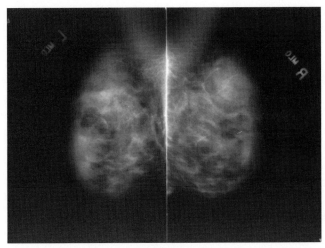

Fig. A

Fig. B

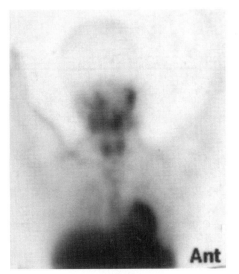

Fig. C

Technique

- 25 to 30 mCi (900 to 1100 MBq) technetium-99m sestamibi administered intravenously in the arm contralateral to the breast lesion.
- Low-energy high-resolution collimator.
- Energy window is 10% centered on 140 keV.
- Lateral views of each breast obtained with the patient prone. The breast to be imaged should be dependent; the contralateral breast should be compressed against the chest wall. Dedicated tables or padded table overlays for this procedure are commercially available. Anterior views including the axillae are then obtained with the patient supine and with her arms elevated.
- Planar images obtained for 10 minutes per view 5 minutes after administration of tracer; start with the lateral views.

Image Interpretation

Oblique mammograms (Fig. A) demonstrate extremely dense and heterogeneous parenchyma, markedly lowering the sensitivity of the study. An abnormality could certainly be present, and the images are essentially noncontributory. The lateral scintimammogram (Fig. B) shows homogeneous breast uptake. Tissue close to the chest wall or not in tangent may be obscured on the lateral view. The anterior view (Fig. C) shows normal cardiac, thyroid, salivary gland, hepatobiliary system, splenic, and bowel activity. The anterior view with higher threshold settings of the image is better used for the evaluation of the axillae. The normal breast has inherently low uptake of sestamibi. Bilateral, flame-shaped activity is more likely due to fibrocystic change. Nipple activity is in the contralateral occasionally seen.

Any focal accumulation of activity greater than that of adjacent breast is considered abnormal. Study conclusion should be normal, probably normal, or abnormal. This examination would be interpreted as normal.

Diagnosis and Clinical Follow-up

Excisional biopsy of the left breast revealed fibrosis.

Discussion

Scintimammography uses "hot spot" localization of the radiopharmaceutical in malignant tissue. Thallium-201 chloride, technetium-99m methylene diphosphonate (MDP), ^{18}FDG and labeled estrogens are some of the agents that have been evaluated for efficacy. The most readily available agent with the most attractive dosimetry is technetium-99m sestamibi. This modality is not recommended as a screening test; rather, it is indicated for the patient with dense parenchyma or postsurgical changes who is difficult to evaluate. There are recognized limitations of mammography and physical examination, and in these situations scintimammography may actually have superior sensitivity for malignancy. Overall reported sensitivity and specificity for sestamibi range from 52 to 76% and from 85 to 94%, respectively.

The advantage of scintimammography is that the tracer does not typically accumulate in normal breast parenchyma or scar tissue. Tumors that are otherwise difficult to detect may be discovered earlier with associated improvement in prognosis. Primary breast cancer and nodal metastases have been detected with encouraging sensitivity and specificity.

Suggested Readings

Diggles L, Mena I, Khalkhali I. Technical aspects of prone dependent-breast scintimammography. *Journal of Nuclear Medicine Technology* 22:165–170, 1994.

Kalkhali I, Mena I, Diggles L. Review of imaging techniques for the diagnosis of breast cancer: A new role of prone scintimammography using technetium-99m sestamibi. *Eur J Nucl Med* 21:357–362, 1994.

Kalkhali I, Mena I, Jouanne E, et al. Prone scintimammography in patients with suspicion of carcinoma of the breast. *J Am Coll Surg* 178:491–497, 1994.

Miraluma (Technetium Tc 99m Sestamibi) Package Insert. Billerica, MA: Dupont Merck Pharmaceutical Company; January 1997.

Palmedo H, Schomburg A, Grunwald F, et al. Technetium-99m-MIBI scintimammography for suspicious breast lesions. *J Nucl Med* 37:626–630, 1996.

Case 83

Clinical Presentation

47-year-old woman with a unilateral left breast implant for hypomastia noticed a thickening in her left breast.

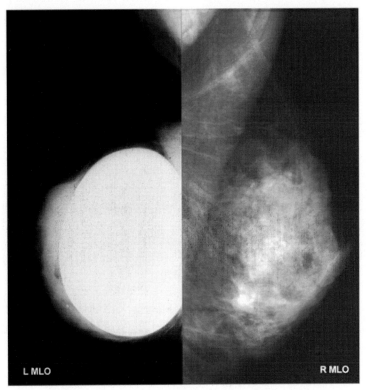

Fig. A

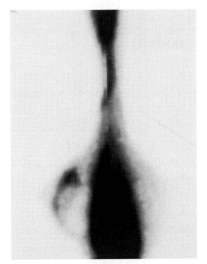

Fig. B

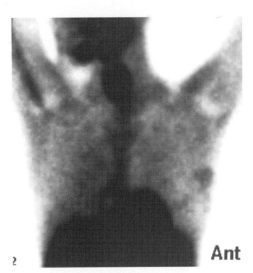

Fig. C

Technique

- 25 to 30 mCi (900 to 1100 MBq) technetium-99m sestamibi administered intravenously in the arm contralateral to the breast lesion.
- Low-energy high-resolution collimator.
- Energy window is 10% centered on 140 keV.
- Lateral views of each breast obtained with the patient prone. The breast to be imaged should be dependent; the contralateral breast should be compressed against the chest wall. Dedicated tables or padded table overlays for this procedure are commercially available. Anterior views including the axillae are then obtained with the patient supine and with arms elevated.
- Planar images obtained for 10 minutes per view 5 minutes after administration of tracer; start with the lateral views.

Image Interpretation

Oblique mammograms (Fig. A) show the unilateral left implant with asymmetrical density surrounding the upper aspect of the implant that could be due to surgical change or capsule formation. The features are not particularly worrisome mammographically and were present on previous mammograms. The quality of the images are degraded because of the presence of the implant.

The lateral (Fig. B) and frontal (Fig. C) scintimammographic images clearly show an intense focus of activity in the upper left breast. No nodal activity is seen. This study was interpreted as abnormal on the left, normal on the right.

Differential Diagnosis

- Breast carcinoma
- False positives are infrequent but can be seen in general benign lesions including fibrocystic changes, fibroadenomas, highly mitotic juvenile adenomas and focal inflammation.

Diagnosis and Clinical Follow-up

Excisional biopsy revealed a 2.5-cm invasive carcinoma. Axillary dissection did not demonstrate nodal involvement.

Discussion

Scintimammography has been shown to detect both invasive and intraductal carcinoma of the breast with high sensitivity and specificity for tumors greater than 1.0 to 1.5 cm. Of particular value may be the high negative predictive value (reported up to 97%) of the study for patients with a sizable abnormality on mammography or physical examination. Nodal involvement has also been revealed with reasonable sensitivity that may help select which patients should undergo axillary dissection.

The method by which cancer accumulates sestamibi is multifactorial and includes uptake of this isonitrile lipophilic cationic complex based on the negative electrochemical gradient of mitochondria.

Patients with screening studies difficult to interpret as well as those with palpable abnormalities would derive the most benefit from scintimammography. Neoadjuvant chemotherapy is occasionally used for locally advanced disease, and assessment of response is another potential role for scintimammography.

Suggested Readings

Carvalho PA, Chiu ML, Kronauge JF. Subcellular distribution and analysis of technetium-99m-MIBI in isolated perfused rat hearts. *J Nucl Med* 33:1516–1522, 1992.

Kalkhali I, Cutrone J, Mena I, et al. Technetium-99m-sestamibi scintimammography of breast lesions: Clinical and pathological follow-up. *J Nucl Med* 36:1784–1789, 1995.

Khalkhali I, Cutrone JA, Mena I, et al. Scintimammography: The complementary role of Tc-99m sestamibi prone breast imaging for the diagnosis of breast carcinoma. *Radiology* 196:421–426, 1995.

Waxman AD, Ramanna L, Memsic LD, et al. Thallium scintigraphy in the evaluation of mass abnormalities of the breast. *J Nucl Med* 34:18–23, 1993.

Case 84

Clinical Presentation

57-year-old woman presenting with a left axillary mass and a right breast mass.

Technique

- 25 to 30 mCi (900 to 1100 MBq) technetium-99m sestamibi administered intravenously in the arm contralateral to the breast lesion when possible or via a pedal vein.
- Low-energy high-resolution collimator.
- Energy window is 10% centered on 140 keV.
- Lateral views of each breast obtained with the patient prone. The breast to be imaged should be dependent; the contralateral breast should be compressed against the chest wall. Dedicated tables or padded table overlays for this procedure are commercially available. Anterior views including the axillae are then obtained with the patient supine and with her arms elevated.
- Planar images obtained for 10 minutes per view 5 minutes after administration of tracer; start with the lateral views.

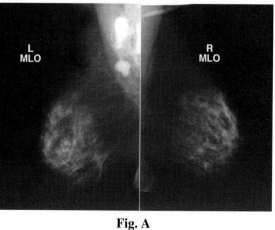

Fig. A

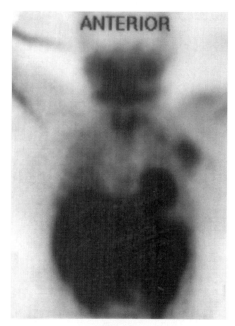

Fig. C

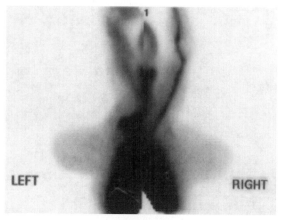

Fig. B

Image Interpretation

Oblique mammograms (Fig. A) show predominantely fatty breasts with enlarged lymph nodes in the left axilla. No parenchymal abnormality is seen. Lateral (Fig. B) and frontal (Fig. C) scintimammograms clearly define a focus of intense radiopharmaceutical accumulation in the left axilla without focal activity seen in either breast.

The study was interpreted as abnormal axillary activity suggestive of metastatic disease or axillary primary. Both breasts were interpreted as normal.

Differential Diagnosis

* Axillary metastasis such as from breast cancer.
* Axillary neoplasm such as lymphoma.
* Inflammation or infection of axillary tissues.

Diagnosis and Clinical Follow-up

A left modified radical mastectomy was performed. Innumerable small foci (1.0 to 3.0 mm) of poorly differentiated invasive ductal carcinoma were present throughout the entire left breast. Axillary dissection yielded 15 out of 15 positive lymph nodes.

Discussion

Limitations and benefits of breast scintigraphy are simultaneously demonstrated in this case. Solitary or multiple tumors smaller than 1.0 to 1.5 cm are less routinely depicted. Diffuse breast involvement is less visible because of a reduction of the normal contrast between normal breast and cancer, and loss of the target configuration. For these reasons the left breast parenchyma is normal in appearance.

Axillary disease detection with scintimammography has been reported with high sensitivity (84%) and specificity (91%). In addition, abnormal activity has been reported in supraclavicular, internal mammary, and mediastinal lymph nodes.

With the decision to perform axillary dissection becoming less routine, information from this study would be helpful in patient selection. The surgical procedure is a diagnostic rather than therapeutic exercise as a means of predicting prognosis. Consequently, nodal sampling may be either encouraged or obviated by scintimammography.

Suggested Readings

Peller PJ, Khedkar NY, Martinez CJ. Breast tumor scintigraphy. *Journal of Nuclear Medicine Technology* 24:198–203, 1996.

Taillefer R, Robidoux A, Lambert R, et al. Technetium-99m-sestamibi prone scintimammography to detect primary breast cancer and axillary lymph node involvement. *J Nucl Med* 36:1758–1765, 1995.

Case 85

Clinical Presentation

22-year-old patient presenting with a history of neuroblastoma. Indium-111 pentetreotide (OctreoScan®) was requested for staging (Figs. A and B). Five months later, after chemotherapy, a metaiodobenzylguanidine (MIBG) study was requested for restaging (Fig. C).

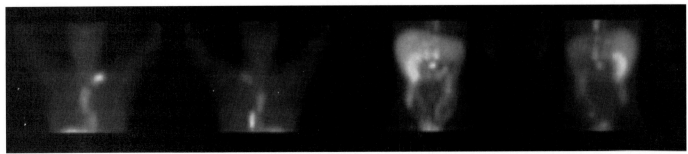

Fig. A

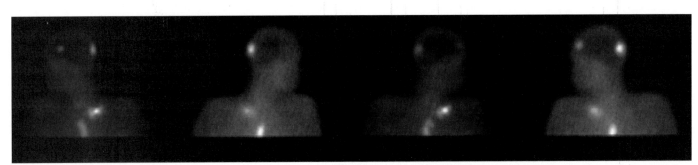

Fig. B

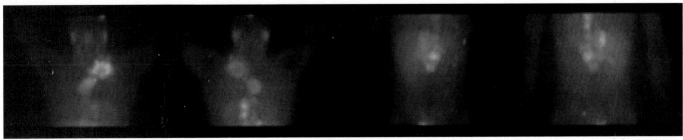

Fig. C

Technique

Indium-111 Pentetreotide

- Indium-111 pentetreotide is administered intravenously at a dose of 6 mCi (222 MBq).
- To enhance renal clearance, patients are asked to drink fluids.
- Images at 4 and 24 hours with large field of view (LFOV) gamma camera.
- Medium-energy collimator.
- Photopeaks of 172 keV and 247 keV and 15% window.
- Planar views include anterior and posterior spot views of the chest, abdomen, and pelvis (1.5 M counts or 15 min/view using 256×256 matrix).
- Anterior and posterior whole body images (8 cm/min at 4 hours and 5 cm/min at 24 hours using 256×1024 matrix).
- Single photon emission computed tomography (SPECT) images of the abdomen at 4 hours and at 24 hours (if needed) and chest at 24 hours, using 64×64 matrix, 64 images for 360 degrees, 50 sec/image at 4 hours, and 70 sec/image at 24 hours. SPECT reconstruction is as per manufacturer.

I-123 and I-131 MIBG

- Patient preparation includes (1) withholding potentially interfering medications such as tricyclic antidepressants, antihypertensives, sympathomimetics, cough and cold preparations sold over the counter that often contain either phenylpropanolamine or pseudoephedrine, and drugs such as cocaine and (2) thyroid blockade with saturated potassium iodide solution (1 drop three times a day for a total of 5 days, starting 48 hours prior to, or at least on the day of, the injection of radiolabeled MIBG and continuing for 3 days after the injection).
- Radiopharmaceutical is 10 mCi (370 MBq) of sodium iodide I-123 MIBG or 0.5 to 1 mCi (18.5 to 37 MBq) of I-131 MIBG injected intravenously. The doses are reduced per body surface area for pediatric patients.
- Images are obtained at 24 hours for I-123 MIBG and 48 hours for I-131 MIBG using a LFOV camera equipped with a high-energy (I-131 MIBG) or low-energy, high-resolution (I-123 MIBG) collimator; the 20% window is centered at 364 keV (I-131 MIBG) or 159 keV (I-123 MIBG). Planar acquisition includes anterior and posterior spot views of the body (15 minutes or 1.5 to 2 M counts/image, 256×256 matrix) or whole body images, or both. SPECT images can also be obtained with I-123 MIBG (50 to 70 sec/step if possible or at least 20 sec/step, 360 degrees, 64×64 matrix).

Image Interpretation

Anterior and posterior views of the chest and abdomen (Fig. A) obtained 4 hours after the injection of In-111 pentetreotide demonstrate abnormal uptake extending from the left supraclavicular region, down the chest along the paravertebral region bilaterally, and into the abdomen to the level of the cisterna chyli. An additional focus is seen in the left posterior pelvis.

Lateral views of the head (Fig. B) obtained 24 hours after the injection of the radiopharmaceutical show two additional foci in the skull. Again noted are the supraclavicular and chest foci already described in Figure A. Note the physiological thyroid uptake commonly seen at 24 hours. Pituitary uptake is also physiological.

- *(continued)* Focal activity in the region of the gallbladder fossa may represent physiological biliary excretion of the tracer. Repeat images may demonstrate migration of the tracer into the small bowel.

- Benign thyroid adenoma has also been shown to accumulate In-111 pentetreotide.

- Sites of recent surgery can show increased tracer activity on In-111 pentetreotide scanning. This is thought to be related to the presence of activated leukocytes expressing somatostatin receptors.

- Impaired renal function can cause an increase in background activity.

- Somewhat less consistent results have been reported in carcinoid tumors, medullary thyroid carcinomas, and paragangliomas. The heterogeneity of uptake can be explained by the variable expression of *a*mine *p*recursor *u*ptake (and) *d*ecarboxylation (APUD) function by different types of tumor.

- Tumors with high cell turnover (rapid cell uptake but also rapid secretion) exhibit faint images.

- There have been reports of discordant findings between In-111 pentetreotide and MIBG scanning. These may be related to technique. However, these agents are targeting two different metabolic processes and discrepant results may indicate differences in the biology of the tumors in these patients. Prospective correlative studies are needed to further investigate the reason behind these discrepancies.

Figure C shows anterior and posterior views of the chest and abdomen obtained 5 months later with I-123 MIBG. The sites of abnormal MIBG uptake essentially match those demonstrated 5 months earlier by In-111 pentetreotide, but the tumor burden has markedly increased in the interval.

Differential Diagnosis

- Neuroendocrine tumors expressing somatostatin-receptor subtype 2 (SSR2) (see *Discussion*).
- Non-neuroendocrine, non-neural crest tumors including melanomas, breast carcinomas, and Merkel's cell tumors.
- Granulomatous diseases and autoimmune diseases.

Diagnosis and Clinical Follow-up

Metastatic neuroblastoma. The In-111 pentetreotide scan (Figs. A and B) demonstrated extensive metastatic disease involving the soft tissues as well as the skeleton. The patient underwent salvage chemotherapy but failed to respond.

Five months later, I-131 labeled MIBG therapy was considered, and a request was made to restage the patient. Given the planned therapy, an I-123 labeled MIBG study was performed instead of In-111 pentetreotide to assess the tumor avidity for MIBG. In this patient, the results of the I-123 MIBG study matched the sites demonstrated by In-111 pentetreotide, but the tumor burden had markedly increased in the interval. The patient went on to receive a therapeutic dose of I-131 labeled MIBG.

Discussion

Somatostatin is an endogenous cyclic tetradecapeptide composed of 14 linked amino acids configured by a cysteine-cysteine-disulfide bridge. Although somatostatin is an effective inhibitor of peptide release, its short half-life in circulation (1 to 3 minutes) prevents its use as a therapeutic agent. Octreotide (Sandostatin®), an octapeptide somatostatin analogue is more potent than somatostatin, has a longer half-life (90 to 120 minutes), and is used to control some of the symptoms exhibited by patients with neuroendocrine tumors, such as flushing and diarrhea. When conjugated to pentetic acid (DTPA) it can be easily labeled with In-111, and the compound is cleared primarily via the kidneys (80 to 98%).

There are five human somatostatin-receptor (SSR) subtypes. In-111 pentetreotide seems to have the highest affinity for SSR2, but it also binds to SSR5. Receptors with a high affinity for somatostatin have been found in neuroblastomas as well as pheochromocytomas, and tumors of the gastroenteropancreatic axis such as insulinoma, gastrinoma, carcinoid tumor, glucagonoma, vipoma, and nonfunctional islet cell tumor. Other neural crest tumors with a high density of somatostatin receptors include small cell lung carcinoma, medullary thyroid carcinoma, paraganglioma, meningioma, astrocytoma, medulloblastoma, pituitary adenoma, and paraganglioma.

In-111 pentetreotide does not have a high affinity for all five receptor subtypes, and SSR2 may be expressed to a lower degree in some tumors compared with others. This is especially true in insulinoma and medullary thyroid carcinoma, which may explain the lower detection rate in those cases. Therefore, a negative study in a patient with a known neuroendocrine tumor does not imply that there is no active tumor. It merely means that the cells are not expressing a high level of SSR2. Conversely, if a baseline study demonstrates high avidity within the tumor, a follow-up study can be performed after the patient has been placed on octreotide therapy. Decreased uptake would be suggestive of response to octreotide. There may also be dedifferentiation of receptors in medullary thyroid carcinomas and carcinoid tumors. Endogenous somatostatin production, as seen in pheochromocytoma and medullary thyroid carcinoma, may competitively inhibit binding of radiolabeled octreotide to the receptor sites. Exogenous administration of octreotide therapy could theoretically have a similar result.

A history of radiation therapy may result in nonspecific uptake within and along the radiation port that may persist for a long time. A concurrent common cold or influenza may also result in false-positive uptake in the lungs. Focal hypoxia in the lung, with resultant reactive hyperplasia of neuroendocrine cells, may show increased tracer activity mimicking tumor.

Therapeutic applications using somatostatin analogues radiolabeled with beta and Auger electron-emitting isotopes are currently in clinical trials. In-111 pentetreotide has also been suggested for the evaluation of non-Hodgkin's and Hodgkin's lymphomas. In our experience, comparison with Ga-67 imaging favors the latter. However, both techniques may provide some useful biological and biochemical information and should be studied in a controlled fashion before making any conclusions.

MIBG, originally developed as an adrenal medullary imaging agent, is a radio-iodinated analogue of norepinephrine (NE) obtained by combining the benzyl portion of bretylium tosylate with the guanidine group of guanethidine monosulfate. It can be labeled with I-123 or I-131, the former being more advantageous for imaging. Only I-131 MIBG is available commercially. MIBG is thought to have uptake and storage mechanisms similar to those of NE, hence its strong affinity for adrenergic tissue. Unlike NE, MIBG is not bound to the postsynaptic receptor and is not metabolized by either monoamine oxidase or catechol O-methyltransferase. MIBG is secreted from or diffuses out of the cell and is then recirculated by entering the cell again via the uptake-1 mechanism and passive diffusion.

The normal distribution includes salivary glands, nasal region, neck muscles (in children), lung, heart, liver, spleen, thyroid (if not appropriately blocked), kidneys, bladder (the route of excretion), gastrointestinal tract, and normal adrenal gland (40% in children, less than 20% in adults with I-131 MIBG, more frequently seen with I-123 MIBG).

MIBG scanning can be successfully applied to the diagnosis of pheochromocytoma (true-positive rate [TPR] of 87% and true-negative rate [TNR] of 99%) and neuroblastoma (TPR 94%, TNR 100%). It is also used in the evaluation of myocardial NE receptors.

The cardiac uptake of MIBG is related to the level of catecholamines in circulation. High cardiac uptake is commonly seen with low circulating catecholamine levels. In that case, uptake in the adrenal region is most likely physiological.

Suggested Readings

Farahati J, Muller SP, Coennen HH, et al. Scintigraphy of neuroblastoma with radioiodinated m-iodobenzylguanidine. In: Treves ST, ed. *Pediatric Nuclear Medicine,* 2nd ed. New York: Springer-Verlag, 1995:528–541.

Jais P, Terris B, Ruszniewski P, et al. Somatostatin receptor subtype gene expression in human endocrine gastroentero-pancreatic tumors. *Eur J Clin Invest* 27:639–644, 1997.

Krenning EP, Kwekkeboom DJ, Pauwels S, Kvols LK, Reubi JC. Somatostatin receptor imaging. In : Freeman LM, ed. *Nuclear Medicine Annual.* New York: Raven Press, 1995:1–50.

Krenning EP, Kwekkeboom DJ, Bakker WH, et al. Somatostatin receptor scintigraphy with [^{111}In-DTPA-D-Phe^1]-and [^{123}I-tyr^3]-octreotide. The Rotterdam experience with more than 1000 patients. *Eur J Nucl Med* 20:716–731, 1993.

Kwekkeboom DJ, Lamberts SW, Habbema JD, et al. Cost-effectiveness analysis of somatostatin receptor scintigraphy. *J Nucl Med* 37:886–892, 1996.

Kwekkeboom DJ, Krenning EP. Radiolabeled somatostatin analog scintigraphy in oncology and immune diseases: An overview. *Eur Radiol* 7:1103–1109, 1997.

Mozley D, Kim CK, Mohsin J, et al. The efficacy of I-123-MIBG as a screening test for pheochromocytoma. *J Nucl Med* 35:1138–1144, 1994.

OctreoScan Kit for the preparation of In-111 pentetreotide: Package insert. Mallinckrodt Medical, Inc., St. Louis, MO, 1994.

Reubi JC. Neuropeptide receptors in health and disease: The molecular basis for in vivo imaging. *J Nucl Med* 36:1825–1835, 1995.

Von Moll L, McEwan JA, Shapiro B, et al. I-131-MIBG of neuroendocrine tumors other than pheochromocytoma and neuroblastoma. *J Nucl Med* 28:979–988, 1987.

Woltering EA, O'Dorisio MS, O'Dorisio TM. The role of radiolabeled somatostatin analogs in the management of cancer patients. *Principles & Practice of Oncology (PPO Updates)* 9:1–16, 1995.

Case 86

Clinical Presentation

56-year-old man presenting with a history of gastrinoma, status post-resection, liver transplant, and chemotherapy, and complaining of rib pain. Indium-111 pentetreotide (OctreoScan®) study was requested for restaging.

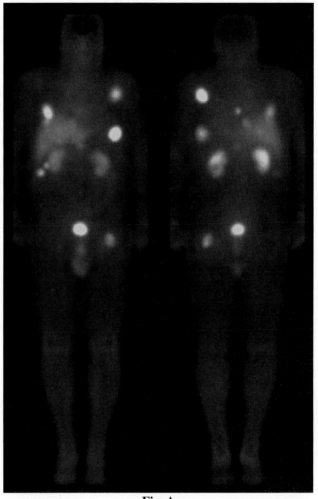

Fig. A

Technique

- Indium-111 pentetreotide is administered intravenously at a dose of 6 mCi (222 MBq).
- To enhance renal clearance, patients are asked to drink fluids.
- Images are obtained at 4 hours and 24 hours with a large field of view (LFOV) gamma camera equipped with a medium-energy collimator, photopeaks centered over 172 keV and 247 keV, and a 15% window. The planar acquisition includes anterior and posterior spot views of the chest, abdomen, and pelvis (1.5 M counts or 15 min/view using a 256 × 256 matrix) followed by anterior

and posterior whole body planar images (8 cm/min at 4 hours and 5 cm/min at 24 hours using a 256 × 1024 matrix). Single photon emission computed tomography (SPECT) images of the abdomen (at 4 hours, and 24 hours if needed) and chest (at 24 hours) are obtained using a 64 × 64 matrix, 64 images for 360 degrees, 50 sec/image at 4 hours and 70 sec/image at 24 hours. SPECT reconstruction parameters are per manufacturer.

Image Interpretation

Anterior and posterior whole body images (Fig. A) obtained at 4 hours demonstrate multiple focal areas of high pentetreotide avidity throughout the body, including multiple ribs, the thoracic spine, and the left femur. In addition, focal uptake is seen in the abdomen inferior to the left hepatic lobe. SPECT (not shown) showed that the other foci superimposed upon the liver were consistent with rib metastases.

Differential Diagnosis

- Primary and metastatic neuroendocrine tumors expressing somatostatin-receptor subtype 2 (SSR2) (see *Discussion*)
- Non-neuroendocrine, non-neural crest tumors (melanomas, breast carcinomas, and Merkle's cell tumors)
- Granulomatous diseases and autoimmune diseases

Diagnosis and Clinical Follow-up

The diagnosis was gastrinoma. The findings were consistent with widespread metastatic disease. Correlative radiographs of the ribs and left femur demonstrated lytic lesions corresponding to the focal areas of uptake seen on the scan and consistent with metastases.

Discussion

Somatostatin is an endogenous cyclic polypeptide hormone of 14 amino acids that inhibits secretion of growth hormone. Octreotide is an 8 amino acid analogue of somatostatin, with its structure altered to resist enzymatic degradation. Octreotide can be conjugated to pentetic acid (DTPA), allowing labeling with the radionuclide In-111. In-111–labeled pentetreotide binds to somatostatin receptors in tissues throughout the body and in tumors with a high density of somatostatin receptors.

There are five human somatostatin-receptor (SSR) subtypes and In-111 pentetreotide seems to have the highest affinity for SSR2, but it also binds to SSR5. Receptors with a high affinity for somatostatin have been found in tumors of the gastroenteropancreatic axis such as gastrinoma, insulinoma, carcinoid tumor, glucagonoma, vipoma, and nonfunctional islet cell tumor. Other neural crest tumors with a high density of SSRs include pheochromocytoma, small cell lung carcinoma, medullary thyroid carcinoma, paraganglioma, meningioma, astrocytoma, medulloblastoma, neuroblastoma, pituitary adenoma, and paraganglioma.

A technetium-99m–labeled somatostatin analog has been recently approved by the FDA for the staging of small cell lung carcinoma.

- *(continued)* Since the main route of excretion is renal, impaired renal function can cause an increase in background activity.

- Focal hypoxia in the lung, with resultant reactive hyperplasia of neuroendocrine cells, may show increased tracer activity mimicking tumor.

- Therapeutic applications using somatostatin analogues radiolabeled with beta and Auger electron-emitting isotopes are currently in clinical trials.

- In-111 pentetreotide has also been suggested for the evaluation of non-Hodgkin's and Hodgkin's lymphomas. In our experience, comparison with Ga-67 imaging favors the latter. However, both techniques may provide some useful biological and biochemical information and should be compared in a controlled fashion.

Suggested Readings

Jais P, Terris B, Ruszniewski P, et al. Somatostatin receptor subtype gene expression in human endocrine gastroentero-pancreatic tumors. *Eur J Clin Invest* 27:639–644, 1997.

Janson ET, Westlin JE, Eriksson B, et al. [111In-DTPA-D-Phel] octreotide scintigraphy in patients with carcinoid tumors: The predictive value for somatostatin analogue treatment. *Eur J Endocrinol* 131:577–581, 1994.

Krenning EP, Kwekkeboom DJ, Bakker WH, et al. Somatostatin receptor scintigraphy with [^{111}In-DTPA-D-Phe^1]- and [^{123}I-tyr^3]-octreotide. The Rotterdam experience with more than 1000 patients. *Eur J Nucl Med* 20:716–731, 1993.

Krenning EP, Kwekkeboom DJ, Pauwels S, Kvols LK, Reubi JC. Somatostatin receptor imaging. In: Freeman LM, ed. *Nuclear Medicine Annual.* New York: Raven Press, Ltd., 1995:1–50.

Kwekkeboom DJ, Lamberts SW, Habbema JD, et al. Cost-effectiveness analysis of somatostatin receptor scintigraphy. *J Nucl Med* 37:886–892, 1996.

Kwekkeboom DJ, Krenning EP. Radiolabeled somatostatin analog scintigraphy in oncology and immune diseases: An overview. *Eur Radiol* 7:1103–1109, 1997.

Octreoscan Kit for the Preparation of Indium In-111 Pentetreotide, St. Louis, MO: Mallinckrodt Medical, Inc., 1994.

Case 87

Clinical Presentation

50-year-old woman presenting with obstructive jaundice. A computed tomography (CT) scan of the abdomen revealed an obstructing mass in the head and uncinate process of the pancreas. Biopsy demonstrated neuroendocrine tumor. A staging indium-111 pentetreotide scan was ordered to evaluate for distant metastases.

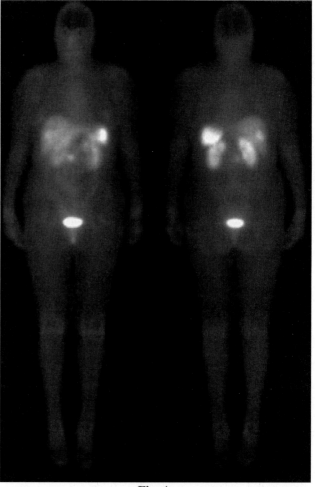

Fig. A

Technique

- Indium-111 pentetreotide (OctreoScan®) is administered intravenously at a dose of 6 mCi (222 MBq).
- To enhance renal clearance, patients are asked to drink fluids.

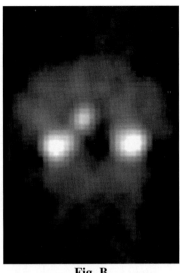

Fig. B

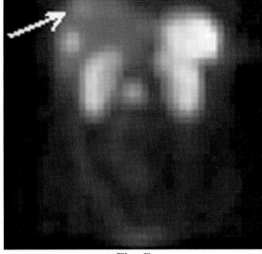

Fig. C

- Images are obtained at 4 hours and 24 hours with a large field of view (LFOV) gamma camera equipped with a medium-energy collimator and photopeaks centered over 172 keV and 247 keV and a 15% window. The planar acquisition includes anterior and posterior spot views of the chest, abdomen, and pelvis (1.5 M counts or 15 min/view using a 256×256 matrix) followed by anterior and posterior whole body planar images (8 cm/min at 4 hours and 5 cm/min at 24 hours using a 256×1024 matrix). Single photon emission computed tomography (SPECT) images of the abdomen (at 4 hours, and 24 hours if needed) and chest (at 24 hours) are obtained using a 64×64 matrix, 64 images for 360 degrees, 50 sec/image at 4 hours and 70 sec/image at 24 hours. SPECT reconstruction parameters are per manufacturer.
- The study was correlated with a recent CT scan of the abdomen.

Image Interpretation

Anterior and posterior whole body planar images obtained 4 hours after tracer injection (Fig. A) demonstrate a focus of increased tracer accumulation in the mid-abdomen. An additional focus of increased activity is seen in the lateral aspect of the right hepatic lobe.

An axial SPECT image at the level of the mid-abdominal abnormality (Fig. B) shows that the focus of increased tracer activity is in the region of the pancreatic head.

A three-dimensional volumetric reconstruction of the abdominal SPECT images (Fig. C) confirms the presence of the pancreatic and right hepatic lesions and also demonstrates a third focus of abnormal tracer uptake at the hepatic dome (arrow).

Differential Diagnosis

- Primary and metastatic neuroendocrine tumors that express somatostatin receptors subtype 2 (SSR2) such as glucagonomas, vipomas, carcinoid tumors, non-functioning islet cell tumors of the pancreas, and insulinomas.
- Paragangliomas, pheochromocytomas, neuroblastomas, medullary thyroid carcinomas, tumors of the anterior pituitary, small cell lung carcinomas.
- Other diseases in which activated leukocytes are present.

- *(continued)* Focal activity in the region of the gallbladder fossa may represent physiological biliary excretion of the tracer. Repeat images may demonstrate migration of the tracer into the small bowel.

- Somatostatin analogues radiolabeled with beta and Auger electron-emitting isotopes are currently being assessed in clinical trials as therapeutic agents for carcinoid and other neuroendocrine tumors.

Diagnosis and Clinical Follow-up

Findings were consistent with metastatic carcinoid tumor. The patient underwent surgery to relieve the biliary obstruction, and the surgical exploration revealed a mass in the head and uncinate process of the pancreas, a palpable nodule in the right hepatic lobe, and a second nodule at the hepatic dome. Biopsies of these areas demonstrated neuroendocrine tumor consistent with carcinoid tumor.

Discussion

Somatostatin is an endogenous cyclic polypeptide hormone of 14 amino acids that inhibits secretion of growth hormone and has been shown to slow the growth of neuroendocrine tumors. Octreotide is an 8 amino acid analogue of somatostatin, with its structure altered to resist enzymatic degradation. Octreotide can be conjugated to pentetic acid (DTPA), allowing labeling with the radionuclide indium-111. In-111 pentetreotide binds to somatostatin receptors in tissues throughout the body and in tumors expressing somatostatin receptors subtype 2 (SSR2).

Normal uptake of tracer is seen in the thyroid, liver, gallbladder, spleen, kidneys, bladder, and pituitary gland. Ninety-eight percent of the tracer is excreted by the kidneys, and approximately 2% is excreted via the hepatobiliary system.

Suggested Readings

Jais P, Terris B, Ruszniewski P, et al. Somatostatin receptor subtype gene expression in human endocrine gastroentero-pancreatic tumors. *Eur J Clin Invest* 27:639–644, 1997.

Janson ET, Westlin JE, Eriksson B, et al. [111In-DTPA-D-Phe1] octreotide scintigraphy in patients with carcinoid tumors: The predictive value for somatostatin analogue treatment. *Eur J Endocrinol* 131:577–581, 1994.

Krenning EP, Kwekkeboom DJ, Reubi JC, et al. 111In-octreotide scintigraphy in oncology, *Digestion* 54(suppl 1):84–87, 1993.

Krenning EP, Kooij PP, Pauwels S, et al. Somatostatin receptor: Scintigraphy and radionuclide therapy, *Digestion* 57(suppl 1):57–61, 1996.

Kvols LK. Somatostatin-receptor imaging in human malignancies: A new era in the localization, staging, and treatment of tumors. *Gastroenterology* 105:1909–1914, 1993.

Kwekkeboom DJ, Lamberts SW, Habbema JD, et al. Cost-effectiveness analysis of somatostatin receptor scintigraphy. *J Nucl Med* 37:886–892, 1996.

Kwekkeboom DJ, Krenning EP. Radiolabeled somatostatin analog scintigraphy in oncology and immune diseases: An overview. *Eur Radiol* 7:1103–1109, 1997.

Kwekkeboom DJ, Krenning JP. Somatostatin receptor scintigraphy in patients with carcinoid tumors. *World J Surg* 20:157–161, 1996.

Octreoscan Kit for the Preparation of Indium In-111 Pentetreotide, St. Louis, MO: Mallinckrodt Medical, Inc., 1994.

Case 88

Clinical Presentation

58-year-old woman referred 4 years after surgery for colorectal carcinoma for follow-up computed tomography (CT) of the abdomen and pelvis because of a rising level of carcinoembryonic antigen (CEA) (27.2 ng/mL) without clinical symptoms of recurrent tumor. She presented 4 years earlier with a history of rectal bleeding that had lasted 6 months. A barium enema at that time showed a 5-cm polypoid mass in the anterior wall of the rectosigmoid junction. Staging studies were negative for metastases. The patient underwent an abdominal perineal resection and sigmoid colostomy. Pathology revealed a moderately differentiated adenocarcinoma, stage T3N0Mx, Dukes'-Kirklin B2. Her postoperative course was uneventful, and her postoperative CEA was 2.7 ng/mL (normal value for nonsmoker, 0 to 3 ng/mL).

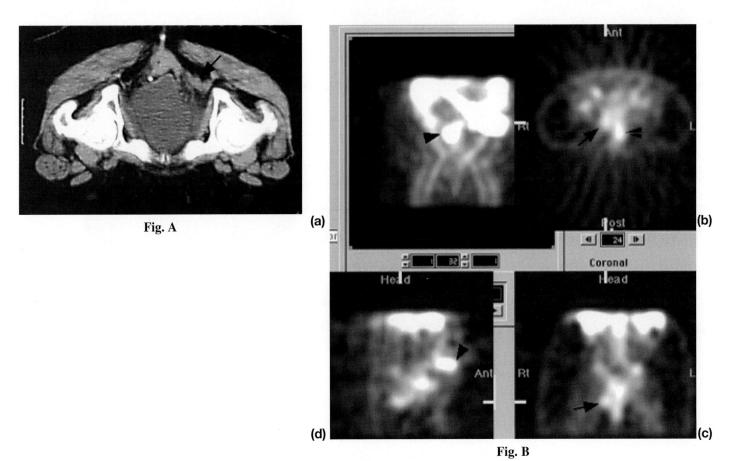

Fig. A

(a)   (b)

(d)   (c)

Fig. B

PEARLS/PITFALLS

- Recurrence of colorectal tumor is seen in up to 40% of patients with Dukes' stage B or C within 18 months post-surgery and is limited to a single site in 75% of patients: liver (33%), lung (22%), local (20%), intra-abdominal (18%).

- Almost 30% of patients with recurrent colorectal tumor do not have elevated serum CEA levels, which does not preclude positive immunoscintigraphy.

- Delayed images are helpful in the case of slow antibody clearance from the circulation and are feasible up to 10 days post-injection.

- Monoclonal antibody fragments may be better for detection of liver metastases because their degradation and excretion is mostly renal.

- Human antimurine antibodies (HAMA) may be induced in up to 40% of patients (as opposed to 1% with Tc-99m-arcitumomab [CEA-Scan®]), but they return to normal levels in 50% of patients in 4 to 12 months. HAMA production may, however, interfere with future use of murine antibody–based therapeutic products or diagnostic tests, and may theoretically increase the risk of allergic reaction. *(continued)*

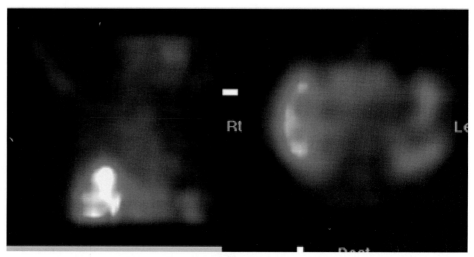

Fig. C

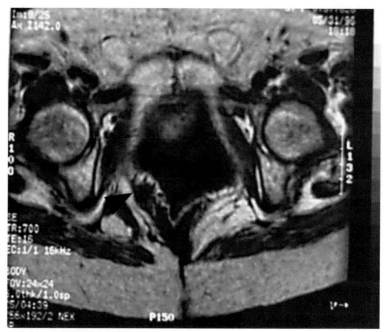

Fig. D

Technique

- Indium-111 satumomab pendetide (OncoScint®), 1 mg, labeled with 5 mCi (185 MBq) of indium-111 is administered intravenously over 5 minutes. The patient is then monitored for 15 minutes.
- Images are typically obtained 2 to 3 days post-injection and followed with delayed images at 24-hour intervals, if needed. Planar images and single photon emission computed tomography (SPECT) are acquired on a large field of view gamma camera equipped with medium-energy parallel hole collimators. Energy windows are set at 171 keV and 245 keV. Total body static images (0.5 M to 1M counts) in anterior and posterior views and SPECT images (360 degrees of rotation for single-headed or 180 to 360 degrees for dual-headed camera; 64 or 32 stops; 50 sec/stop) from the skull base through the pubic symphysis are typically obtained.

- *(continued)* In our case, immunoscintigraphy predicted locoregional recurrence of the tumor more accurately than did CT and MRI, whose interpretations were equivocal or misleading.

- Indium-111 satumomab pendetide is primarily metabolized in the liver, and metabolites remain bound to the cytosol. Liver metastases are therefore usually seen as cold defects, as opposed to "hot" spots. MRI and CT are generally the favored imaging modalities for detection of liver metastases, but antibody scintigraphy is very helpful in the detection of extrahepatic involvement, such as pelvic or nodal disease; in the characterization of equivocal morphological findings; and for the detection of occult distant disease. Best results are reported for masses larger than 2 cm and with a serum CEA level higher than 2.5 ng/mL.

- PET imagings with F-18-fluorodeoxyglucose has also shown excellent results in the evaluation of recurrent rectal cancer.

- Images are interpreted in conjunction with other imaging modalities, particularly CT or magnetic resonance imaging (MRI).

Image Interpretation

CT of the abdomen and pelvis (Fig. A) demonstrates nodular soft tissue density in the right ischiorectal fossa (*arrow*). Scarring cannot be differentiated from early local recurrence of the tumor. Indium-111-satumomab pendetide was ordered to further characterize this abnormality.

Images performed 72 hours post injection (Fig. B) demonstrate abnormal uptake in the right perirectal region. Volume-rendered image of midabdomen and pelvis (a), axial cut of lower pelvis (b), coronal cut of pelvis and abdomen (c), and sagittal image (d) demonstrate abnormal focal uptake of the tracer in the right perirectal soft tissues, suggesting local recurrence of the tumor in the right ischiorectal fossa (*arrow*). Normal excretion of the activity is noted in the large bowel (much less intense in the excluded portion of distal rectosigmoid, double *arrowhead*). Intense uptake is seen at the colostomy site (*arrowhead*).

Volume-rendered image of the liver (Fig. D) in the right anterior oblique view (left) and axial slice through the liver (right) demonstrate heterogeneity of uptake (with negative concurrent CT and MRI).

The MRI performed 4 months later (Fig. C) shows a low signal intensity band of tissue in the right perirectal fat that was interpreted as scarring secondary to prior surgery and pelvic irradiation.

Differential Diagnosis

- Scarring and inflammatory changes secondary to prior surgery and pelvic irradiation
- Physiological tracer within the bowel or colostomy site
- Recurrent or residual tumor

Diagnosis and Clinical Follow-up

Findings suggestive of recurrent rectal cancer are confirmed in the follow-up of this patient. In the course of 6 months following the indium-111 satumomab pendetide (OncoScint®) study, the patient developed recurrent disease in the anterior abdominal wall at the colostomy site, which was resected. Pathology showed the same histological type of tumor as the original primary site. Ten months later, the patient developed multiple rapidly progressing liver metastases and recurrent pelvic disease with tumor infiltrating the presacral soft tissues. The patient received chemotherapy, and her disease has stabilized.

Discussion

Monoclonal antibody imaging of colorectal carcinoma represents a valuable diagnostic modality because it increases the sensitivity and specificity of conventional imaging modalities (CT and MRI). OncoScint® (indium-111 satumomab pendetide) is a murine monoclonal antibody (B72.3) raised against the cell surface mucine-like glycoprotein antigen TAG-72 that is found on a variety of epithelial malignancies, including 83% of colorectal and 97% of ovarian carcinomas. Oncoscint® is labeled with indium-111 chloride (physical half-life is 67 hours). The antibody, an intact IgG, has a biologic half-life of 30 to 60 hours. Dominquez et al (1996) compared blind interpretation of Oncoscint® to CT in patients with recurrent colorectal carcinoma. The results were also correlated with surgical findings. Oncoscint® showed a higher sensitivity than CT did (60 versus 47%) but a lower positive predictive value (82 versus 100%). The need for combined interpretation of all imaging modalities is emphasized by the fact that immunoscintigraphy alone would have affected patient management positively in only 13%, had no effect in 67%, and generated misleading information in 20%.

In postsurgical follow-up and in the setting of rising CEA, combined imaging may identify a subgroup of patients who may benefit from surgical management. Approximately 25% of first colorectal cancer recurrences are isolated locoregional failures, and an additional 15 to 20% are metastatic deposits that are potentially resectable, which increases 5-year disease-free survival to 30%. On the other hand, patients who are presumed to be candidates for resection of isolated metastases but are then shown to have disseminated occult disease may be spared unnecessary surgical intervention. More accurate restaging including intraoperative radioimmunolocalization of metastatic foci has been shown to improve survival.

Suggested Readings

August DA, Ottow RT, Sugarbaker PH. Clinical perspectives on human colorectal cancer metastases. *Cancer Metastasis Rev* 3:303–324, 1984.

Dominquez JM, Wolff BG, Nelson H, et al. 111In-CYT-103 scanning in recurrent colorectal cancer—does it affect standard management? *Dis Colon Rectum* 39:514–519, 1996.

Moffat FL, Pinsky CM, Hammershaimb L, et al. Clinical utility of external immunoscintigraphy with the IMMU-4 Technetium-99m Fab' antibody fragment in patients undergoing surgery for carcinoma of the colon and rectum: Results of a pivotal, phase III trial. *J Clin Oncol* 14:2295–2305, 1996.

Nabi HA, Erb DA, Cronin VR. Superiority of SPECT to planar imaging in the detection of colorectal carcinoma with In-111 monoclonal antibodies. *Nucl Med Commun* 16:631–639, 1995.

OncoScint CR/OV Kit (satumomab pendetide): Package insert. Princeton, NJ: Cytogen Corporation; December 30, 1992.

OncoScint (satumomab pendetide) Imaging, Colorectal Carcinoma, Recurrent Disease. Available: http://nuc-med-read.uthscsa.edu/williams/NucMed/tum03.htm

Patt YZ. Radioactive immunodiagnosis (RAID) in patients with colorectal cancer and rising serum CEA. *New Perspectives in Cancer Diagnosis and Management* 1:33–39, 1993.

Prati U, Roveda L, Antoni A, et al. Radioimmunoassisted follow-up and surgery vs traditional examinations and surgery after radical excision of colorectal cancer. *Anticancer Res* 15:1081–1085, 1995.

Stomper PC, D'Souza DJ, Bakshi SP, et al. Detection of pelvic recurrence of colorectal carcinoma: Prospective, blinded comparison of Tc-99m-IMMU-4 Monoclonal antibody scanning and CT. *Radiology* 197:688–692, 1995.

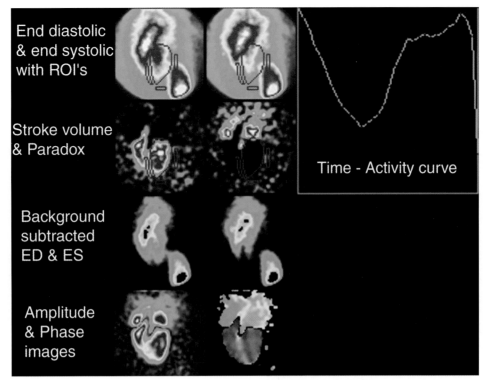

Color Plate 1.   Case 50, Fig. A. (See page 121.)

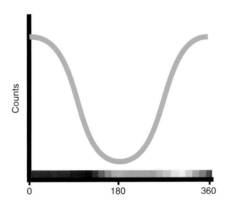

Color Plate 2.   Case 50, Fig. C. (See page 124.)

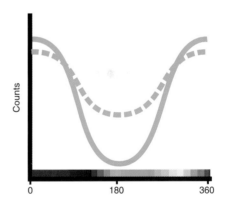

Color Plate 3.   Case 50, Fig. D. (See page 124.)

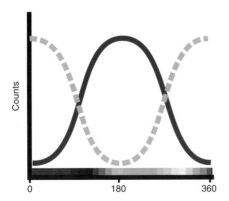

Color Plate 4.   Case 50, Fig. E. (See page 124.)

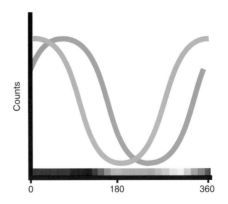

Color Plate 5.   Case 50, Fig. F. (See page 124.)

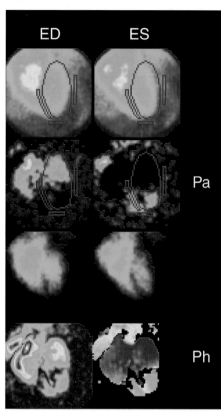

ED   ES

Pa

Ph

Color Plate 6.   Case 51, Fig. A. (See page 125.)

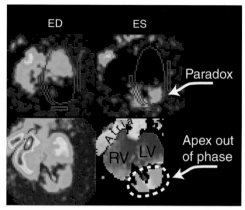

ED   ES

Paradox

Apex out of phase

Atria

RV LV

Color Plate 7.   Case 51, Fig. B. (See page 126.)

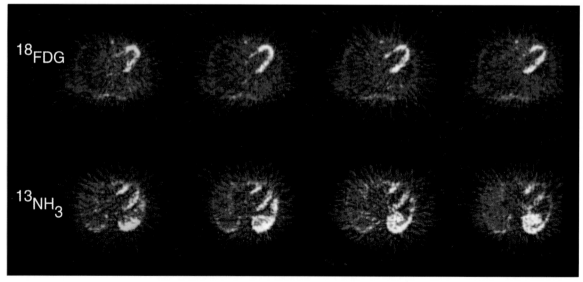

^{18}FDG

^{13}NH$_3$

Color Plate 8.   Case 52, Fig. A. (See page 127.)

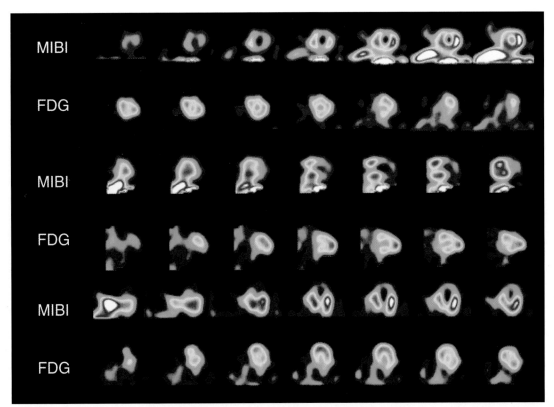

Color Plate 9. Case 53, Fig. A. (See page 129.)

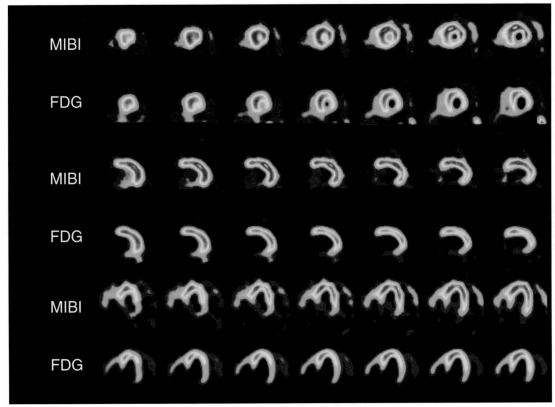

Color Plate 10. Case 54, Fig. A. (See page 131.)

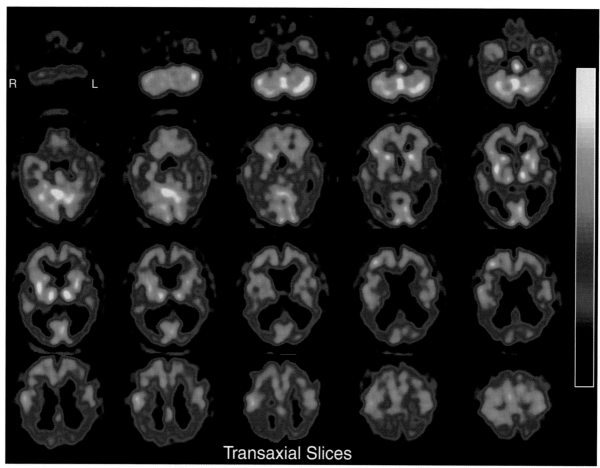

Transaxial Slices

Color Plate 11.   Case 137, Fig. A. (See page 383.)

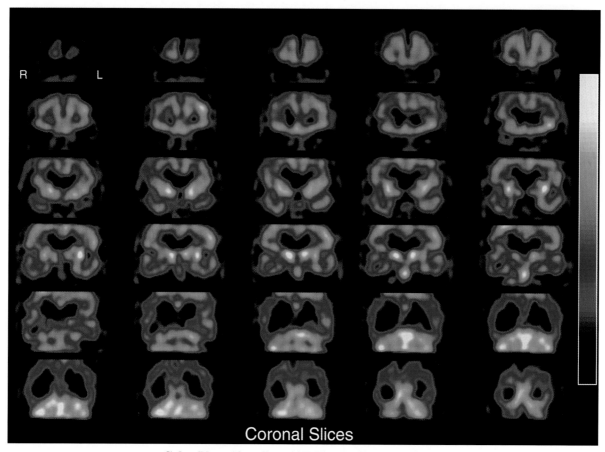

Coronal Slices

Color Plate 12.   Case 137, Fig. B. (See page 383.)

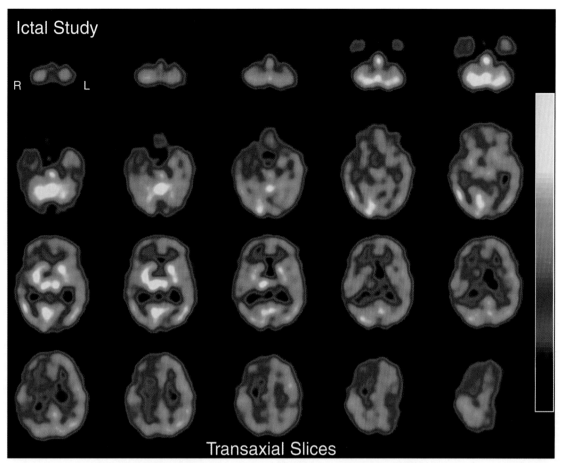

Color Plate 13.   Case 138, Fig. A. (See page 386.)

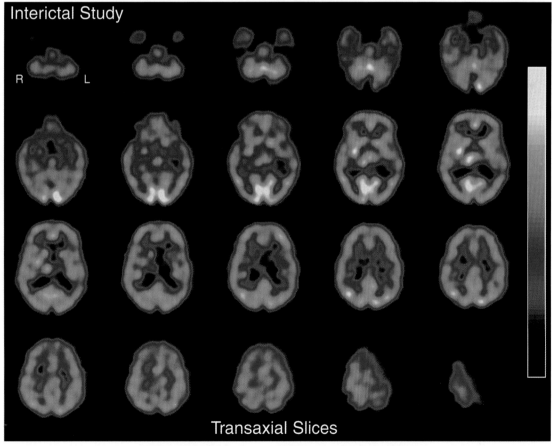

Color Plate 14.   Case 138, Fig. B. (See page 387.)

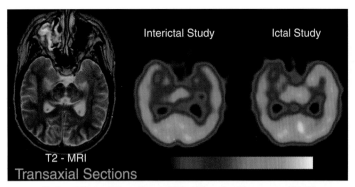

Interictal Study   Ictal Study

T2 - MRI
Transaxial Sections

Color Plate 15.   Case 138, Fig. C. (See page 387.)

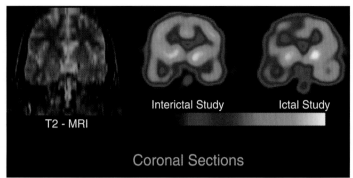

Interictal Study   Ictal Study

T2 - MRI

Coronal Sections

Color Plate 16.   Case 138, Fig. D. (See page 387.)

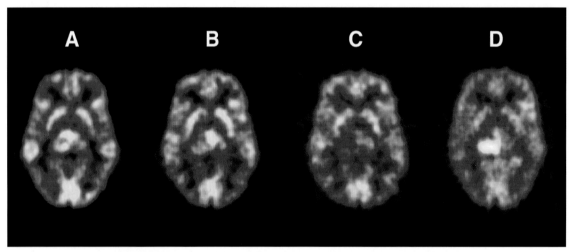

A   B   C   D

Color Plate 17.   Case 139, Figs. A, B, C, D. (See page 389.)

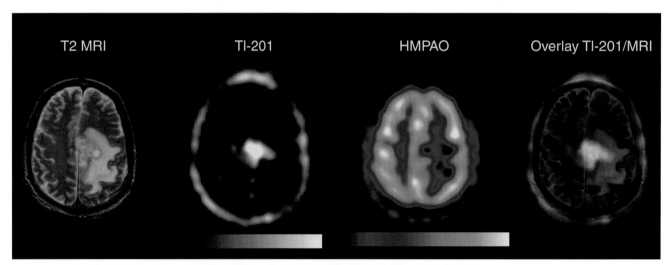

T2 MRI   TI-201   HMPAO   Overlay TI-201/MRI

Color Plate 18.   Case 140, Fig. A. (See page 393.)

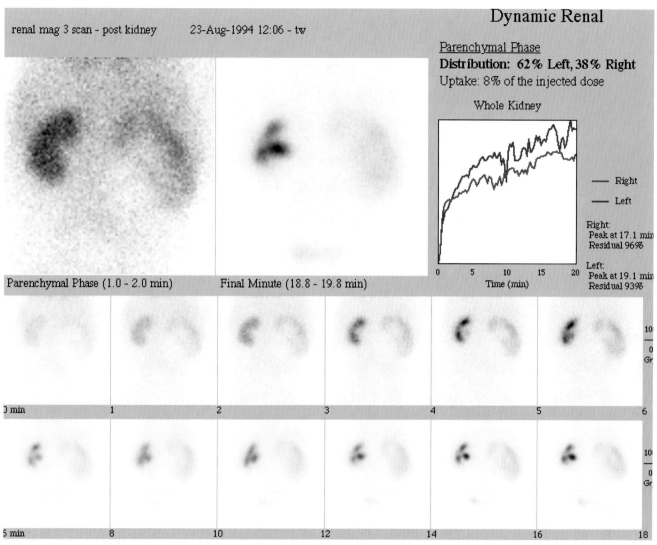

Dynamic Renal

renal mag 3 scan - post kidney   23-Aug-1994 12:06 - tw

Parenchymal Phase
Distribution: 62% Left, 38% Right
Uptake: 8% of the injected dose

Whole Kidney

—— Right
—— Left

Right:
Peak at 17.1 min
Residual 96%

Left:
Peak at 19.1 min
Residual 93%

Parenchymal Phase (1.0 - 2.0 min)   Final Minute (18.8 - 19.8 min)

Color Plate 19.   Case 169, Fig. A. (See page 480.)

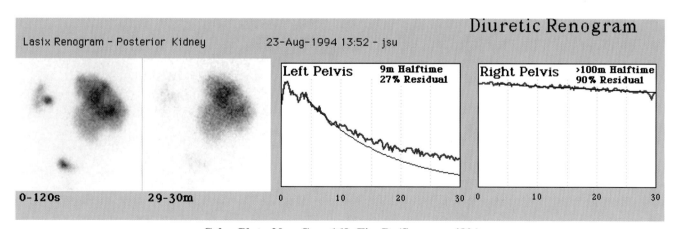

Diuretic Renogram

Lasix Renogram - Posterior Kidney   23-Aug-1994 13:52 - jsu

Left Pelvis   **9m Halftime**
                    27% Residual

Right Pelvis   **>100m Halftime**
                    90% Residual

0-120s   29-30m

Color Plate 20.   Case 169, Fig. B. (See page 480.)

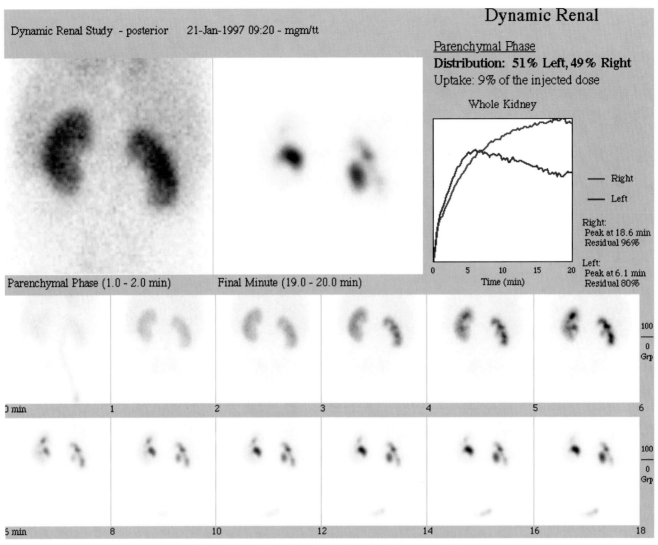

Color Plate 21.   Case 169, Fig. C. (See page 482.)

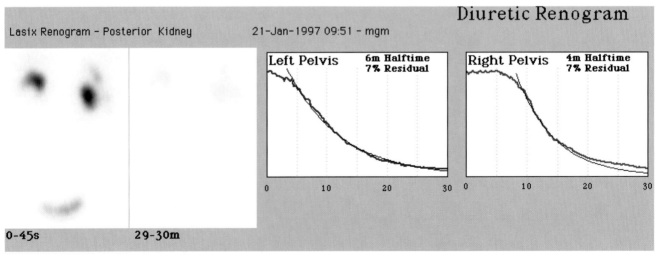

Color Plate 22.   Case 169, Fig. D. (See page 482.)

Case 89

Clinical Presentation

52-year-old woman who is a heavy smoker with negative medical history was referred for a complete work up because of an incidental finding of markedly elevated carcinoembryonic antigen (CEA) at 170 ng/mL (normal value for smoker, 0 to 5 ng/mL). All other laboratory tests were within normal limits. She indicated mild fatigue in the recent past that brought her in for a regular medical check up. Upper and lower gastrointestinal (GI) endoscopies demonstrated multiple polyps on the mucosa of the stomach and large bowel. Biopsies showed that all the polyps were hyperplastic, but no adenomatous polyps were found.

Computed tomography (CT) of the abdomen and pelvis (not shown) revealed no definite evidence of primary tumor or metastatic disease. Barium enema revealed several small polyps.

Technetium-99m-arcitumomab (CEA-Scan®) was ordered to search for an occult primary tumor in the setting of a polyposis syndrome.

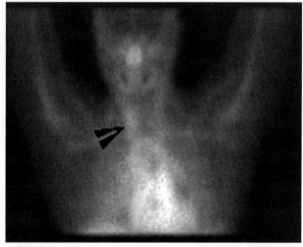

Fig. A

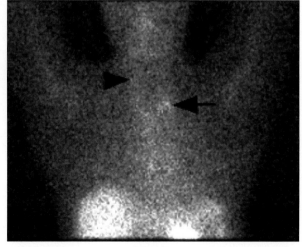

Fig. B

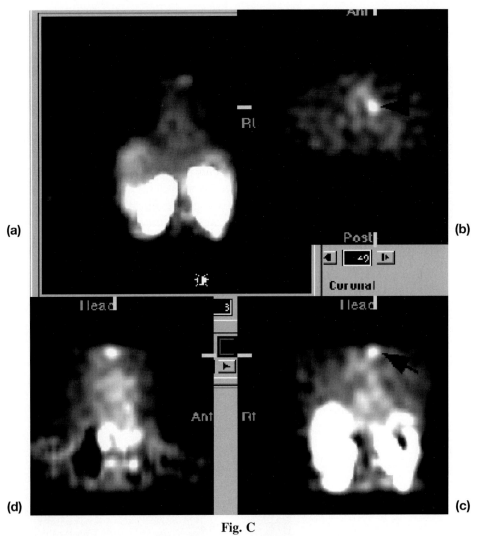
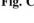

(a)

(b)

(d)

(c)

Fig. C

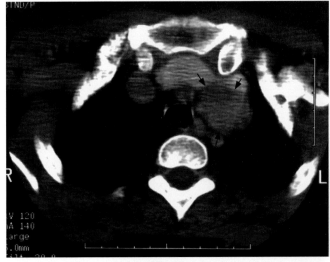

Fig. D

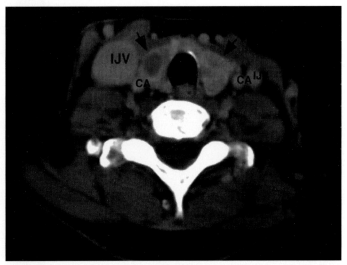

Fig. E

Technique

- Tc-99m arcitumomab, 1.25 mg, labeled with 30 mCi (1110 MBq) of tc-99m administered intravenously over 5 minutes. Patient is then monitored for 15 minutes.
- Planar images and single photon emission computed tomography (SPECT) are acquired at 3 to 6 hours and 24 hours after injection on a large field of view gamma camera equipped with low-energy, high-resolution parallel hole collimators. Energy windows set at 140 keV (20% window). Total body static images (0.5M to 1M counts) in anterior and posterior views and SPECT images (360 degrees of rotation for single-headed or 180 to 360 degrees for dual-headed camera; 64 or 32 stops) from the skull base through the pubic symphysis are typically obtained at 3 to 6 hours and 24 hours after injection.
- Images are interpreted in conjunction with other imaging modalities, particularly CT or magnetic resonance imaging (MRI).

Image Interpretation

Early images obtained 6 hours after injection of the tracer (Fig. A) showed no definite focal abnormality and the activity in the right neck (*arrowhead*) is most likely consistent with normal blood pool activity. Images obtained 24 hours after injection (Fig. B) demonstrated clearance of the blood pool activity on the right, but residual uptake on the left (*arrowhead*). The left upper anterior mediastinal abnormality is better visualized with SPECT (Fig. C). The SPECT of the chest 24 hours post-injection demonstrates intense focal abnormal uptake in the anterior mediastinum on the left, at the level of manubrium sterni (*arrow*). The display format includes in clockwise sequence starting in left upper corner: (a) volume-rendered image of chest and upper abdomen, (b) axial cut of the upper chest, (c) coronal cut of anterior thorax, and (d) sagittal image in the plane of the dominant lesion. (Bars indicate positions of the cuts in other planes.)

Axial CT of the chest at the level of the manubrium (Fig. D) demonstrates a 3 cm × 3 cm × 4 cm nodule (*arrows*) impinging on the left brachiocephalic vein, which is opacified with intravenous contrast.

Correlative axial CT of the neck through the thyroid (Fig. E) demonstrates multiple nodules and cysts, possibly multinodular goiter (*arrows*). Prominent jugular vein on the right may partly explain the uptake as seen in the right neck on Fig. B suggesting blood pool activity.

Arcitumomab guided further workup with neck and chest CT. In the corresponding location, a 3 cm × 3 cm × 4 cm mass was found in the anterior mediastinum (Fig. D). Multiple nodules and several cysts were also seen in the thyroid gland (Fig. E). No other distant metastases were demonstrated.

Differential Diagnosis

- Primary tumor expressing CEA
- Metastasis from a primary tumor expressing CEA
- Infectious or inflammatory site
- Iatrogenic etiology such as uptake in a scar post surgery or biopsy
- Blood pool activity

Diagnosis and Clinical Follow-up

The findings on arcitumomab scintigraphy yielded further work-up with neck and chest CT. The mass seen in the anterior mediastinum on CT was surgically removed and histological examination showed a well-differentiated neuroendocrine neoplasm most consistent with medullary carcinoma of the thyroid (MTC). Bronchoscopy and mediastinoscopy with sampling of multiple mediastinal lymph nodes were negative. The cells within the mass were strongly reactive for CEA and chromogranin and negative for calcitonin, which is seen in approximately 20% of MTC. Total thyroidectomy was also performed. Pathological examination of the thyroid revealed multifocal tumor of the same histology, with the largest nodule being 0.3 cm. Neck lymph nodes were negative for tumor. Patient has remained on hormone supplemental therapy, clinically free of the disease.

Discussion

Monoclonal anti-CEA antibodies play an increasingly promising role in the imaging of CEA-expressing cancers. Their most frequent application is the diagnosis of recurrent colorectal carcinoma (CRC). Technetium 99m arcitumomab is a murine monoclonal Fab' antibody fragment generated from IMMU-4 directed against the CEA surface antigen found in colorectal carcinomas, but also in other tumors, such as medullary carcinoma of the thyroid and non–small cell lung carcinoma in variable concentration. The agent has a short biological half-life, 13.4 hours, and rapid blood clearance, which improves target-to-background ratios. Small fragment size promotes renal excretion. About 30% of the agent is excreted in the urine over the first 24 hours after injection. A variety of tumors express CEA including non–small cell lung cancer, pancreatic cancer, ovarian cancer, and breast cancer. CRC and MTC show a higher tumor to whole body activity ratio than other tumors.

Our case illustrates the usefulness of total body imaging with the finding of an unsuspected CEA-producing primary tumor in a patient who was presumed to be at high risk for CRC in the setting of suspected polyposis syndrome or lung cancer, or both, because of the history of heavy smoking.

MTC represents 1 to 5% of all thyroid tumors and is often associated with amyloid deposition in the primary or secondary tumor. MTC spreads rapidly to lymph nodes (50%), lung, liver, and bone. The 10-year survival is 90% without nodal metastases, 42% with nodal metastases. MTC may be associated with multiple endocrine neoplasia, type IIA (MEN IIA) (pheochromocytoma + parathyroid hyperplasia) or MEN IIB (without a parathyroid component).

An inverse relationship between tumor mass and absolute uptake of antibody has been reported that is related in part to monoclonal anti-CEA antibody accessibility, tumor perfusion, vascularization, and interstitial pressure. In CRC, 60% of lesions < 1 cm were detected, which may be very promising for the detection of unknown primary tumor. Moffat et al (1996) demonstrated much higher imaging accuracy of CEA-Scan® compared with conventional imaging (61% versus 33%) in patients with an occult cancer in the setting of abnormal CEA and history of prior CRC.

Imaging for MTC is indicated in MEN II or if recurrent disease is suspected in patients with rising calcitonin levels. Monoclonal anti-CEA antibodies have been used with variable success, including more recently a bispecific anti-CEA/anti-In-111–labeled diethylenetriamine pentaacetic acid (DTPA) dimer.

Other radiopharmaceuticals such as OctreoScan® can diagnose MTC because these tumors also express somatostatin receptors. Iodine 123 or iodine 131

- *(continued)* Reading of scans without morphological correlation should be avoided.

- Blood pool activity may create false-positive readings.

- Iatrogenic sites of uptake may be seen in a scar after surgery or colostomy site.

- Know the postsurgical anatomy; the bladder moves backwards after rectal ampule resection; segmental resection of the bowel changes usual bowel distribution.

- Injection via central lines and catheters may produce artifacts, and infiltration of the tracer may lead to axillary lymph node visualization.

- Negative results using arcitumomab in patients with a history of colorectal cancer do not exclude disease. One may also consider using satumomab pendetide in the follow-up of those patients to evaluate extrahepatic involvement if no HAMA are present. The longer biological and physical half-lives of satumomab pendetide may help in diagnosing small tumor burdens that may not be visualized by arcitumomab because of its shorter physical and biological half-lives.

- PET imaging with F-18-fluorodeoxyglucose has shown excellent results in the evaluation of recurrent colorectal cancer.

metaiodobenzylguanidine (MIBG) may also be useful in the detection of an associated pheochromocytoma in MEN II.

Suggested Readings

Arcitumomab (CEA-Scan). Available: http://nuc-med-read.uthscsa.edu/williams/NucMed/TUM08.htm

Behr TM, Sharkey RM, Juweid ME, et al. Variables influencing tumor dosimetry in radioimmunotherapy of CEA-expressing cancers with anti-CEA and antimucin monoclonal antibodies. *J Nucl Med 38:409–418, 1997.*

Dahnert W. Disease entities of ear, nose and throat disorders. In Grayson TH, Eckhart C, eds. *Radiology Review Manual.* Baltimore: Williams & Wilkins, 1991:188.

Moffat FL, Pinsky CM, Hammershaimb L, et al. Clinical utility of external immunoscintigraphy with the IMMU-4 Technetium-99m Fab' antibody fragment in patients undergoing surgery for carcinoma of the colon and rectum: Results of a pivotal, phase III trial. *J Clin Oncol 14:2295–2305, 1996.*

Nabi HA, Erb DA, Cronin VR. Superiority of SPET to planar imaging in the detection of colorectal carcinoma with In-111 monoclonal antibodies. *Nucl Med Commun 16:631–639, 1995.*

Peltier P, Curtet C, Chatal J-F, et al. Radioimmunodetection of medullary thyroid cancer using a bispecific anti-CEA/anti-indium-111-labeled DTPA dimer. *J Nucl Med 34: 1267–1273, 1993.*

Vekermans M-C, Urbain J-L, Charkes ND. Advances in thyroid cancer imaging. *New Perspectives in Cancer Diagnosis and Management 4:58–67, 1997.*

Case 90

Clinical Presentation

73-year-old man is found to have an elevated prostate-specific antigen (PSA) level on routine screening. An ultrasound-guided transrectal biopsy of the prostate was performed and demonstrated prostate cancer of Gleason grade 9. A bone scan showed no evidence of skeletal metastases. Actual computed tomography (Fig. A) shows a questionable lymph node (*arrow*) near the aortic bifurcation. ProstaScint® is requested to evaluate extraprostatic disease.

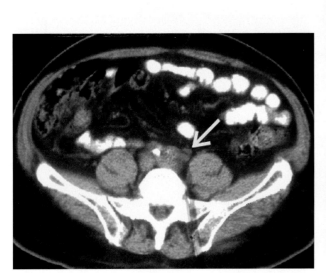

Fig. A

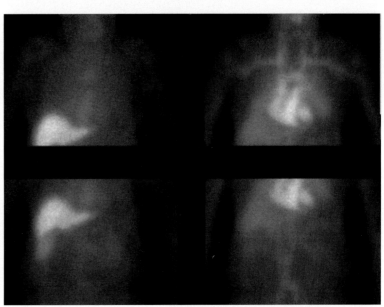

Fig. B

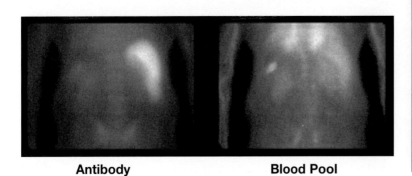

Antibody   **Blood Pool**

Fig. C

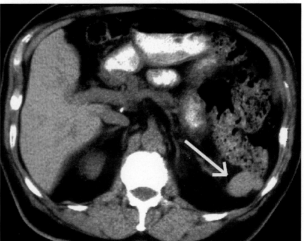

Fig. D

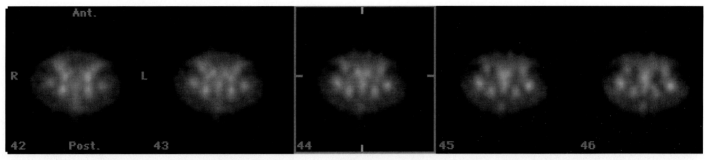

Fig. E

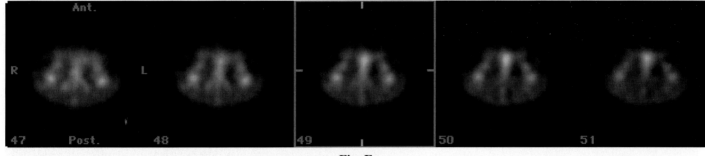

Fig. F

Technique

• 5.0 mCi indium-111–labeled capromab pendetide (ProstaScint®) intravenously, and then monitor the patient for 15 minutes.

• Approximately 96 hours post-injection, images preobtained using a dual acquisition technique following technetium-99m radiolabeling of autologous red blood cells (RBCs) to delineate blood pool activity.

• Whole-body planar images are obtained as well as single photon emission computed tomography (SPECT) images of the abdomen and pelvis. SPECT of other regions are also acquired as needed, based on findings on planar images.

• If necessary, the patient may return for delayed images at 144 hours. This can be useful in confirming bowel excretion of tracer. In such a case, the uptake will have disappeared or changed in position and configuration.

Image Interpretation

Planar anterior capromab pendetide images of the chest and abdomen (Fig. B on the left) show slightly higher hepatic uptake than expected but no focal abnormal capromab uptake. The accompanying planar anterior technetium-99m–labeled RBC images of the chest and abdomen (Fig. B on the right) show normal blood pool activity. Posterior planar capromab pendetide images of the abdomen (Fig. C on the left) show a vague region of tracer uptake in the left upper quadrant. The technetium-99m–labeled RBC image (Fig. C on the right) shows that this focus has high blood pool activity. Review of the CT shows a splenulus at this location (Fig. D).

Axial capromab pendetide SPECT images of the lower pelvis down to the base of the penile shaft (Figs. E and F) show blood pool activity in the femoral vessels and the base of the penile shaft as well as physiologic uptake within skeletal structures. Increased capromab pendetide uptake is seen in the prostate bed in this patient, who had not had a prostatectomy at the time of imaging.

- *(continued)* As a whole antibody, capromab pendetide is excreted in the bowel, and activity from the colon or small bowel can mimic uptake in retroperitoneal or mesenteric lymph nodes. SPECT imaging or delayed imaging, or both, can be useful in differentiating intestinal activity from nodal activity.

- The role of capromab pendetide imaging in the evaluation and management of patients with prostate cancer is currently in development. Two indications for capromab imaging are stated by the manufacturer of ProstaScint®, Cytogen (Princeton, NJ), based on data from phase III clinical trials. The first indication is for the detection of metastases in patients with newly diagnosed prostate cancer who are thought to be at high risk for metastases by PSA level, Gleason score, or other clinical factors. If a bone scan, CT scan, or MRI or a combination of these, shows no evidence of metastases or if they are equivocal, a ProstaScint® scan may be of use in identifying occult metastases. Such a finding would affect the patient's stage and management. The second indication for ProstaScint®, one that seems to be more widely agreed on, is in the setting of post-prostatectomy patients with a rising PSA level, a negative bone scan, and a negative CT or MRI. In these cases, if disease is believed to be confined to the prostatic fossa, salvage radiation therapy of the pelvis is contemplated. If, however, distant metastases are present, systemic therapy would be instituted. The ProstaScint® scan may be useful in determining if distant occult metastases are present, and therefore which treatment modality should be used.

246

Diagnosis and Clinical Follow-up

There was no scintigraphic evidence of metastatic disease in the questionable lymph node or outside the prostatic bed.

Discussion

Technetium-99m radiolabeling of RBCs is performed on the first day of imaging 96 hours after the injection of capromab pendetide to delineate the blood pool activity. These images are useful because capromab pendetide, as a whole antibody, will demonstrate persistent physiological blood pool activity. The technetium-99m RBC images can demonstrate that a positive finding on the capromab pendetide images may be due to blood pool activity rather than activity within a tumor site.

Capromab pendetide is a whole murine monoclonal antibody that is directed against prostate membrane specific antigen (PMSA), a transmembrane glycoprotein expressed by prostate epithelial cells. PMSA expression is higher in prostate adenocarcinoma cells than in nonmalignant cells, and it is higher in metastatic lesions than in primary lesions. Capromab pendetide may be useful in the evaluation or post-prostatectomy patients with rising PSA who have an otherwise negative or equivocal workup for metastases. A potential role for capromab pendetide, as seen in this case, is in the staging of newly diagnosed prostate cancer. This remains controversial.

Suggested Readings

Kahn D, Williams RD, Manyak MJ, et al. 111-Indium capromab pendetide in the evaluation of patients with residual or recurrent prostate cancer after radical prostatectomy. *J Urol* 159:2041–2046, 1998.

Kahn, Williams RD, Hasman MK, et al. Radioimmunoscintigraphy with In-111-labeled capromab pendetide predicts prostate cancer response to salvage radiotherapy after failed radical prostatectomy. *J Clin Oncol* 16:284–289, 1998.

Lamb HM, Faulds, D. Capromab pendetide: A review of its use as an imaging agent in prostate cancer. *Drugs Aging* 12:293–304, 1998.

ProstaScint® (Kit for the Preparation of Indium-111 Capromab Pendetide): A Guide for Interpretation. Princeton, NJ: Cytogen Corp., 1997.

Saitoh H, Hidda M, Shimbo T, et al. Metastatic patterns of prostate cancer. *Cancer* 54:3078–3084, 1984.

Case 91

Clinical Presentation

64-year-old man presenting with pleuritic chest pain.

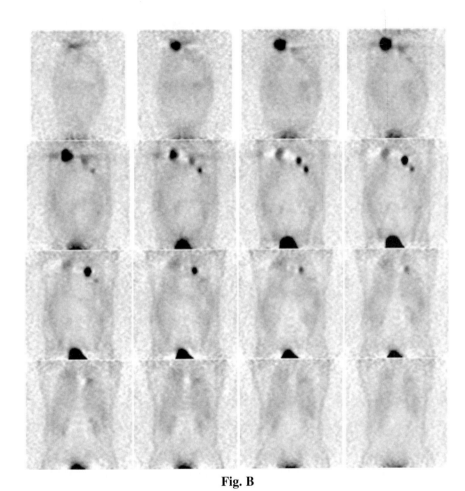

Fig. B

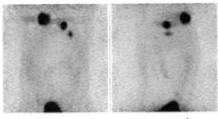

Anterior   Lateral

Fig. A

Technique

- Patient is instructed to take nothing by mouth for 8 hours prior to the study.
- 5 mCi ^{18}FDG intravenously.
- Image at 1.25 hours supine with arms up.
- Images obtained using dual-headed gamma camera with coincidence detection capabilities.

Image Interpretation

Reprojection anterior and lateral images (Fig. A) and coronal slices (Fig. B) demonstrate three foci of uptake. The largest in the right chest wall, with two smaller foci in the left upper lobe of the lung.

Differential Diagnosis

• Pulmonary neoplastic disease, either primary or secondary
• Coccoidomycosis
• Histoplamosis
• Sarcoidosis
• Rheumatoid arthritis-associated lung disease

Diagnosis and Clinical Follow-up

Biopsy demonstrated non–small cell lung cancer. Patient was started on chemotherapy.

Discussion

Positron-emission tomography (PET) imaging of non–small cell lung cancer is emerging as a sensitive, specific test for the staging of this disease. In several studies, it has been shown to be more sensitive than anatomic imaging studies such as computed tomography (CT). This improved sensitivity may prevent thoracotomy in patients with otherwise undetectable metastatic disease.

Suggested Readings

Guhlmann A, Storck M, Kotzerke J, et al. Lymph node staging in non–small cell lung cancer: Evaluation by [18F]FDG positron emission tomography (PET). *Thorax* 52:438–441, 1997.

Kubota K, Matsuzawa T, Fujiwara T, et al. Differential diagnosis of lung tumor with positron emission tomography: A prospective study. *J Nucl Med* 31:1927–1932, 1990.

Schiepers C. Role of positron emission tomography in the staging of lung cancer. *Lung Cancer* 17 (Suppl 1):S29–35, 1997.

Valk PE, Pounds TR, Hopkins DM, et al. Staging non–small cell lung cancer by whole-body positron emission tomographic imaging. *Ann Thorac Surg* 60:1573–1581, 1995.

Case 92

Clinical Presentation

59-year-old man with stage III non–small cell lung cancer. Computed tomography (CT) of the chest demonstrates a large mass with a necrotic center in the right upper lobe.

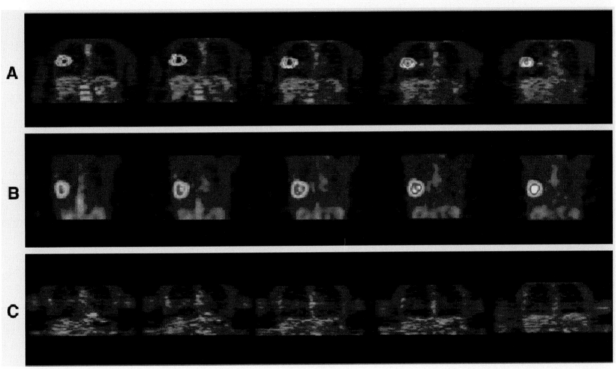

Fig. A

Technique

^{18}FDG Positron Emission Tomography (PET)

- Patient preparation: nothing by mouth for 8-12 hours before administration of the radiopharmaceutical. Switch all glucose-containing intravenous solutions to normal saline on the day before imaging.
- 10 mCi ^{18}FDG, administered intravenously 45 minutes prior to image acquisition.
- Imaging device: whole-body PET camera with in-plane and axial resolutions of 5.0 mm full width half maximum (FWHM), 9.5 cm field of view, 15 contiguous slices of 6.5-mm separation, and sensitivity of approximately 5000 cps/mCi.
- Image acquistion: ten-minute acquisitions in four bed positions are taken (9.5 cm each), starting at the neck and extending to the lower chest.
- Transmission measurements: transmission measurements should be five-minute acquisitions at the same bed positions using a rotating pin source containing gallium-68.

- Image reconstruction: image reconstruction is by conventional filtered-back projection algorithm to an in-plane resolution of 7 mm FWHM. All projection data are corrected for nonuniformity of detector response, dead time, random coincidences, attenuation, and scattered radiation. The transmission data are used for attenuation correction.

^{18}FDG Single Photon Emission Computed Tomography (SPECT)

- Patient preparation same as it is for PET.
- Radiopharmaceutical same as it is for PET.
- Imaging device is a dual-head gamma camera.
- Ultra-high-energy collimator.
- Energy window is 20% centered at 511 keV.
- Image acquisition is immediately after completion of the PET study; 360 degree acquisition (180 degrees per head) with 128 projections. Each projection is acquired for 20 seconds.
- Image reconstruction is order of 7, Butterworth filter, with a cutoff of 0.5 times the Nyquist frequency.

Image Interpretation

Prior to therapy, the ^{18}FDG PET images (Fig. A. A.) demonstrated a large area of abnormal tracer accumulation in the chest corresponding to the lesion detected by CT. The periphery of this lesion showed intensely increased tracer uptake, indicating metabolically active tumor. In contrast, the center of the tumor had reduced ^{18}FDG uptake consistent with necrosis. In addition, a small area of mildly increased ^{18}FDG uptake was detected in the region of the right hilum. This lesion was not identified by CT. The ^{18}FDG SPECT images (Fig. A. B.) showed a pattern of tracer accumulation similar to that of the PET study. Anatomic definition of the tumor margins was poorer, the region of necrosis was not well-visualized, and the hilar lesion was not detected. After therapy, the PET images demonstrated a marked reduction in tumor accumulation of ^{18}FDG uptake (Fig. A. C.), indicating a favorable response.

Differential Diagnosis

- Pulmonary neoplastic disease, either primary or secondary
- Coccoidomycosis
- Histoplamosis
- Sarcoidosis
- Rheumatoid arthritis-associated lung disease

Diagnosis and Clinical Follow-up

Six months after completion of therapy, the patient remained free of symptoms, and a repeat CT demonstrated significant reduction in tumor size and extent.

Discussion

^{18}FDG PET and SPECT studies were performed to (1) evaluate the presence of additional lesions, particularly involvement of hilar lymph nodes; (2) characterize the metabolic state of the lesion; and (3) provide a baseline for monitoring the effect of radiation therapy. Based on the results of the PET study, the radiation field was extended to include the hilar lesion.

Suggested Readings

Gupta NC, Frank AR, Dewan NA, et al. Solitary pulmonary nodules: Detection of malignancy with PET with 2-[F-18]-fluoro-2-deoxy-D-glucose. *Radiology* 184:441–444, 1992.

Kubota K, Yamada K, Yoshioka S, et al. Differential diagnosis of idiopathic fibrosis from malignant lymphadenopathy with PET and F-18 fluorodeoxyglucose. *Clin Nucl Med* 17:361–363, 1992.

Sokoloff L, Reivich M, Kennedy C, et al. The ^{14}C-deoxyglucose method for the measurement of local cerebral glucose utilization: Theory, procedure and normal values in the conscious and anesthetized albino rat. *J Neurochem* 28:897–916, 1977.

Warburg O. On the origin of cancer cell. *Science* 123:309–314, 1956.

Case 93

Clinical Presentation

49-year-old man presenting with a large esophageal mass detected by computed tomography (CT) and determined to be esophageal cancer by biopsy.

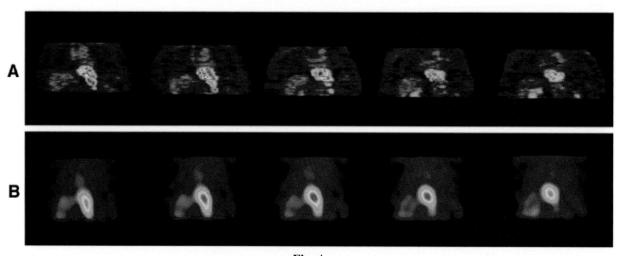

Fig. A

Technique

^{18}FDG Positron Emission Tomography (PET)

- Patient preparation: patient should take nothing by mouth for 8-12 hours before administration of the radiopharmaceutical. Switch all glucose-containing intravenous solutions to normal saline on the day before imaging.
- 10 mCi ^{18}FDG, administered intravenously 45 minutes prior to image acquisition.
- Imaging device: whole-body PET camera with in-plane and axial resolutions of 5.0 mm full width half maximum (FWHM), 9.5 cm field of view, 15 contiguous slices of 6.5-mm separation, and sensitivity of approximately 5000 cps/mCi.
- Image acquisition: ten-minute acquisitions in seven bed positions are taken (9.5 cm each), starting at the neck and extending to the lower chest.
- Transmission measurement: should be 5-minute acquisitions at the same bed positions using a rotating pin source containing gallium-68.
- Image reconstruction: should be by conventional filtered-back projection algorithm to an in-plane resolution of 7 mm FWHM. All projection data are corrected for nonuniformity of detector response, dead time, random coincidences, attenuation, and scattered radiation. The transmission data are used for attenuation correction.

^{18}FDG Single Photon Emission Computed Tomography (SPECT)

• Patient preparation same as it is for PET.
• Radiopharmaceutical same as it is for PET.
• Imaging device is a dual-head gamma camera equipped with ultra-high-energy collimators.
• Energy window is 20% centered at 511 keV.
• Image acquisition immediately after completion of the PET study; 360-degree acquisition (180 degrees per head) with 128 projections. Each projection is acquired for 20 seconds.
• Image reconstruction is order of 7, Butterworth filter, with a cutoff of 0.5 times the Nyquist frequency.

Image Interpretation

The ^{18}FDG PET images (Fig. A. A.) demonstrated an intense focus of increased accumulation surrounding the esophagus and extending from the midchest to the upper abdomen. There was no evidence of increased ^{18}FDG accumulation in hilar or mediastinal lymph nodes. The ^{18}FDG SPECT images (Fig. A. B.) showed a similar pattern of tracer accumulation; anatomic definition of the tumor margins was poorer, however.

Differential Diagnosis

• Esophageal cancer or other malignancy in the mediastinum
• Sarcoidosis
• Abscess or other inflammatory lesion

Diagnosis and Clinical Follow-up

The diagnosis was esophageal cancer. The patient is currently undergoing treatment with a combination of radiation and chemotherapy. A follow-up PET study is planned after completion of therapy.

Discussion

^{18}FDG PET and SPECT studies were performed to: evaluate the presence of additional lesions, particularly involvement of lymph nodes; characterize the metabolic state of the lesion; and provide a baseline for monitoring the effect of radiation therapy. Compared with conventional single photon radionuclide procedures, PET has several advantages: (1) Resolution and sensitivity are considerably higher; (2) implementation of corrections for photon attenuation and scatter are straightforward; (3) the images are quantitative; (4) a variety of radiopharmaceuticals that do not have single photon analogs are available; and (5) the short physical half-lives of many of the radiopharmaceuticals facilitate repetitive studies.

Currently, numerous PET radiopharmaceuticals are available for tumor detection and therapeutic monitoring, including water O-15, butanol O-15, and ammonia N-13 for measuring perfusion; ^{18}FDG for studying glucose metabolism; methionine C-11 and tyrosine F-18 for evaluating amino acid transport and protein synthesis; thymidine C-11 for studying cell proliferation; and numerous C-11

• *(continued)* Incorrect identification of abdominal accumulations of [18]FDG (frequently with unusual configurations) may result from errors in attenuation correction caused by intestinal motion between transmission and emission imaging. Comparison of attenuation-corrected images and uncorrected images can be useful for resolving this issue.

and F-18–labeled receptor ligands. Despite this plurality of tracers, however, [18]FDG has become the "work horse" of clinical PET. The central role of [18]FDG in PET is based on both fundamental aspects of tissue metabolism and practical considerations. On the theoretical side, it is well-established that rapidly dividing tumor cells have accelerated glucose use under anaerobic conditions. Explanations for this phenomenon ("Pasteur effect") include both increased hexokinase activity in tumor cells and increased concentrations of glucose transport proteins. On the practical side, there are at least three reasons for the prominent status of [18]FDG: (1) Current synthetic methods for preparing [18]FDG yield sufficient quantities of tracer for numerous studies; (2) compared with other PET radiopharmaceuticals, the fact that [18]FDG is a "trapped tracer" greatly simplifies imaging procedures; and (3) since ^{18}F has a relatively long half-life (110 minutes) compared with other PET agents, regional distribution facilities can supply imaging centers without on-site cyclotrons. Because of the accelerated anaerobic metabolism associated with neoplasia, it is expected that virtually all types of tumor will have increased [18]FDG accumulation. Important information about tumors of the lung, head and neck, musculoskeletal system, breast, bladder, pituitary, colon, liver, thyroid, and lymphoid tissue has been reported. These measurements have been of significant value in the evaluation of malignant degeneration, prognosis, and recurrence after radiation or chemotherapy. Specifically, PET has been useful for staging lung cancer, differentiating recurrent lung cancer from scar after radiation therapy, staging axillary nodes in breast cancer, differentiating recurrent colorectal cancer from scar, staging primary head and neck cancer, and determining the effect of therapy on these tumors and delineating the degree of malignancy of soft tissue sarcomas.

Recent developments in PET camera design have greatly expanded the clinical usefulness of [18]FDG PET in oncology. For example, scanners with 15- to 25-cm fields of view, full three-dimensional image acquisition capabilities, and the ability for simultaneous acquisition of emission and transmission data are currently available.

Suggested Readings

Adler LP, Blair HF, Makley JT, et al. Noninvasive grading of musculoskeletal tumors using PET. *J Nucl Med* 32:1508–1512, 1991.

Bailet JW, Abemayor E, Jabour BA, et al. Positron emission tomography: A new, precise imaging modality for detection of primary head and neck tumors and assessment of cervical adenopathy. *Laryngoscope* 102:281–288, 1992.

Di Chiro G. Positron emission tomography using [^{18}F] fluorodeoxyglucose in brain tumors. A powerful diagnostic and prognostic tool. *Invest Radiol* 22:360–371, 1987.

Francavilla TL, Miletich RS, Di Chiro G, et al. Positron emission tomography in the detection of malignant degeneration of low-grade gliomas. *Neurosurgery* 24:1–5, 1989.

Joensuu H, Ahonen A. Imaging of metastases of thyroid carcinoma with fluorine-18 fluorodeoxyglucose. *J Nucl Med* 28:910–914, 1987.

Patronas NJ, Di Chiro G, Kufta C, et al. Prediction of survival in glioma patients by means of positron emission tomography. *J Neurosurg* 62:816–822, 1985.

Phelps ME, Huang SC, Hoffman EJ, et al. Tomographic measurements of local cerebral glucose metabolism in humans with (F-18)-2-fluoro-2-deoxy-D-glucose: Validation of method. *Ann Neurol* 6:371–388, 1979.

Strauss LG, Clorius JH, Schlag P, et al. Recurrence of colorectal tumors: PET evaluation. *Radiology* 170:329–332, 1989.

Valk PE, Budinger TF, Levin VA, et al. PET of malignant cerebral tumors after interstitial brachytherapy. Demonstration of metabolic activity and correlation with clinical outcome. *J Neurosurg* 69:830–838, 1988.

Wahl R, Cody R, Hutchins G, Mudgett E. Positron emission tomographic scanning of primary and metastatic breast carcinoma with the radiolabeled glucose analog 2-deoxy-2[^{18}F]fluoro-D-glucose. *N Engl J Med* 324:200, 1991.

Case 94

Clinical Presentation

51-year-old woman developed a right neck mass that was biopsied and demonstrated poorly differentiated adenocarcinoma. Positron-emission tomography (PET) was performed to assess for extent of disease in the chest.

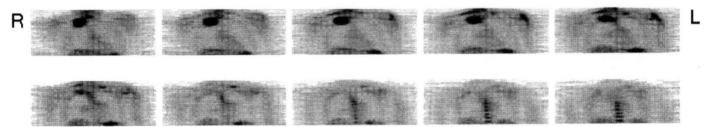

R   L

Fig. A

Technique

- Patient preparation: Patient should take nothing by mouth for at least 4 hours.
- 13 mCi of ^{18}FDG administered intravenously.
- Attenuation-corrected PET imaging (Scanditronix 4096 with field of view of 9.75 cm and spatial resolution of 6.00 mm full width half maximum) of the chest was performed 45 minutes after ^{18}FDG injection.

Image Interpretation

The coronal PET images (anterior to posterior) show a large hypermetabolic mass in the right lung apex corresponding to the primary tumor. A small focus of increased FDG uptake is also seen in the left supraclavicular region that on the sagittal view appeared as a continuous curvilinear region following the contour of the posterior upper chest wall, probably representing muscular uptake.

Differential Diagnosis

- Other histological types of primary lung cancer (e.g., squamous cell carcinoma)
- Lymphoma
- Sarcoma
- Metastatic tumor
- Infectious (e.g., bacterial, fungal, granulomatous, etc.) conditions
- Noninfectious (e.g., sarcoid) inflammatory conditions

Diagnosis and Clinical Follow-up

Poorly differentiated right upper lobe (RUL) adenocarcinoma. The patient underwent RUL wedge resection of the Pancoast tumor followed by radiation and chemotherapy.

PEARLS/PITFALLS

- PET is highly sensitive for detection of malignancy.

- Malignancy is highly unlikely in patients with negative PET.

- PET may be falsely positive in inflammatory conditions, including granulomatous disease.

- PET obviates the need for confirmatory mediastinoscopy and transbronchial or transthoracic biopsy in some patients. PET is the imaging method of choice in follow-up of patients with lung cancer.

Discussion

Several investigators have demonstrated the diagnostic value of ^{18}FDG PET in assessing solitary pulmonary nodules. High sensitivity (about 96%) has been reported, whereas specificity is variable depending on the local prevalence of granulomatous disease that also shows high ^{18}FDG uptake. Malignancy is highly unlikely in patients with negative PET. ^{18}FDG PET can also be used for staging of non–small cell lung cancer (NSCLC) by assessing the hila, the mediastinum, and the extrathoracic sites. Follow-up evaluation post-therapy is another important use of ^{18}FDG PET in lung cancer.

Suggested Readings

Hagberg RC, Segall GM, Stark P, et al. Characterization of pulmonary nodules and mediastinal staging of bronchogenic carcinoma with F-18 fluorodeoxyglucose positron emission tomography. *Eur J Cardiothorac Surg* 12:92–97, 1997.

Lowe VJ, Fletcher JW, Gobar L, et al. Prospective investigation of positron emission tomography in lung nodules. *J Clin Oncol* 16:1075–1084, 1998.

Valk PE, Pounds TR, Hopkins DM, et al. Staging lung cancer by PET imaging. *Ann Thorac Surg* 60:1573–1582, 1995.

Case 95

Clinical Presentation

65-year-old man with a history of squamous cell lung cancer status post–upper lobectomy presented with an abnormal follow-up chest computed tomography (CT) that demonstrated a right hilar mass. Positron emission tomography (PET) was performed for further evaluation of recurrent disease.

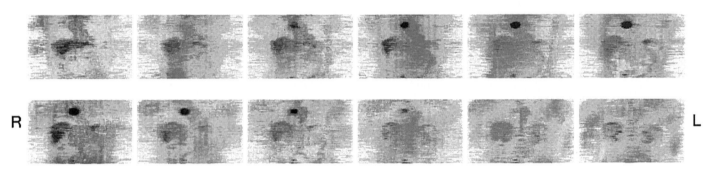

R   L

Fig. A

Technique

- Patient preparation: Patient should take nothing by mouth for at least 4 hours.
- 11 mCi of ^{18}FDG administered intravenously.
- Attenuation-corrected PET imaging (Scanditronix 4096 with field of view of 9.75 cm and spatial resolution of 6.00 mm full width half maximum) of the chest was performed 45 minutes after ^{18}FDG injection.

Image Interpretation

Coronal PET images (from anterior to posterior) of the chest (Fig. A) show a focal area of abnormal hypermetabolism in the right hilum that is highly suspicious for recurrent disease. No other abnormalities were seen.

Differential Diagnosis

- Other histological types of primary lung cancer (e.g., adenocarcinoma)
- Lymphoma
- Sarcoma
- Metastic tumor
- Infectious (e.g., bacterial, fungal, granulomatous, etc.) conditions
- Noninfectious (e.g., sarcoid) inflammatory conditions

Diagnosis and Clinical Follow-up

The patient underwent bronchoscopy with right bronchial washings that demonstrated moderately differentiated squamous cell carcinoma.

Discussion

Follow-up evaluation post-therapy is an important use of FDG PET in lung cancer. PET has high sensitivity for detection of recurrent or metastatic lung cancer. It is particularly useful in differentiating recurrence of malignancy if there is residual fibrotic scar at the original site of disease. Recurrent disease is highly unlikely in patients with negative PET.

Suggested Readings

Duhaylongsod FG, Lowe VJ, Patz EF, et al. Detection of primary and recurrent lung cancer by means of F-18 fluorodeoxyglucose positron emission tomography (FDG-PET). *J Thorac Cardiovasc Surg* 110:139–140, 1995.

Bury T, Dowlati A, Paulus P, et al. Staging of non-small cell lung cancer by whole-body 18FDG-PET. *Eur J Nucl Med* 23:204–206, 1996.

Bury T, Paulus P, Dowlati A, et al. Staging of the mediastinum: Value of positron emission tomography imaging in non-small cell cancer. *Eur Resp J* 9:2560–2564, 1996.

Case 96

Clinical Presentation

70-year-old man presenting with hiccups. An upper gastrointestinal series demonstrated a mass in the distal esophagus. Computed tomography (CT) showed diffuse wall thickening in the distal esophagus. Positron emission tomography (PET) was performed for further evaluation.

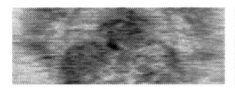 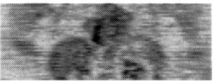 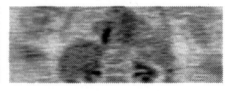

L

Fig. A

Technique

- Patient preparation: Patient should take nothing by mouth for at least 4 hours.
- 11 mCi of ^{18}FDG administered intravenously.
- Attenuation-corrected PET imaging (Scanditronix 4096 with field of view of 9.75 cm and spatial resolution of 6.00 mm full width half maximum) of the chest was performed 45 minutes after FDG injection.

Image Interpretation

Series of coronal PET images (from anterior to posterior) of the chest (Fig. A) show abnormal hypermetabolism in the posterior lower mediastinum. No other abnormalities were seen.

Differential Diagnosis

- Lymphoma
- Gastroesophageal junction carcinoma
- Metastatic tumor
- Infectious or noninfectious esophagitis

Diagnosis and Clinical Follow-up

The patient underwent esophagoscopy with biopsy of the mass that demonstrated moderately differentiated adenocarcinoma. He then underwent left thoracoabdominal esophagogastrectomy and pyloromyotomy.

Discussion

^{18}FDG PET is able to visualize the primary tumor and the extent of disease, including hepatic metastases. Evaluation post-therapy is another important use of ^{18}FDG PET in esophageal cancer.

Suggested Readings

Flanagan FL, Dehdashti F, Siegel BA, et al. Staging of esophageal cancer with 18F-fluorodeoxyglucose positron emission tomography. *AJR* 168:417–424, 1997.

Fukunaga T, Okazumi S, Koide Y, et al. Evaluation of esophageal cancers using fluorine-18-fluorodeoxyglucose PET. *J Nucl Med* 39:1002–1007, 1998.

Luketich JD, Schauer PR, Meltzer CC, et al. Role of positron emission tomography in staging esophageal cancer. *Ann Thorac Surg* 64:765–769, 1997.

Case 97

Clinical Presentation

66-year-old man with a history of pancreatic adenocarcinoma initially presents with painless jaundice. He underwent Whipple's procedure followed by radiation and chemotherapy. Positron-emission tomography (PET) was performed 1 year later for tumor surveillance.

R
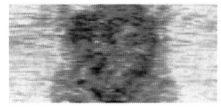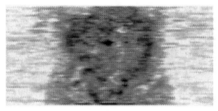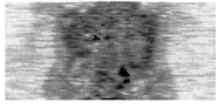

Fig. A

Technique

- Patient preparation: Patient should take nothing by mouth for at least 4 hours.
- 11 mCi of ^{18}FDG administered intravenously.
- Attenuation-corrected PET imaging (Scanditronix 4096 with field of view of 9.75 cm and spatial resolution of 6.00 mm full width half maximum) of the chest was performed 45 minutes after ^{18}FDG injection.

Image Interpretation

Series of coronal PET images (from anterior to posterior) of the abdomen and pelvis (Fig. A) show a small intense focus posterior to the left hepatic lobe in the epigastric area suspicious for recurrence. The multiple foci of diminished activity in the liver corresponded to known cysts. No lymphadenopathy was noted.

Differential Diagnosis

- Cholangioadenocarcinoma
- Hepatoma
- Carcinoma of Vater's ampulla
- Duodenal cancer
- Lymphoma
- Sarcoma
- Metastatic tumor
- Infectious or noninfectious pancreatitis

Diagnosis and Clinical Follow-up

A computed tomography (CT) scan performed after the PET scan showed abnormal soft tissue around the superior mesenteric artery. The patient was later admitted to the hospital with upper gastrointestinal bleed and underwent multiple endoscopies for coagulation of ulcers. The clinical course, however, became complicated with the development of pneumonia and peritonitis that ultimately resulted in death. A limited autopsy was performed. Ductal pancreatic adenocarcinoma was noted at the pancreatico-jejunostomy post-therapy anastomosis corresponding to the PET and CT soft tissue abnormalities.

Discussion

^{18}FDG PET is useful for differentiation of posttherapy changes from residual or recurrent disease in patients after Whipple procedure. PET may also be useful at the time of initial diagnosis for assessing the extent of disease, including detection of liver and nodal metastasis.

Suggested Readings

Friess H, Langhans J, Ebert M, et al. Diagnosis of pancreatic cancer by 2[18F]-fluoro-2-deoxy-D-glucose positron emission tomography. *Gut* 365:771–777, 1995.

Hawkins R. Pancreatic tumors: Imaging with PET. *Radiology* 95:320–322, 1995.

Zimny M, Bares R, Fass J, et al. Fluorine-18 fluorodeoxyglucose positron emission tomography in the differential diagnosis of pancreatic carcinoma: A report of 106 cases. *Eur J Med* 24:678–682, 1997.

Case 98

Clinical Presentation

52-year-old woman presents with an enlarging right thigh mass. Both magnetic resonance imaging (MRI) and positron-emission tomography (PET) of the right lower extremity were performed for evaluation.

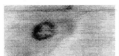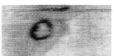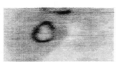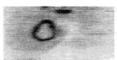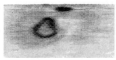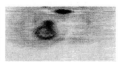

Fig. A

Technique

- Patient preparation: Patient should take nothing by mouth for at least 4 hours.
- 16 mCi of [18]FDG administered intravenously.
- Attenuation-corrected PET imaging (Scanditronix 4096 with field of view of 9.75 cm and spatial resolution of 6.00 mm full width half maximum) of the chest was performed 45 minutes after [18]FDG injection.

Image Interpretation

Coronal PET images (from anterior to posterior) of the lower extremities from the level of symphysis pubis to above the knees (Fig. A) show a large mass with a hypermetabolic rim and central region of diminished activity highly suspicious for malignancy with probable central necrosis.

Differential Diagnosis

- Other histological types of soft tissue sarcoma (e.g., liposarcoma, angiosarcoma)
- Abscess
- Noninfectious myositis with associated necrosis
- Metastatic disease

Diagnosis and Clinical Follow-up

An MRI delineated the anatomic location of the mass to the adductor compartment. The lesion measured approximately 16.2 cm in craniocaudal dimension without bony invasion. An excisional biopsy was performed, and the surgical specimen revealed spindle cell sarcoma.

Discussion

[18]FDG PET has been shown to be useful for preoperative staging, defining extent of disease, assessing recurrence post-therapy, and differential diagnosis of high-grade versus low-grade malignancies.

PEARLS/PITFALLS

- PET provides important information regarding the presence and viability of tumor post-therapy. This information is useful in guiding appropriate management.

- FDG PET may not be able to discriminate benign from low-grade malignant tumors.

Suggested Readings

Griffeth LK, Dehdashti F, McGuire AH, et al. PET evaluation of soft tissue masses with fluorine-18 fluoro-2-deoxy-d-glucose. *Radiology* 182:185–194, 1992.

Kole AC, Nieweg OE, van Ginkel RJ, et al. Detection of local recurrence of soft-tissue sarcoma with positron emission tomography using [18F]fluorodeoxyglucose. *Ann Surg Oncol* 4:57–63, 1997.

Nieweg OE, Pruim J, vanGinkel RJ, et al. Fluorodeoxyglucose PET imaging of soft-tissue sarcoma. *J Nucl Med* 37:257–261, 1996.

Section VI

Inflammation Imaging

Case 99

Clinical Presentation

28-year-old man presenting with a history of a gunshot wound to the tibia. The radiograph of the tibia showed possible osteomyelitis.

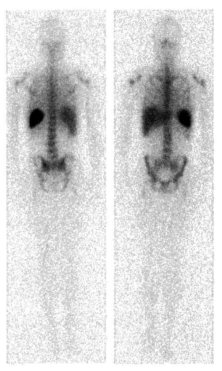

Fig. A

Technique

- Use care in identifying and labeling patient blood samples to ensure that blood products are re-administered to the patient from whom they were taken.

  Follow the procedures of your institution for white blood cell (WBC) collection and labeling with indium-111. An example follows:

- Aspirate 5 mL anticoagulant citrate dextrose solution (ACD) in each of three 20-cc syringes.
- Using a 19-gauge needle, withdraw 15 mL of blood into each of the three syringes.
- Do not use an intravenous line.
- Immediately take blood to the radiopharmacy department for labeling.
- As soon as the labeling is completed, log in the labeled WBC syringes, verify patient name and number, and inject blood into patient within 60 minutes of labeling.
- Image at 24 hours after injection, obtaining anterior and posterior images of the whole body and spot views of the region of interest as necessary.

PEARLS/PITFALLS

- You should be familiar with the normal distribution of labeled WBCs, as noted in Figure A. Bony uptake can be irregular and follows the distribution of red marrow. The proximal extremities in adults often show patchy red marrow distribution. Diffuse lung uptake is normal on early images (< 4 hours).

- In-111 labeled WBCs should be injected as soon as possible following labeling.

- In-111 labeled WBCs can be injected right after bone scan images are obtained in the workup of osteomyelitis. The energy of the bone radiopharmaceutical can be excluded from the WBC images if the gamma camera energy window is set for the higher energy of In-111 gamma photons.

- Labeling of WBCs requires experience and care. Make sure the radiopharmacy is experienced in the handling and labeling of WBCs. Viewing analog images set at only one exposure setting will not allow complete evaluation of both the liver and spleen and the extrasplenic soft tissues. Make certain you view images on a computer system that allows adjustment of background subtraction and pixel intensity. This will allow more complete evaluation of the liver and spleen, which demonstrate intense uptake of the tracer, and the extrasplenic soft tissues that concentrate the tracer less avidly.

- The preferred agent for imaging inflammation is often debated and should be chosen based on individual patient needs and the physician's experience with each of the three most common agents: Ga-67 citrate or WBCs labeled with Tc-99m or In-111.

Image Interpretation

Whole-body images (Fig. A) demonstrate normal tracer distribution. No evidence of abnormal focal uptake is seen in the region of the tibial lesion on spot views (not shown).

Differential Diagnosis

- Normal indium-111 WBC scan
- Poor labeling of WBCs, causing false-negative results
- Injection of WBCs too long after labeling (> 2 hours)

Diagnosis and Clinical Follow-up

The patient continued to recover without evidence of osteomyelitis.

Discussion

Indium 111–labeled WBC imaging is a sensitive, specific test for the diagnosis of focal inflammatory changes. It can be used in both soft tissue infections and osteomyelitis. When white cells are used for the diagnosis of osteomyelitis in bone containing red marrow, it may be necessary to compare the pattern of white cell uptake with that of labeled colloid. Red marrow will normally concentrate labeled WBCs and the difference between normal marrow concentration of labeled white cells and concentration at sites of inflammation may not be great. The colloid will provide information about normal marrow distribution. If the white cells are seen where there is no colloid uptake, infection should be suspected.

Suggested Readings

Alazraki NP. Radionuclide imaging in the evaluation of infections and inflammatory disease. *Radiol Clin North Am* 31:783–794, 1993.

Harbert JC. The musculoskeletal system. In: Harbert JC, Eckelman WC, Neumann RD, eds. *Nuclear Medicine Diagnosis and Therapy*. New York: Thieme, 1996, p. 801–863.

Mountford PJ, Kettle AG, MJ OD, et al. Comparison of technetium-99m-HM-PAO leukocytes with indium-111-oxine leukocytes for localizing intraabdominal sepsis. *J Nucl Med* 31:311–315, 1990.

Schauwecker DS. Osteomyelitis: Diagnosis with In-111-labeled leukocytes. *Radiology* 171:141–146, 1989.

Schauwecker DS. The scintigraphic diagnosis of osteomyelitis. *AJR Am J Roentgenol* 158:9–18, 1992.

Seabold JE, Forstrom LA, Schauwecker DS, et al. Procedure guideline for indium-111-leukocyte scintigraphy for suspected infection/inflammation. Society of Nuclear Medicine. *J Nucl Med* 38:997–1001, 1997.

Case 100

Clinical Presentation

79-year-old woman presents with a recent colostomy for diverticulitis and perforation. She now has an elevated white blood cell (WBC) count and fever.

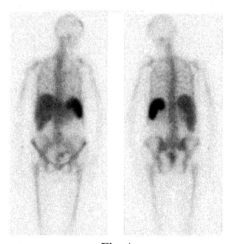

Fig. A

Technique

- Use care in identifying and labeling patient blood samples to ensure that blood products are administered to the patient from whom they were taken.

  Follow the procedures of your institution for WBC collection and labeling with In-111. An example follows:

- Aspirate 5 mL anticoagulant citrate dextrose (ACD) in each of three 20-cc syringes.
- Using a 19-gauge needle, withdraw 15 mL of blood into each of the three syringes.
- Do not use an intravenous line.
- Immediately take blood to the radiopharmacy department for labeling.
- As soon as labeling is completed, log in the labeled WBC syringes, verify patient name and number, and inject into patient as soon as possible or at least within 30 minutes of labeling.
- Image at 24 hours after injection, obtaining anterior and posterior images of the whole body and spot views of the region of interest as necessary.

Image Interpretation

Anterior and posterior whole-body views (Fig. A) show an area of tracer concentration in the left pelvis.

Differential Diagnosis

- Abscess
- Cellulitis
- Diverticulitis
- Ulcerative colitis
- Phlegmon
- Cystitis
- Foreign body (such as indwelling catheter)
- Ostomy
- Postsurgical inflammatory changes
- Active bleeding at the time of tracer injection

Diagnosis and Clinical Follow-up

Computed tomography (CT) scan revealed an 8 cm × 5 cm × 5 cm abscess in the pelvis that was drained under CT guidance.

Discussion

Labeled WBCs are preferred to GA-67 citrate for imaging the abdomen. The normal excretion of gallium into the bowel can hide focal abnormalities, and therefore the use of gallium often requires delayed imaging to clear activity in the bowel. Delayed imaging, however, does not always resolve the question, particularly when there is poor gastrointestinal motility. Indium-111 WBCs are not normally seen in the abdomen up to 24 hours after injection. Any concentration of tracer in the abdomen is therefore easier to detect and more specific for inflammation.

Tc-99m–labeled WBCs, like Ga-67 citrate, will result in tracer in the bowel 3 to 4 hours after injection. The tracer seen in the bowel is likely the breakdown product of the Tc-99m label, which is excreted through the biliary collecting system.

Suggested Readings

Mountford PJ, Kettle AG, MJ OD, et al. Comparison of technetium-99m-HM-PAO leukocytes with indium-111-oxine leukocytes for localizing intraabdominal sepsis. *J Nucl Med* 31:311–315, 1990.

O'Neill H, Stack JP, Malone LA, et al. Complementary role of computerised tomography and indium-111 labelled leucocytes in the management of sepsis. *Eur J Radiol* 9:134–136, 1989.

Case 101

Clinical Presentation

36-year-old woman with a history of subacute bacterial endocarditis presenting with fever of unknown origin (FUO).

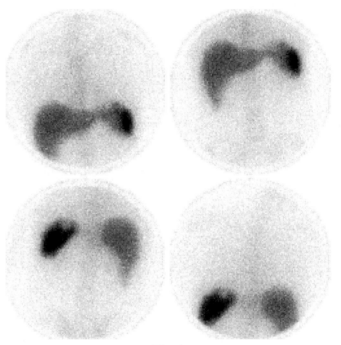

Fig. A

Technique

- Use care in identifying and labeling patient blood samples to ensure that blood products are administered to the patient from whom they were taken.

  Follow the procedures of your institution for white blood cell (WBC) collection and labeling with indium-111. An example follows:

- Aspirate 5 mL anticoagulant citrate dextrose (ACD) in each of three 20-cc syringes.
- Using a 19-gauge needle, withdraw 15 mL of blood into each of the three syringes.
- Do not use an intravenous line.
- Immediately take blood to the radiopharmacy for labeling.
- As soon as labeling is completed, log in the labeled WBC syringes, verify patient name and number, and inject into patient as soon as possible or at least within 30 minutes of labeling.
- Image at 24 hours after injection, obtaining anterior and posterior images of the whole body and spot views of the region of interest as necessary.

Image Interpretation

Planar images (Fig. A) show a defect in the upper pole of the spleen.

Differential Diagnosis

- Cyst
- Abscess
- Hemorrhage
- Infarct
- Extrinsic compression
- Hemangioma
- Metastasis

Diagnosis and Clinical Follow-up

Ultrasound showed a lesion in the upper pole of the spleen with central liquefaction consistent with abscess. Antibiotics were started based on the results of the blood cultures. The splenic defect decreased in size over the next several weeks.

Discussion

Because of the normally intense tracer uptake in the spleen, inflammatory lesions cannot be identified unless they are accompanied by a space-occupying process, such as the abscess with central liquefaction seen in this case. The spleen size and contour should therefore always be assessed when imaging radiolabeled WBCs.

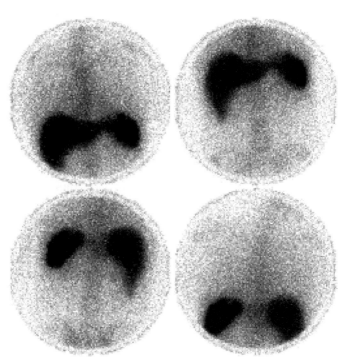

Fig. B

The digital image data should be evaluated on a computer system that allows adjustment of background subtraction and pixel intensity. If the only images available are adjusted for optimal evaluation of extrasplenic soft tissues, the spleen is often too intense to allow resolution of any contour abnormalities. Figure B shows the same images seen in Figure A but adjusted for evaluation of extrasplenic soft tissues. The splenic abscess is no longer visible.

Suggested Readings

Alazraki NP. Radionuclide imaging in the evaluation of infections and inflammatory disease. *Radiol Clin North Am* 31:783–794, 1993.

Datz FL. Abdominal abscess detection: Gallium, 111ln-, and 99mTc-labeled leukocytes, and polyclonal and monoclonal antibodies. *Semin Nucl Med* 26:51–64, 1996.

Mansfield JC, Giaffer MH, Tindale WB, Holdsworth CD. Quantitative assessment of overall inflammatory bowel disease activity using labelled leucocytes: A direct comparison between indium-111 and technetium-99m HMPAO methods. *Gut* 37:679–683, 1995.

Mountford PJ, Kettle AG, MJ OD, et al. Comparison of technetium-99m-HM-PAO leukocytes with indium-111-oxine leukocytes for localizing intraabdominal sepsis. *J Nucl Med* 31:311–315, 1990.

Seabold JE, Forstrom LA, Schauwecker DS, et al. Procedure guideline for indium-111-leukocyte scintigraphy for suspected infection/inflammation. Society of Nuclear Medicine. *J Nucl Med* 38:997–1001, 1997.

Case 102

Clinical Presentation

68-year-old woman presenting with metastatic ovarian cancer and fever of unknown origin.

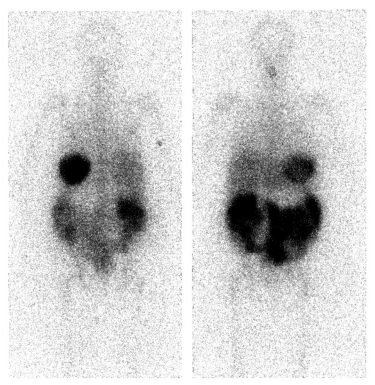

Fig. A

Technique

- Use care in identifying and labeling patient blood samples to ensure that blood products are administered to the patient from whom they were taken.

  Follow the procedures of your institution for white blood cell (WBC) collection and labeling with indium-111. An example follows:

- Aspirate 5 mL anticoagulant citrate dextrose (ACD) in each of three 20-cc syringes.
- Using a 19-gauge needle, withdraw 15 mL of blood into each of the three syringes.
- Do not use an intravenous line.
- Immediately take blood to the radiopharmacy for labeling.
- As soon as labeling is completed, log in the labeled WBC syringes, verify patient name and number, and inject into patient as soon as possible or at least within 30 minutes of labeling.
- Image at 24 hours after injection, obtaining anterior and posterior images of the whole body and spot views of the region of interest as necessary.

Image Interpretation

The 24-hour images (Fig. A) demonstrate intense tracer uptake in the abdomen in a pattern suggesting peritoneal localization.

Differential Diagnosis

- Peritonitis
- Metastatic disease
- Crohn's disease

Diagnosis and Clinical Follow-up

A computed tomography (CT) scan demonstrated diffuse studding of metastatic disease throughout the peritoneum. A small loculated perisplenic fluid collection was noted and drained with no organisms seen, no growth on culture, and no resolution of fever following drainage. Additional extensive workup for fever demonstrated no evidence of infection. Fever did not respond to empiric course of antibiotics.

The final diagnosis was "tumor fever" caused by the disseminated metastatic disease to the peritoneum.

Discussion

This is a very unusual case, demonstrating diffuse uptake of the labeled WBCs throughout the abdominal cavity. The pattern is similar to the distribution of the peritoneum. With the known disseminated peritoneal spread of disease and the lack of other causative organism, the diagnosis (by exclusion) was of tumor fever. It is not surprising that the extensive inflammation in the abdomen would be responsible for fever.

Suggested Readings

Lamki LM, Kasi LP, Haynie TP. Localization of indium-111 leukocytes in noninfected neoplasms. *J Nucl Med* 29:1921–1926, 1988.

Schmidt KG, Rasmussen JW, Wedebye IM, et al. Accumulation of indium-111-labeled granulocytes in malignant tumors. *J Nucl Med* 29:479–484, 1988.

Case 103

Clinical Presentation

26-year-old man presents with Crohn's disease.

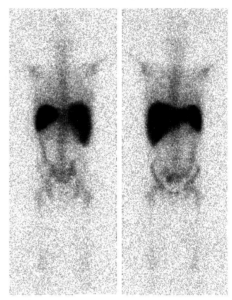

Fig. A

Technique

- Use care in identifying and labeling patient blood samples to ensure that blood products are administered to the patient from whom they were taken.

  Follow the procedures of your institution for white blood cell (WBC) collection and labeling with indium-111. An example follows:

- Aspirate 5 mL anticoagulant-citrate-dextrose (ACD) in each of three 20-cc syringes.
- Using a 19-gauge needle, withdraw 15 mL of blood into each of the three syringes.
- Do not use an intravenous line.
- Immediately take blood to the radiopharmacy for labeling.
- As soon as labeling is completed, log in the labeled WBC syringes, verify patient name and number, and inject into patient as soon as possible or at least within 30 minutes of labeling.
- Image at 24 hours after injection, obtaining anterior and posterior images of the whole body and spot views of the region of interest as necessary.

Image Interpretation

The 24-hour whole-body images (Fig. A) show tracer uptake from the splenic flexure to the sigmoid.

Differential Diagnosis

- Inflammatory bowel disease
- Gastrointestinal hemorrhage
- Diverticulitis
- Bowel infarction
- Swallowed WBCs

Diagnosis and Clinical Follow-up

Barium enema showed mucosal irregularity from the splenic flexure down the descending colon and narrowing of the sigmoid, consistent with inflammatory bowel disease (IBD).

Discussion

Radiolabeled WBCs can provide important information about the extent of inflammation in IBD. Both technetium-99m– and indium-111–labeled WBCs can provide information about bowel uptake and demonstrate localized abscesses or peritonitis.

Suggested Readings

Arndt JW, van der Sluys Veer A, Blok D, et al. Prospective comparative study of technetium-99m-WBCs and indium-111-granulocytes for the examination of patients with inflammatory bowel disease. *J Nucl Med* 34:1052–1057, 1993.

Even-Sapir E, Barnes DC, Martin RH, et al. Indium-111-white blood cell scintigraphy in Crohn's patients with fistulae and sinus tracts. *J Nucl Med* 35:245–250, 1994.

Giaffer MH, Tindale WB, Holdsworth D. Value of technetium-99m HMPAO-labelled leucocyte scintigraphy as an initial screening test in patients suspected of having inflammatory bowel disease. *Eur J Gastroenterol Hepatol* 8:1195–1200, 1996.

Mansfield JC, Giaffer MH, Tindale WB, et al. Quantitative assessment of overall inflammatory bowel disease activity using labelled leucocytes: A direct comparison between indium-111 and technetium-99m HMPAO methods. *Gut* 37:679–683, 1995.

Miller JH. The role of radionuclide-labeled cells in the diagnosis of abdominal disease in children. *Semin Nucl Med* 23:219–230, 1993.

Case 104

Clinical Presentation

28-year-old woman with a history of Crohn's disease presents with abdominal pain and fevers.

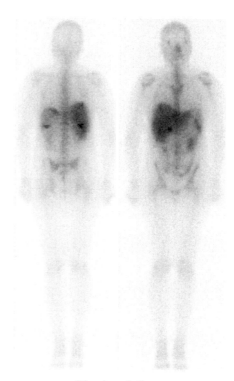

Fig. A—3 days

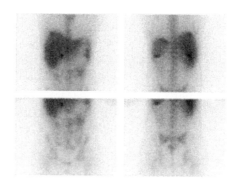

Fig. B—6 days

Technique

- 6 mCi of gallium-67 citrate intravenously.
- Whole-body planar images or spot views of the whole body and SPECT imaging are generally obtained at 3 days; delayed images may be obtained up to 14 days post-injection.
- Medium-energy collimator.

PEARLS/PITFALLS

- Delayed images over several days will help to distinguish normal bowel activity from focal inflammatory disease.

- SPECT images of the abdomen will also help to distinguish tracer concentration in the bowel from surrounding tissues and have significantly decreased the number of patients called back for delayed images in some institutions.

- Gallium movement in the cecum is often sluggish. Delayed clearance of tracer from the cecum over several days should not be read as abnormal unless there is other evidence of local inflammation.

- Bowel cleansing procedures such as enemas and laxatives to improve clearance of gallium from the colon are advocated by some investigators, but the relative risks and benefits of these procedures are not clear.

- Energy windows are 20% centered on the 93.3 keV, 184.5 keV, and 296 keV photopeaks.

Image Interpretation

Initial whole body images obtained 3 days after tracer injection (Fig. A) and delayed images obtained at 6 days (Fig. B) demonstrate focally increased tracer accumulation in the region of the liver and the spleen. The delayed images show that several sites of uptake in the abdomen do not show interval movement.

Differential Diagnosis

- Abdominal abscesses
- Ulcerative colitis
- Lymphoma
- Diverticulitis
- Bilateral pyelonephritis
- Active gastrointestinal hemorrhage at the time of tracer injection

Diagnosis and Clinical Follow-up

Patient had a history of colonic perforation. Computed tomography (CT) scan demonstrated evidence of abscesses in the regions of gallium uptake. Needle biopsy revealed purulent material. Surgical resection of multiple abscess cavities was performed.

Discussion

Normal bowel excretion of the tracer makes detection of abdominal sites of infection more difficult with gallium than with labeled white blood cells. Delayed images of the abdomen over several days, however, often show movement of gallium normally excreted in the bowel, distinguishing it from sites of inflammatory uptake that do not show movement over time. In this patient, the focal sites of uptake are not in a pattern consistent with normal tracer accumulation in the bowel. This pattern of tracer uptake suggests focal inflammatory disease even in the first set of images.

Suggested Readings

Datz FL. Abdominal abscess detection: Gallium, 111In-, and 99mTc-labeled leukocytes, and polyclonal and monoclonal antibodies. *Semin Nucl Med* 26:51–64, 1996.

Gerzof SG, Oates ME. Imaging techniques for infections in the surgical patient. *Surg Clin North Am* 68:147–165, 1988.

Case 105

Clinical Presentation

41-year-old man presenting with abdominal pain and fever of unknown origin (FUO).

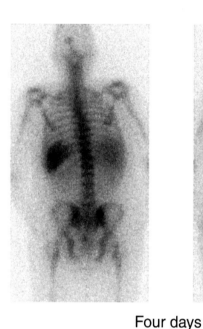
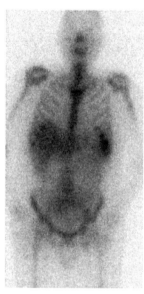

Four days
Fig. A

Six days

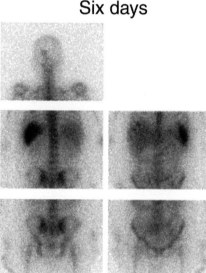

Posterior   Anterior
Fig. B

Technique

- 6 mCi of gallium-67 citrate intravenously.
- Whole-body planar images or spot views of the whole body and SPECT imaging are generally obtained at 3 days; delayed images may be obtained up to 14 days post-injection.
- Medium-energy collimator.
- Energy windows are 20% centered on the 93.3 keV, 184.5 keV, 296 keV photopeaks.

Image Interpretation

Images at 4 days (Fig. A) and 6 days (Fig. B) post-injection of tracer demonstrate increased tracer uptake in the spleen, a defect at the top of the spleen, and a focus of abnormal tracer concentration in the posterior aspect of the head to the left of midline.

Differential Diagnosis

- Multiple abscesses
- Metastatic disease

- Toxoplasmosis
- Cerebritis
- Osteomyelitis of the skull

Diagnosis and Clinical Follow-up

A computed tomography (CT) scan demonstrated a 3-cm enhancing lesion in the left occipitoparietal area of the brain and a second 3-cm lesion in the right subinsular cortex. No bone involvement was noted. Two craniotomies were performed at the two sites which revealed two abscesses, which were drained. The patient recovered after antibiotic therapy.

Discussion

The advantage of radioisotopic imaging of FUO is that the entire body can be surveyed. In this case, no localizing symptoms suggesting brain involvement were present. If anatomic imaging had been used to survey the abdomen and pelvis, the splenic lesion might have been diagnosed as the cause of the FUO, with no further investigation. This strategy could have led to problems in this patient if either abscess in the brain had evolved to result in a neurological deficit. Additional oblique views or SPECT views of the head might have resulted in better localization and differentiation of the brain lesions in this patient.

Suggested Readings

Orsolon P, Bagni B, Talmassons G, et al. Evaluation of a patient with a brain abscess caused by nocardia asteroides infection with Ga-67 and Tc-99m HMPAO leukocytes. *Clin Nucl Med* 22:407–408, 1997.

Waxman AD, Siemsen JK. Gallium scanning in cerebral and cranial infections. *Am J Roentgenol* 127:309–314, 1976.

Case 106

Clinical Presentation

36-year-old man with a history of intravenous drug abuse presenting with right hip and flank pain radiating down his right leg.

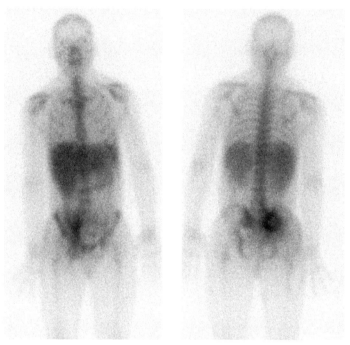

Fig. A

Technique

- 6 mCi of gallium-67 citrate intravenously.
- Whole-body planar images or spot views of the whole body and SPECT imaging are generally obtained at 3 days; delayed images may be obtained up to 14 days post-injection.
- Medium-energy collimator.
- Energy windows are 20% centered on the 93.3 keV, 184.5 keV, and 296 keV photopeaks.

Image Interpretation

Intense tracer uptake is noted in the region of the right sacroiliac joint (Fig. A). Faint tracer uptake is also noted in the soft tissues of the right buttock.

Differential Diagnosis

- Osteomyelitis
- Soft tissue infection or inflammation
- Acute trauma
- Malignancy

PEARLS/PITFALLS

- In osteomyelitis, the gallium scan demonstrates more extensive and more intense uptake when compared with the pattern of uptake seen with bone tracers.

- Gallium scans are often positive at sites of trauma. It is difficult to distinguish noninfectious from infectious causes of local inflammation.

- The value of the combined bone and gallium scans versus MRI for the diagnosis of osteomyelitis has been debated. In difficult cases, all three studies may be needed to make the most accurate diagnosis.

- The usefulness of bone scan and gallium scan for the diagnosis of osteomyelitis in the diabetic foot has been questioned. Because of the extensive bone trauma that can occur in the diabetic foot with resulting inflammatory changes, the most reliable indicator of osteomyelitis may be combined bone and labeled WBC scans.

Diagnosis and Clinical Follow-up

Findings consistent with osteomyelitis. A correlative bone scan (see Case 17) demonstrates increased tracer uptake in the same region. Magnetic resonance imaging (MRI) of the region demonstrates local sacroiliac bone destruction and edema of adjacent gluteus muscles.

Discussion

Three-phase bone scans have a high sensitivity and specificity for osteomyelitis when plain radiographs are normal. When the three-phase bone scan results are equivocal or when the radiographs are not normal, gallium scanning can be useful in distinguishing normal bone remodeling secondary to trauma from repair secondary to underlying osteomyelitis.

In this case, the bone scan was not completely consistent with osteomyelitis because the flow phase of the bone scan was normal. This was probably because the scan was done in an anterior projection, which was thought to be optimal for viewing the hips. The gallium scan shows intense tracer accumulation at the site of the abnormality noted on bone scan and is more intense than the bone tracer uptake suggesting a primary inflammatory process.

Suggested Readings

Etchebehere EC, Etchebehere M, Gamba R, et al. Orthopedic pathology of the lower extremities: Scintigraphic evaluation in the thigh, knee, and leg. *Semin Nucl Med* 28:41–61, 1998.

Johnson JE, Kennedy EJ, Shereff MJ, et al. Prospective study of bone, indium-111-labeled white blood cell, and gallium-67 scanning for the evaluation of osteomyelitis in the diabetic foot. *Foot Ankle Int* 17:10–16, 1996.

Palestro CJ, Torres MA. Radionuclide imaging in orthopedic infections. *Semin Nucl Med* 27:334–345, 1997.

Streek PV, Carretta RF, Weiland FL, et al. Upper extremity radionuclide bone imaging: The wrist and hand. *Semin Nucl Med* 28:14–24, 1998.

Section VII

Imaging in Acquired Immunodeficiency Syndrome

Case 107

Clinical Presentation

30-year-old man positive for human immunodeficiency virus (HIV+) presenting with shortness of breath and cough. His symptoms were not relieved with a 6-week course of antibiotics. Three bronchoscopies with transbronchial biopsies were negative.

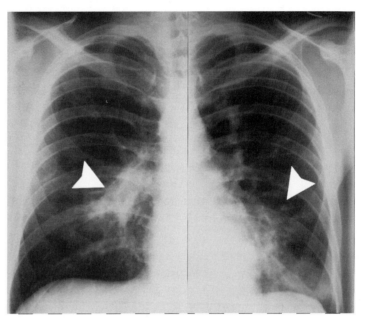

Fig. A

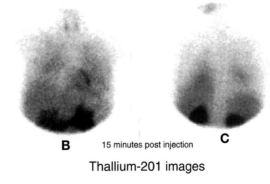

B   15 minutes post injection   C

Thallium-201 images

3 hours post injection

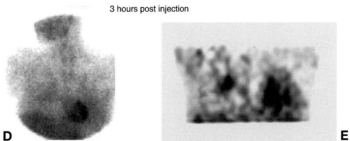

D   E

Figs. B, C, D, E

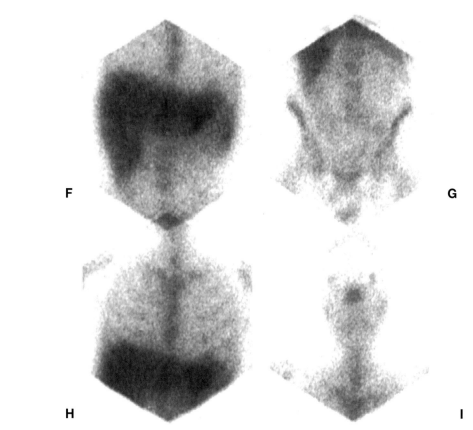

F   G

H   I

Figs. F, G, H, I

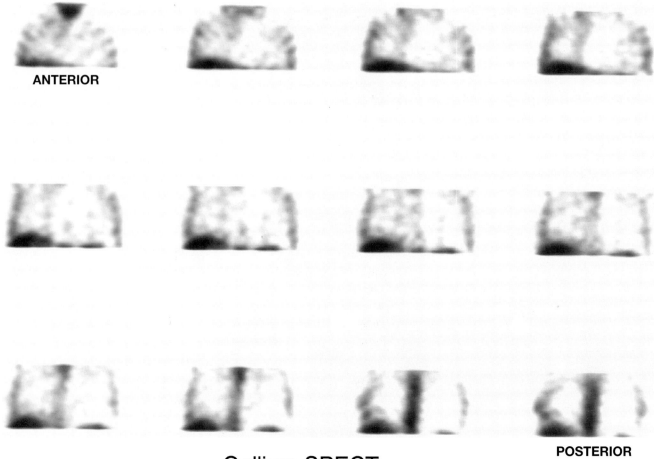

ANTERIOR

POSTERIOR

Gallium SPECT

Fig. J

PEARLS/PITFALLS

- Correlation with findings on other studies is important.

- The thallium-201 scan must be performed prior to the gallium-67 scan, because downscatter from the higher gallium-67 energies into the thallium-201 window will degrade the images.

- Inflammation or edema can cause early uptake of thallium which will subside on delayed images.

- Pulmonary gallium-67 uptake can be seen at 24 hours in normal studies; normal lung tissue will clear by 48 hours.

Technique
Thallium-201 Scan

- 3 mCi of thallium-201 thallous chloride administered intravenously.
- High-resolution or low-energy all-purpose collimator.
- Energy windows are 20% centered on 71 keV and 168 keV.
- Imaging time for statics is 0.5 million counts for the chest image; all others are for the same time.
- Single photon emission computed tomography (SPECT) is performed as 64 stops, 30 to 40 seconds/stop.
- Early static images are obtained starting at 15 minutes after injection. Delayed static and tomographic views are obtained at 3 hours.

Gallium-67 Scan

- 8 to 10 mCi of gallium-67 citrate administered intravenously.
- Medium-energy collimator.
- Energy windows are 20% centered on the 93.3 keV, 184.5 keV, and 296 keV photopeaks.
- Imaging time for statics is 10 minutes per image.
- SPECT is performed as 64 stops, 30 to 40 seconds/stop.
- Static and SPECT views are generally obtained 3 days post-injection. Follow-up views to allow clearing of bowel uptake may be obtained up to 14 days post-injection.

Image Interpretation

The chest X-ray in Figure A demonstrates infiltrates in the left lower and right lower lobes. The thallium-201 study shows bilateral lower lobe uptake in the early images obtained 15 minutes post-injection (Fig. B, anterior chest; Fig. C, posterior chest). An anterior chest image (Fig. D) and a single coronal slice (Fig. E) demonstrate persistent uptake in the delayed (3-hour) images.

Anterior liver (Fig. F), abdomen (Fig. G), chest (Fig. H), and head (Fig. I) images were obtained 72 hours after injection of gallium-67 citrate. Coronal SPECT slices of the chest are displayed in Figure J. All images demonstrate normal uptake of gallium; there are no foci of increased uptake in the chest.

Differential Diagnosis

(lung uptake of thallium-201)

- Kaposi's sarcoma
- Cytomegalovirus pneumonia
- Left ventricular failure
- Lung cancer (usually not diffuse tracer uptake)
- Tuberculosis
- Lymphangitic carcinomatosis

Diagnosis and Clinical Follow-up

A biopsy obtained during bronchoscopy 1 week later was positive for pulmonary Kaposi's sarcoma.

Discussion

Kaposi's sarcoma occurs frequently in patients with acquired immunodeficiency syndrome (AIDS). Identification of skin lesions is not difficult, but pulmonary lesions pose a diagnostic dilemma because radiographic findings are variable and nonspecific.

Increased thallium-201 uptake has been described in several tumor types (breast, lymphoma, thyroid, etc.), including Kaposi's sarcoma. Although thallium-201 is a potassium analog and is known to be transported into cells, the exact mechanism for preferential concentration in tumors is unknown.

Patients with AIDS are also predisposed to develop non-Hodgkin's lymphoma, which is also thallium-201 avid. To distinguish lymphoma from Kaposi's sarcoma, a follow-up gallium-67 study is performed. Lymphoma tumors are both thallium-201 and gallium-67 avid, whereas Kaposi's sarcoma only concentrates thallium-201.

Gallium-67 citrate is taken up by several tumors (lymphomas, melanomas, osteosarcoma, etc.) and also localizes in sites of infection and inflammation. Gallium is an iron analog that is incorporated into leukocytes and bacteria and binds to lactoferrin and bacterial siderophores in sites of infection and inflammation. As an iron analog, gallium-67 citrate also binds to transferrin in the plasma. The mechanism of uptake in tumors is most likely related to the expression of transferrin receptors and the binding of the gallium-67 citrate–transferrin complex.

Suggested Readings

Getz JM, Bekerman C. Diagnostic significance of Tl-201-Ga-67 discordant pattern of biodistribution in AIDS. *Clin Nuc Med* 19:1117–1118, 1993.

Gomez MDV, Beiras JMC, Gallardo FG, Verdejo J. Thallium and gallium scintigraphy in pulmonary Kaposi's sarcoma in an HIV-positive patient. *Clin Nuc Med* 19:467–468, 1994.

Lee VW, Fuller JD, O'Brien MJ, et al. Pulmonary Kaposi sarcoma in patients with AIDS: Scintigraphic diagnosis with sequential thallium and gallium scanning. *Radiology* 180:409–412, 1991.

Lee VW, Rosen MP, Baum A, et al. AIDS-related Kaposi sarcoma: Findings on thallium-201 scinitgraphy. *AJR Am J Roentgenol* 151:1233–1235, 1988.

Tsan MF. Mechanism of gallium-67 accumulation in inflammatory lesions. *J Nucl Med* 26:88–92, 1985.

Case 108

Clinical Presentation

32-year-old man positive for human immunodeficiency virus (HIV+) presents with cough and fever.

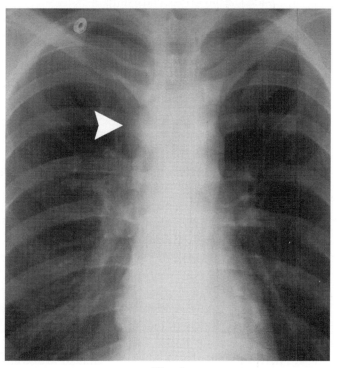

Fig. A

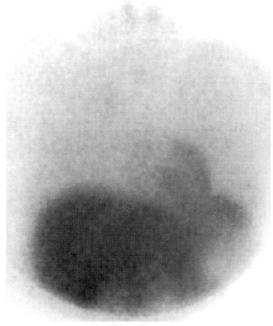

Fig. B—Thallium

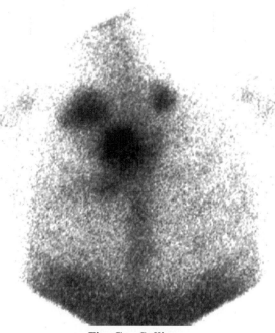

Fig. C—Gallium

Technique

Thallium-201 Scan

- 3 mCi of thallium-201 thallous chloride administered intravenously.
- High-resolution or low-energy all-purpose collimator.
- Energy windows are 20% centered on 71 keV and 168 keV.
- Imaging time for statics is 0.5 million counts for the chest image; all others are for the same time.
- Single photon emission computed tomography (SPECT) is performed as 64 stops, 30 to 40 seconds/stop.
- Early statics are obtained starting at 15 minutes after injection. Delayed static and tomographic views are obtained at 3 hours.

Gallium-67 Scan

- 8 to 10 mCi of gallium-67 citrate administered intravenously.
- Medium-energy collimator.
- Energy windows are 20% centered on the 93.3 keV, 184.5 keV, and 296 keV photopeaks.
- Imaging time for statics is 10 minutes per image.
- SPECT is performed as 64 stops, 30 to 40 s/stop.
- Static and SPECT views are generally obtained 3 days post injection. Follow-up views to allow clearing of bowel uptake may be obtained up to 14 days post-injection.

Image Interpretation

The chest X-ray in Figure A demonstrates widening of the superior mediastinal and azygous lymph nodes (*arrow*). A 3-hour thallium image of the anterior chest is normal (Fig. B). A 48-hour gallium-67 image of the anterior chest (Fig. C) demonstrates intense increased uptake in mediastinal and supraclavicular nodes.

Differential Diagnosis

- Mycobacterial infection (*Mycobacterium tuberculosis* and *Mycobacterium avium intracellulare*)
- Lymphoma
- Lung cancer
- Sarcoidosis

Diagnosis and Clinical Follow-up

A follow-up biopsy and culture obtained during bronchoscopy was positive for *M. tuberculosis*.

Discussion

Gallium-67 citrate is known to concentrate at sites of infection, inflammation and in some tumors. Localization is dependent on intact blood supply. Gallium-67 citrate is an iron analog, binding to lactoferrin and bacterial siderophores. Thallium-201 is not retained at sites of inflammation or infection. Thallium-201 is known to concentrate in certain tumors, including lymphoma and Kaposi's sar-

PEARLS/PITFALLS

- Correlation with findings on other imaging modalities is important.

- The thallium-201 scan must be performed prior to the gallium-67 scan because downscatter from the higher gallium-67 energies into the thallium-201 window will degrade the images.

- The 3-hour thallium images are more important than the early images.

- Pulmonary gallium uptake can be seen at 24 hours in normal studies; the lungs will normally clear by 48 hours.

coma. Uptake is dependent on an intact blood supply, although the exact mechanism for preferential concentration in tumors is unknown.

Opportunistic infections are common among immunodeficient patients. The chest X-ray and computed tomography (CT) appearance are nonspecific and cannot be easily differentiated from pulmonary Kaposi's sarcoma. The early thallium-201 uptake at 15 to 30 minutes post-injection in lung infections is variable and may be confusing but will decrease in the delayed (3-hour) scan. The importance of delayed thallium-201 imaging, therefore, cannot be overemphasized.

Pathogens that are particularly gallium-67 citrate–avid include the mycobacteria (*M. tuberculosis* and *M. avium-intracellulare*), *Pneumocystis carinii pneumonia* (PCP), and common bacteria such as *Streptococcus pneumoniae* and *Haemophilus influenzae*. Focal nodal uptake is more common in mycobacterial infections; diffuse intense pulmonary uptake is more common in untreated cases of PCP. Gallium-67 has variable avidity for common viral agents such as cytomegalovirus and fungal pathogens such as cryptococcus and coccidioidomycosis. Gallium-67 has no known avidity for *Candida albicans*.

The studies in this case are consistent with an infectious process because the lesions are gallium-67 citrate and not thallium-201 avid. The nodal pattern of uptake is consistent with a mycobacterial infection (although *Cryptococcus* can present in the same manner).

Suggested Readings

Kramer, EL, The immunocompromised patient. In: Murray IPC, Ell PJ, eds. *Nuclear Medicine in Clinical Diagnosis and Treatment*. London: Churchill Livingstone, 1994.

Lee VW, Cooley TP, Fuller JD, Ward RJ, Farber HW. Pulmonary mycobacterial infections in AIDS: Characteristic pattern of thallium and gallium scan mismatch. *Radiology* 193:389–392, 1994.

Lee VW, Panageas E, Turnbull BA. Radionuclide evaluation of the chest in AIDS. In: Thrall JH, ed. *Current Practice of Radiology*. St. Louis, MO: Mosby, 1993.

Case 109

Clinical Presentation

28-year-old man positive for human immunodeficiency virus (HIV+) presents with an abdominal mass.

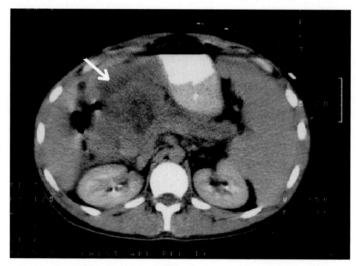

Fig. A

Thallium - 201

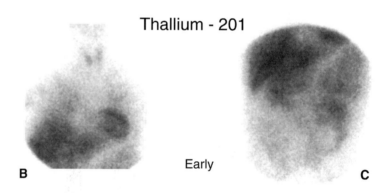

Early

B

C

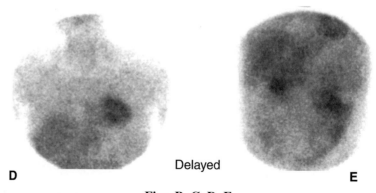

Delayed

D

E

Figs. B, C, D, E

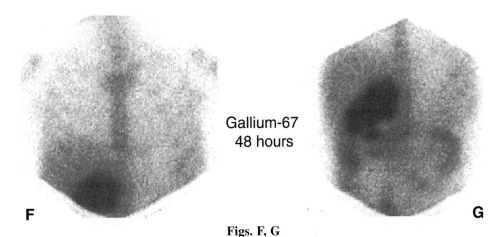

Gallium-67
48 hours

Figs. F, G

Technique

Thallium-201 Scan

- 3 mCi of thallium-201 thallous chloride administered intravenously.
- High-resolution or low-energy all-purpose collimator.
- Energy windows are 20% centered on 71 keV and 168 keV.
- Imaging time for statics is 0.5 million counts for the chest image; all others are for the same time.
- Single photon emission computed tomography (SPECT) is performed as 64 stops, 30 to 40 seconds/stop.
- Early statics are obtained starting at 15 minutes after injection. Delayed static and tomographic views are obtained at 3 hours.

Gallium-67 Scan

- 8 to 10 mCi of gallium-67 citrate administered intravenously.
- Medium-energy collimator.
- Energy windows are 20% centered on the 93.3 keV, 184.5 keV, and 296 keV photopeaks.
- Ten minutes per image.
- SPECT is performed as 64 stops, 30 to 40 seconds/stop.
- Static and SPECT views are generally obtained 3 days post-injection. Follow-up views to allow clearing of bowel uptake may be obtained up to 14 days post-injection.

Image Interpretation

The computed tomography scan in Figure A demonstrates a large mass in the head of the pancreas (*arrow*). The early thallium-201 images (Figs. B and C) show increased uptake in the right side of the chest and in the upper right abdomen. Delayed thallium-201 images (Figs. D and E) show clearance of the chest uptake and persistence of the abdominal uptake. The 48-hour gallium images of the chest (Fig. F) and abdomen (Fig. G) demonstrate intense increased uptake in the region of the head of the pancreas, concordant with the thallium-201 uptake.

Differential Diagnosis

(abdominal gallium and thallium uptake)

- Lymphoma
- Other malignancy
- Reactive lymph nodes
- Infection
- Cellulitis
- Crohn's disease
- Diverticulitis

Diagnosis and Clinical Follow-up

A follow-up biopsy was consistent with non-Hodgkin's lymphoma.

Discussion

Thallium-201 is known to concentrate in Kaposi's sarcoma and non-Hodgkin's lymphomas. Gallium-67 citrate localizes in lymphomas, with a greater affinity for the higher grade lymphomas (intermediate and high grades), but it will not localize in Kaposi's sarcoma (see Case 107).

Lymphoma is more prevalent in patients with acquired immunodeficiency syndrome than it is in the general population. Immunoblastic lymphoma, primary central nervous system lymphoma, and Burkitt's lymphoma are the most commonly encountered forms.

Suggested Readings

Kramer, EL. The immunocompromised patient. In: Murray IPC, Ell PJ, eds. *Nuclear Medicine in Clinical Diagnosis and Treatment.* London: Churchill Livingstone, 1994.

Lee VW, Panageas E, Turnbull BA. Radionuclide evaluation of the chest in AIDS. In: Thrall JH, ed. *Current Practice of Radiology.* St. Louis, MO: Mosby, 1993.

Case 110

Clinical Presentation

31-year-old HIV-seropositive man presents with a fever. A gallium scan was requested for further evaluation.

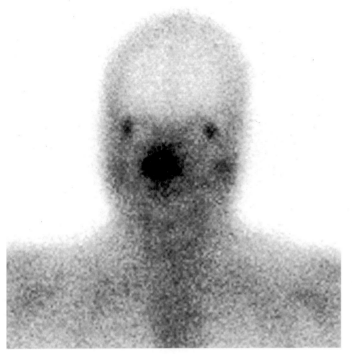

Fig. A

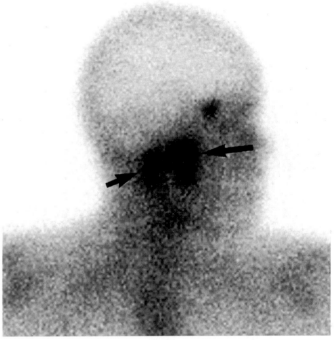

Fig. B

Technique

- 10 mCi of gallium-67 citrate intravenously.
- Medium-energy collimator.
- Energy window is 20% at 93, 184, and 296 keV.
- Planar and single photon emission computed tomography (SPECT) images are obtained 72 hours after tracer injection. Planar image is 1M counts per view; SPECT is 64 stops at 25 sec/stop, 360-degree rotation. No specific preparation is required.

Image Interpretation

Anterior view of the head and neck and upper chest (Fig. A) shows gallium uptake in the nasal region and salivary glands. Right lateral view of the head and neck (Fig. B) reveals normal tracer uptake in the parotid gland (*arrow*). In addition, there is a focus of increased uptake medially, in the posterior pharynx (*large arrow*).

- Focal nodal uptake in the chest, axilla, neck, or groin may suggest the diagnosis of lymphoma. Mycobacterial infections are another likely possibility, however.

- Uptake in a pattern suggestive of small bowel or mesenteric lymph node involvement may also be seen in both lymphoma and mycobacterial infection, particularly *Mycobacterium avium intracellulare*.

- Delayed images and/or SPECT may help differentiate physiological excretion of gallium into the bowel from pathologic involvement.

- Leukocytes labeled with technetium-99m HMPAO or indium-111 oxine may be useful in the differential diagnosis.

Differential Diagnosis

- Lymphoma
- Infection

Diagnosis and Clinical Follow-up

Biopsy of the nasopharyngeal mass revealed B-cell lymphoma. Patient was treated accordingly.

Discussion

AIDS-related lymphomas may differ clinically from non-AIDS lymphomas. Lymphomas in AIDS patients are more frequently non-Hodgkin's lymphomas and often B-cell lymphomas. Extranodal disease is more frequent, and the disease is usually more advanced on initial presentation. The high avidity of these lymphomas for gallium-67 citrate has been useful in their early detection.

Suggested Readings

Ferrozzi F, Bova D, Campodonico F, et al. AIDS related malignancies. *Eur Radiol* 55:477, 1995.

Nyberg DA, Jeffery RB, Federle MP, et al AIDS-related lymphomas; evaluation by abdominal CT. *Radiology* 159:59–63, 1986.

Schoeppel SL, Hoppe RT, Dorfman RF, et al. Hodgkin's disease in homosexual men with generalized lymphadenopathy. *Ann Intern Med* 102:68–70, 1985.

Case 111

Clinical Presentation

39-year-old man presenting with AIDS and multiple bone pain. Computed tomography (CT) of the pelvis showed lytic lesion in the left bone. A gallium-67 scan was requested for further evaluation.

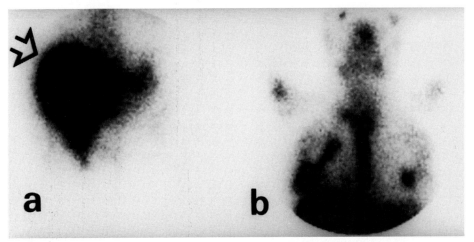

Fig. A

Technique

- 10 mCi gallium-67 citrate intravenously.
- Use medium-energy collimator.
- Energy window is 20% at 93, 184, and 296 keV.
- Imaging is performed 72 hours after tracer injection (1M counts/view).

Image Interpretation

Posterior view of the pelvis (Fig. Aa) shows extensive, intense tracer uptake in the left pelvis (*open arrow*). Anterior chest (Fig. Ab) shows multiple focal areas of intense tracer uptake involving several ribs as well as the right sterno-clavicular junction, sternum, and right humeral head.

Differential Diagnosis

- Skeletal lymphoma
- Multifocal osteomyelitis
- Metastatic skeletal disease

Diagnosis and Clinical Follow-up

Biopsy from left iliac bone was consistent with non-Hodgkin's lymphoma, B-cell type. Combined radiation as well as systemic chemotherapy were started, and a follow-up gallium scan showed significant improvement in the skeletal lesions.

PEARLS/PITFALLS

- Combined thallium-201 chloride and gallium-67 scans may be useful to differentiate lymphoma from Kaposi's sarcoma. Kaposi's sarcoma lesions are not gallium avid.

- A lytic lesion in a patient with AIDS with a negative gallium scan may represent Kaposi's sarcoma.

- Skeletal lymphoma cannot be differentiated from osteomyelitis on a gallium scan. Leukocytes labeling with either technetium-99m HMPAO or indium-111 oxine may be useful in the differential diagnosis.

- In the follow-up of any patient with skeletal lymphoma, gallium-citrate may remain falsely positive following treatment because of uptake in bony repair. The intensity of uptake is usually lower compared with the primary tumor, but residual disease cannot be totally excluded. In these cases, a combined thallium-201 chloride and gallium-67 scintigraphy may be helpful in evaluating residual disease (which may be thallium and gallium positive) versus bony repair (which will be thallium negative but can remain gallium positive).

Discussion

Primary musculoskeletal lymphoma is a rare disease. Secondary involvement of the bone in patients with Hodgkin's and non-Hodgkin's lymphoma is more common. In patients with AIDS there is no definite evidence of an absolute increase in the incidence of musculoskeletal Hodgkin's disease. This is in contrast to non-Hodgkin's lymphoma in AIDS patients who show more frequent involvement of the skeletal system, a more aggressive behavior, and a poorer response to treatment. Gallium-67 imaging is useful for early detection of skeletal lymphomas.

Suggested Readings

Lee DJ, Sartoris DJ, Musculoskeletal manifestation of human immunodeficiency virus infection. *Radiol Clin North Am* 32:399, 1994.

Nuclear medicine and AIDS. Kramer EL, Sanger JJ. Nuclear Medicine Annual. 1990.

Case 112

Clinical Presentation

38-year-old man with acquired immunodeficiency syndrome (AIDS) presenting with cough and shortness of breath.

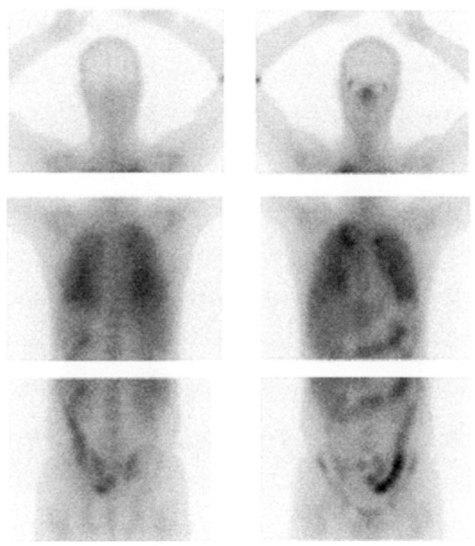

Fig. A

Technique

- 6 mCi of gallium-67 citrate intravenously.
- Whole-body planar images or spot views of the whole body and SPECT imaging are finally obtained at 3 days; delayed images may be obtained up to 14 days post-injection.
- Medium-energy collimator.
- Energy windows are 20% centered on the 93.3 keV, 184.5 keV, and 296 keV photopeaks.

- If the chest film shows a diffuse infiltrative pattern and the gallium scan shows no gallium concentration, Kaposi's sarcoma should be considered. Thallium scanning can be useful for the diagnosis of Kaposi's sarcoma.

- Diffuse pulmonary uptake may also be caused by ARDS, drug reaction, or imaging within 24 hours of tracer injection. The clinical condition of the patient and medical history should be considered before the study is read.

- The frequency with which the diffuse pattern of uptake is noted in PCP is not clear. With the frequent use of early antibiotic therapy, the diffuse pattern of uptake may be more the exception than the rule.

Image Interpretation

Images obtained 3 days after tracer injection (Fig. A) show diffuse, intense tracer uptake throughout the lung fields. There is slightly more intense concentration of tracer at the lung apices, more on the right than on the left. Delayed images at 7 days (not shown) demonstrate clearance of the tracer from the bowel.

Differential Diagnosis

- *Pneumocystis carinii* pneumonia (PCP)
- Acute respiratory distress syndrome (ARDS)
- Pulmonary inflammation secondary to chemotherapy
- Normal finding when imaging is done within 24 hours of tracer injection
- Imaging following lymphangiography
- Tuberculosis
- Pneumoconiosis
- Idiopathic pulmonary fibrosis
- Pulmonary reaction following radiation therapy

Diagnosis and Clinical Follow-up

Sputum analysis showed *Pneumocystis carinii*. The reason for the more intense uptake in the apices in this patient is not known.

Discussion

Gallium scanning can be very useful for documentation of inflammatory changes in the lungs. Anatomical studies, such as chest X-ray and computed tomography (CT) scan, demonstrate changes caused by inflammation but do not provide much information about current inflammatory activity. In patients with AIDS, diffuse lung uptake of gallium which appears more intense than that seen in the liver, is almost pathognomonic for PCP. Antibiotic therapy can change the diffuse pattern of lung uptake to a more patchy distribution, however, particularly in patients on inhalant therapy.

Suggested Readings

Abdel-Dayem HM, Bag R, DiFabrizio L, et al. Evaluation of sequential thallium and gallium scans of the chest in AIDS patients. *J Nucl Med* 37:1662–1667, 1996.

Jules-Elysee KM, Stover DE, Zaman MB, et al. Aerosolized pentamidine: Effect on diagnosis and presentation of *Pneumocystis carinii* pneumonia. *Ann Intern Med* 112:750–757, 1990.

Kroe DM, Kirsch CM, Jensen WA. Diagnostic strategies for *Pneumocystis carinii* pneumonia. *Semin Respir Infect* 12:70–78, 1997.

Woolfenden JM, Carrasquillo JA, Larson SM, et al. Acquired immunodeficiency syndrome: Ga-67 citrate imaging. *Radiology* 162:383–387, 1987.

Case 113

Clinical Presentation

37-year-old man with a history of acquired immunodeficiency syndrome (AIDS) presenting with slight fever and shortness of breath.

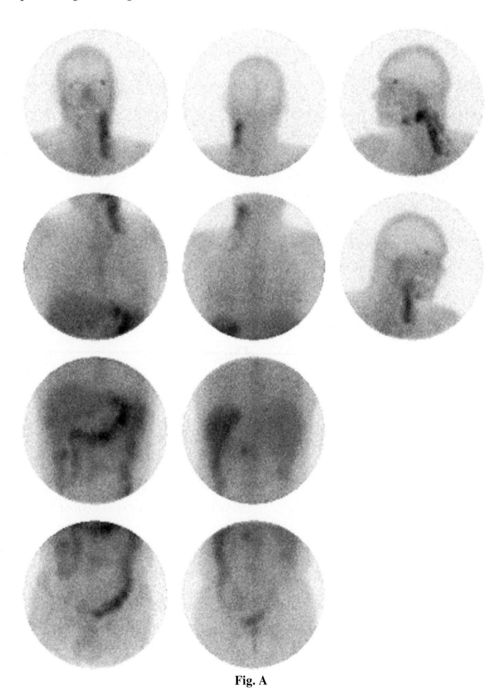

Fig. A

Technique

• Administer 6 mCi gallium-67 citrate intravenously.
• Whole-body planar images or spot views of the whole body and SPECT imaging obtained at 3 days; delayed images may be obtained at up to 14 days post-injection.
• Medium-energy collimator.
• Energy windows are 20% centered on the 93.3 keV, 184.5 keV, and 296 keV photopeaks.

Image Interpretation

Spot views of the anterior and posterior aspects of the body (Fig. A) from the head to the pelvis demonstrate tracer concentration in the left side of the neck and in the large bowel. Delayed images of the abdomen (not shown) show movement of the bowel activity.

Differential Diagnosis

• *Mycobacterium avium-intracellulare* infection
• Lymphoma
• Tuberculosis
• Multiple abscesses

Diagnosis and Clinical Follow-up

Biopsy of the nodes in the left side of the neck demonstrated *M. avium-intracellulare*.

Discussion

Gallium uptake is nonspecific, but the history and physical exam at presentation may help to modify the differential diagnosis. Uptake in a nodal chain in a patient with human immunodeficiency virus suggests lymphoma, tuberculosis, and *M. avium-intracellulare* infection.

Biopsy is probably warranted in most patients with lymphadenopathy because of the nonspecificity of gallium uptake. If the adenopathy is discovered to be lymphoma, gallium scanning can be a valuable tool for following response to therapy, but only if the tumor is known to be gallium positive prior to chemotherapy.

Suggested Readings

Buscombe JR, Buttery P, Ell PJ, et al. Patterns of Ga-67 citrate accumulation in human immunodeficiency virus positive patients with and without *Mycobacterium avium intracellulare* infection. *Clin Radiol* 50:483–488, 1995.

Gomez MV, Gallardo FG, Cobo J, et al. Identification of AIDS-related tuberculosis with concordant gallium-67 and three-hour delayed thallium-201 scintigraphy. *Eur J Nucl Med* 23:852–854, 1996.

Miller RF. Nuclear medicine and AIDS. *Eur J Nucl Med* 16:103–118, 1990.

Santin M, Podzamczer D, Ricart I, et al. Utility of the gallium-67 citrate scan for the early diagnosis of tuberculosis in patients infected with the human immunodeficiency virus. *Clin Infect Dis* 20:652–656, 1995.

Sulavik SB, Spencer RP, Palestro CJ, et al. Specificity and sensitivity of distinctive chest radiographic and/or ^{67}Ga images in the noninvasive diagnosis of sarcoidosis. *Chest* 103:403–409, 1993.

Case 114

Clinical Presentation

45-year-old man presenting with acquired immune deficiency syndrome (AIDS) and a prior history of treated non-Hodgkin's lymphoma of the abdomen. He had a new complaint of left upper quadrant pain. Gallium scan was requested for further evaluation.

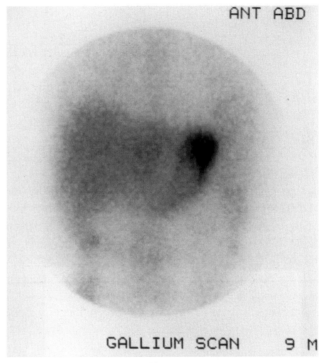

Fig. A

Technique

- 10 mCi of gallium-67 citrate administered intravenously.
- Use a medium-energy collimator.
- Energy window 20% at 93, 184, and 296 keV.
- Imaging for the planar view of the abdomen is 72 hours after tracer injection (1M counts/view).

Image Interpretation

A gallium scan of the anterior view of the upper abdomen (Fig. A) shows increased tracer uptake in the left upper quadrant corresponding to the region of the fundus of the stomach. Delayed follow-up of the abdomen 7 days post-injection of the tracer showed no interval change.

Differential Diagnosis

- Lymphoma
- Cytomegalovirus (CMV)
- Cryptosporidiosis
- Gastritis
- Sarcoma

Diagnosis and Clinical Follow-up

Endoscopy of the upper gastrointestinal tract was performed, and a biopsy of the stomach showed chronic gastritis with viral cytopathological changes and histochemical evidence of CMV infection. There was no evidence of lymphomatous involvement.

Discussion

Occult malignancies of the stomach, such as lymphomas, are gallium-avid and have been described in AIDS patients. Other etiologies of gastric gallium uptake in AIDS patients include CMV infection, cryptosporidiosis, and gastritis secondary to medications.

Suggested Readings

McNeill JA, Llaurado JG. Innocent intramural gastric uptake of Gallium-67 in a case of AIDS. *Clin Nucl Med* 11:123–125, 1986.

Nikpoor N, Drum DE, Aliabadi P. Gastric uptake of Gallium-67 in AIDS. *J Nucl Med* 33:643–645, 1992.

Teixidor HS, Honig CL, Norsoph E, et al. Cytomegalovirus infection of the alimentary canal: Radiological findings with pathologic correlation. *Radiology* 163:317–323, 1987.

Case 115

Clinical Presentation

38-year-old human immunodeficiency virus (HIV)–positive man presenting with abdominal pain, low-grade fever, and diarrhea. Leukocytes labeled with technetium-99m–hexamethyl propylene amine oxime (HMPAO) were requested for further evaluation.

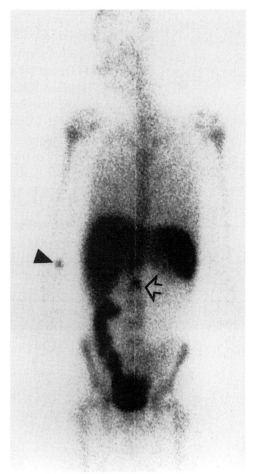

Fig. A

Technique

- 12 mCi of technetium-99m–HMPAO administered intravenously.
- Use a low-energy high-resolution collimator.
- Energy window 20% centered at 140 keV.
- Imaging time 30 minutes, 2 hours, and 3 to 4 hours post-injection of the radio-labeled white blood cells (WBCs).

Image Interpretation

Leukocyte scan in the anterior planar view of the head and neck, chest, abdomen, and pelvis (Fig. A) shows increased tracer uptake in the distal ileum as well as in the ascending colon. There is also a focus of increased uptake in the upper lumbar spine (*open arrow*). Arrowhead indicates the injection site.

Diagnosis and Clinical Follow-up

Endoscopy of the colon showed inflammation of the mucosa, and a biopsy revealed *Salmonella typhimurium*. The patient was treated accordingly.

Discussion

The bowel is one of the least common organs involved with opportunistic infections in patients with acquired immodeficiency syndrome (AIDS). Intestinal mucosal inflammation may be present in the absence of a demonstrable infectious agent, however. Gallium-67 citrate scanning may demonstrate uptake within the mucosal inflammatory process; however, an abnormal gallium-67 citrate scan would not be expected to distinguish between infection and inflammation. Indium-111 oxine or technetium-99m–HMPAO–labeled WBCs are preferable studies for evaluating possible bowel infections.

Suggested Readings

Balthazar EJ, Martino JM. Giant ulcers in the ileum and colon caused by cytomegalovirus in patients with AIDS. *AJR Am J Roentgenol* 166:1275, 1996.

Feczko PJ. Gastrointestinal complications of HIV infection. *Semin Roentgenol* 29:275, 1994.

Murry JG, Evans SJJ, Jeffery PB, et al. Cytomegalovirus colitis in AIDS. *AJR Am J Roentgenol* 165:67, 1995.

Weller V. The gay bowel. *Gut* 26:869–875, 1985.

Case 116

Clinical Presentation

29-year-old human immunodeficiency virus (HIV)–positive male drug addict presenting with low back pain. A gallium scan was requested to evalute symptoms.

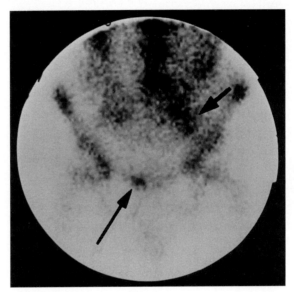

Fig. A

Technique

- Radiopharmaceutical is 5 mCi gallium-67 citrate administered intravenously.
- Use a medium-energy collimator.
- Energy window is 20% centered at 93, 184, and 296 keV.
- Imaging for the planar views (1 M counts per view) at 72 hours after gallium-67 injection. No prior preparation required.

Image Interpretation

Planar anterior gallium scan of the pelvis (Fig. A) shows diffuse increased gallium-67 uptake in the left sacroiliac (SI) region (*short arrow*). There is also a focal increased uptake in the right superior pubic bone (*long arrow*). Anteroposterior radiograph of the pelvis and axial computed tomography (CT) demonstrated widening of the right SI joint and symphysis pubis with destruction of the cortices and new bone formation.

Differential Diagnosis

- Septic arthritis
- Osteomyelitis

Diagnosis and Clinical Follow-up

Aspiration of the SI joint was performed, and the culture was positive for *Streptococcus pneumoniae* organism. The patient was treated with systemic antibiotics and responded to treatment. Later, reconstructive surgery of the pelvis was performed.

Discussion

Arthralgias are a common complaint among HIV-positive patients. Although arthritis such as rheumatoid arthritis, seronegative arthritis such as in Reiter's syndrome, and psoriasis are commonly reported in HIV-positive patients, septic arthritis is not as frequent, except in HIV-positive patients who are also drug abusers.

Suggested Readings

Hughes RA, Row IF, Shan Son D, Keat AC. Septic bone joint and muscle lesions associated with human immunodeficiency virus infection. *Br J Rheumatol* 31:381–388, 1992.

Tehranzadeh J, Stienbach LS. *AIDS Musculoskeletal Manifestations* St. Louis, MO: Warren H. Green, 1994.

Vanarthos W, Ganz WI, Vanarthos JC, et al. Diagnostic uses of nuclear medicine in AIDS. *Radiographics* 12:731–749, 1992.

Case 117

Clinical Presentation

38-year-old man positive for human immunodeficiency virus (HIV) without a history of drug abuse complaining of depression, irritability, and memory loss. A brain perfusion scan was requested for evaluation.

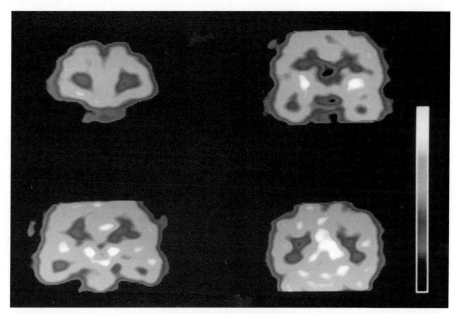

Fig. A—Normal subject

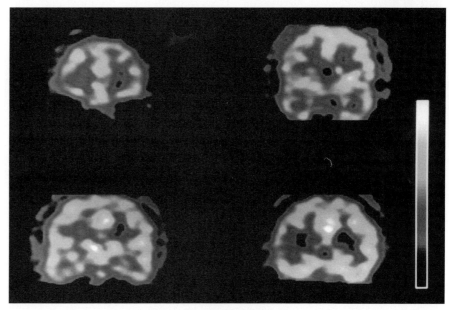

Fig. B—Patient

- Multiple focal cortical defects involving the frontal, temporal, and parietal lobes are common in AIDS dementia complex ADC. In addition, reduced uptake in basal ganglia has been reported. Involvement of the visual cortex and cerebellum is rare.

- Brain perfusion scans of HIV-negative chronic cocaine abusers show similar cortical defects in the frontal, temporal, and parietal lobes. Therefore, the two scintigraphic patterns of ADC and chronic cocaine abusers cannot be distinguished from each other.

- Although conventional magnetic resonance imaging and computed tomography studies are normal in most of these patients, autopsy results in HIV-positive subjects show a high incidence of diffuse and focal brain disease.

- The findings on SPECT are nonspecific. Multiple regional perfusion abnormalities have been seen in chronic fatigue syndrome and systemic lupus erythematosus in addition to the conditions cited before. Therefore, the SPECT findings should not be considered to be of primary diagnostic importance but rather as descriptive data that may be helpful in elucidating the disease process in each of these disorders.

Technique

- 20 mCi technetium-99m–hexamethyl propylene amine oxime (HMPAO) administered intravenously.
- Use a low-energy high-resolution collimator.
- Energy window 20% centered at 140 keV.
- Imaging is 15 minutes post-injection, 360-degree single photon emission computed tomography (SPECT), 30-minute acquisition.

Image Interpretation

Coronal images of a normal subject (Fig. A) show symmetrical distribution of tracer uptake throughout the cortex. Coronal images of the patient (Fig. B) show multiple focal areas of cortical defects involving the frontal, temporal, and parietal lobes.

Differential Diagnosis

- Chronic cocaine abuser
- Acquired immunodeficiency syndrome (AIDS) dementia complex (ADC)
- Chronic fatigue syndrome
- Systemic lupus erythematous

Diagnosis and Clinical Follow-up

Findings in this clinical context are suggestive of ADC.

Discussion

ADC is a devastating complication of HIV infection. Early detection may be difficult because other complications of HIV infection, such as major depression, CNS opportunistic infection, and drug side effects, can mask the signs and symptoms of ADC. Brain perfusion SPECT is a sensitive, but not specific, diagnostic technique in early ADC.

Suggested Readings

Holman BL, Garada B, Johnson KA, et al. A comparison of brain perfusion SPECT in cocaine abuse and dementia complex. *J Nucl Med* 33:1312–1315, 1992.

Schwartz RB, Komaroff AL, Garada BM, et al. SPECT imaging of brain: comparison of findings in patients with chronic fatigue syndrome, AIDS dementia complex and major unipolar depression. *AJR Am J Roentgenol* 162:943–951, 1994.

Case 118

Clinical Presentation

32-year-old female intravenous drug user seropositive for human immunodeficiency virus (HIV) presenting with fever and night sweats. A chest radiograph was negative. A gallium-67 citrate scan was requested to further investigate the symptoms.

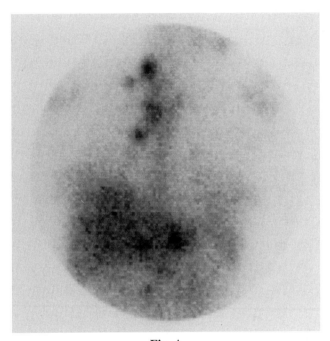

Fig. A

Technique

- 5 mCi gallium-67 citrate administered intravenously.
- Use a medium-energy collimator.
- Energy window 20% at 93, 184, and 296 keV.
- Imaging time is 72 hours after tracer injection, 1M counts per view.

Image Interpretation

The gallium scan shows focal right supraclavicular, mediastinal, and right hilar uptake. There are also positive lymph nodes in the upper abdomen.

Differential Diagnosis

- Lymphoma
- Mycobacterial infection (tuberculosis, MAI)
- Sarcoidosis

Diagnosis and Clinical Follow-up

Histological examination of a supraclavicular lymph node biopsy showed granulomatous mycobacterial lymphadenitis with numerous acid-fast bacilli.

Discussion

Focal lymph node uptake on a gallium-67 scan is frequently associated with mycobacterial infections or lymphoma in HIV-positive patients. Intravenous drug abusers with acquired immunodeficiency syndrome (AIDS) have been a major source of the increase in tuberculosis according to the Centers for Disease Control.

Suggested Readings

Goodman PC. Tuberculosis and AIDS. *Radiol Clin North Am* 33:707, 1995.

Jm J, Song KS, Kang AS, et al. Mediastinal tuberculosis lymphadenitis. *Radiology* 164:115–119, 1987.

Lee VW, Cooly TP, Fuller JD, Ward RJ, Farber HW. Pulmonary Mycobacterial infections in AIDS: Characteristic pattern of thallium and gallium scan mismatched. *Radiology* 193:389, 1994.

Lung N, Prauner MW, Gamsu, G, et al. Pulmonary tuberculosis in AIDS patients, CT findings. *Radiology* 198:687–691, 1996.

Section VIII

Renal Scintigraphy

Case 119

Clinical Presentation

64-year-old man with an 11-cm abdominal aortic aneurysm admitted in preparation for surgery. Within 48 hours, he developed acute renal failure. There was a concern for aortic dissection extending to the renal arteries.

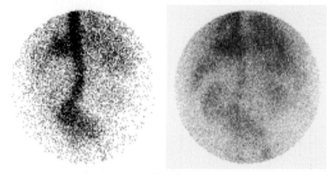

Fig. A

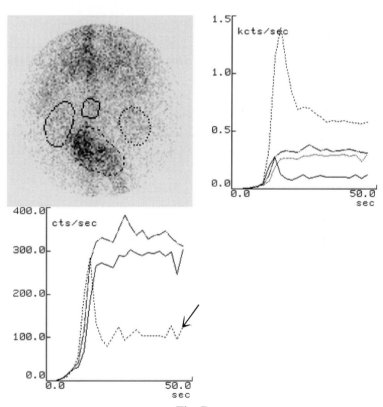

Fig. B

Technique

- 10 mCi technetium-99m diethylene triamine pentaacetic acid (DTPA) intravenously as a bolus.
- Use low-energy all-purpose collimator.
- Energy window 20% centered at 140 keV.
- Imaging time is dynamic sequence: 24 frames at 2 sec/frame; 16 frames at 15 sec/frame; 60 frames at 30 sec/frame.

Image Interpretation

By stepping through the flow phase frame by frame (first 48 seconds in this dynamic setup), one can identify the image where the tracer reaches the abdominal aorta (Fig. A, left). The normal aorta and the large aneurysm are clearly seen, and a blush is noted over both kidneys. The functional image at 1 to 2 minutes (Fig. A, right) shows tracer accumulated in the kidneys. Regions of interest (ROIs) can then be drawn over the normal aorta and the aneurysm seen in the flow phase and over the left and right kidneys seen in the functional images (Fig. B, upper left quadrant). Time activity curves (TACs) for the flow phase were generated (Fig. B, upper right quadrant). The high dominant curve represents the aneurysm, with its large volume of blood. Better resolution of the curves is noted when the aorta curve and the kidney curves are displayed separately (Fig. B, lower left quadrant), allowing the flow through the aorta and kidneys to be compared more easily.

The aorta curve in the bottom left portion of Figure B (*arrow*) has a brisk upstroke and reaches a distinct peak, followed by a decrease as the bolus of tracer passes through the ROI. The kidney curves show a brisk upstroke consistent with the upstroke of the aorta curve followed by gradually increasing activity as the tracer accumulates in the kidneys.

Differential Diagnosis

- Preserved renal blood flow
- Blood flow to spleen mistaken for left kidney flow

Diagnosis and Clinical Follow-up

Preserved renal perfusion was the diagnosis. Surgery was planned initially but was not performed because of circulatory instability and declining renal function. The patient's condition deteriorated further, kidney failure developed, and the patient subsequently died. Autopsy was not performed.

Discussion

Assessment of renal flow is one of the few renal studies that may need to be performed urgently. Such studies can (should) be performed at the bedside if a mobile camera is available. Patients in need of such assessment are often in critical condition and transportation and transfer to imaging tables should be avoided. This patient was indeed in very critical condition with low systolic BP in spite of invasive monitoring and full volume and pressor support. Clinically, it was felt that the failing renal function was due to renal ischemia, either due to involvement of the renal arteries by the aneurysm, or a result of the compromised circulation. The first possibility was potentially correctable. The result of the perfusion study was quite clear and changed patient management significantly.

An alternate approach would be angiography. However, contrast agents are often nephrotoxic and pose an unnecessary risk.

Suggested Reading

Britton KE, Maisey MN, Hilson AJW. Renal radionuclide studies. In: Maisey MN, Britton KE, Gilday DL, eds. *Clinical Nuclear Medicine*. London: Chapman and Hall, pp. 93–133, 1990.

Case 120

Clinical Presentation

41-year-old woman presenting with a long history of bilateral kidney stones and infections. In recent years, symptoms were mainly in the form of fevers and intermittent left flank pain. Ultrasound showed a small left kidney without signs of obstruction. Nephrectomy was being considered in this patient if left renal function did not contribute significantly to overall renal function.

FUNCTION IMAGES

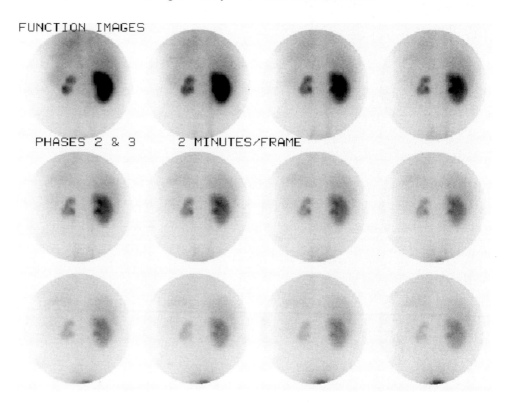

PHASES 2 & 3   2 MINUTES/FRAME

DIFFERENTIAL UPTAKES

LEFT (%)   13.1
RIGHT (%)   86.9

Fig. A

PEARLS/PITFALLS

- Assessment of function in absolute units (ERPF or glomerular filtration rate) with a plasma sample technique or camera-based method as used here adds an extra dimension when evaluating many clinical problems.

- The combined information from the images, dynamic ciné display, and functional curves and the calculated values make a complete set of data. The elements of each component of the study complement each other, providing an overall picture of renal physiology.

- Digital images and computer analysis are a must. Analog imaging alone is not acceptable.

- Split function must be calculated from data obtained at the time when uptake best reflects function. This time differs for filtered and tubular agents. Filtered agents such as technetium-99m–labeled pentetic acid (DTPA) are best measured at 90 to 150 seconds; tubular agents such as technetium-99m–labeled MAG-3 are best measured at 60 to 120 seconds after bolus injection. *(continued)*

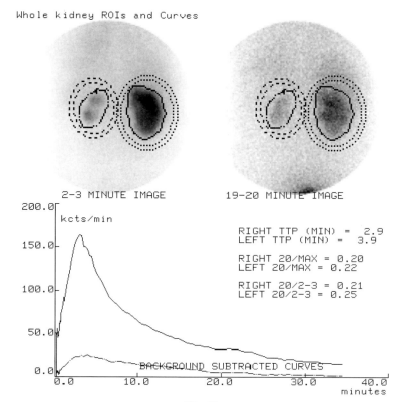

Fig. B

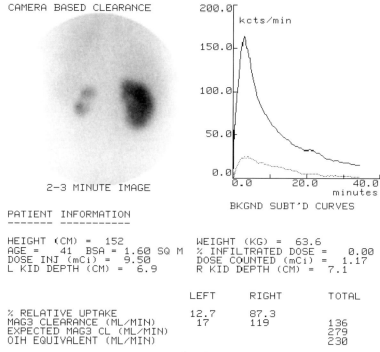

Fig. C

Technique

- 10 mCi technetium-99m mercaptoacetyltriglycine (MAG-3) intravenously.
- Use low-energy all-purpose collimator.
- Energy window 20% centered at 140 keV.
- Imaging time is a dynamic sequence: 24 frames at 2 sec/frame; 16 frames at 15 sec/frame; 60 frames at 30 sec/frame.

- *(continued)* Both glomerular (filtered) agents such as DTPA and predominantly secreted (tubular) agents such as MAG-3 (> 90% tubular elimination and < 10% filtration) and iodine-123–labeled iodohippurate sodium (hippuran) can be used and are probably equally good for assessment of split function in most patients. In patients with known moderate to markedly decreased function, tubular agents are preferred because image quality is improved, resulting in functional curves with less noise. MAG-3 has generally replaced iodine-123–labeled iodohippurate sodium as the tubular agent of choice.

- Technetium-99m–labeled 2,3-dimercaptosuccinic acid (DMSA), a 100% tubular agent, is useful for split function assessment and detection of cortical structural abnormalities and allows for single photon emission computed tomography. The use of DMSA has declined markedly because of its inconsistent availability.

Image Interpretation

Images from the functional phase, 2 min/frame, starting at 1 minute after injection (Fig. A) show very little functional tissue on the left side, mainly as two "islands" in the upper and mid portion of the kidney. A very small pelvis can be identified medial to the lower island, which drains normally. The parenchymal appearance is not that of cortical thinning; therefore, there is no evidence of obstruction. The right kidney is relatively enlarged and has normal uptake and elimination phases (Fig. B). Split function analysis shows the left kidney to perform 13% of the total renal function and the right kidney to perform 87%. Total function, expressed as effective renal plasma flow (ERPF), is moderately reduced at 136 mL/min, which is 50% of expected considering age, gender, and body surface area (Fig. C). The expected total function is 279 mL/min. Therefore, each kidney should ideally clear about 140 mL/min (range 126 to 154, presuming 50% ± 5% normal split function). Thus, the right kidney function is within normal limits for a single kidney.

Differential Diagnosis

- Chronic, severe left renal pyelonephritis
- Congenital left renal abnormality
- Infarcted left kidney
- More acute causes of a diminished left kidney, such as trauma, hemorrhage, or neoplastic disease would not explain the relative hypertrophy of the right kidney

Diagnosis and Clinical Follow-up

Chronic pyelonephritis was the diagnosis. Left nephrectomy was performed to relieve the symptoms. Creatinine did not increase significantly.

Discussion

Assessment of split function is one of the most common indications for radionuclide renal studies. When introduced more than 20 years ago, the method was validated against individual kidney function assessment with continuous inulin infusion to steady state and simultaneous sampling from each ureter, a cumbersome, invasive method. The radionuclide study, on the other hand, is no more invasive than an antecubital injection of tracer, and the reproducibility is very good (± 2%).

The left kidney abnormality in this patient is not of the obstructive type (no cortical thinning pattern and the intrarenal and extrarenal collecting systems are not dilated). Scarring after infection with loss of functional tissue is the most likely etiology; congenital abnormality is also a possibility.

Suggested Reading

Britton KE, Maisey MN, Hilson AJW. Renal radionuclide studies. In: Maisey MN, Britton KE, Gilday DL, eds. *Clinical Nuclear Medicine*. London: Chapman and Hall, 1990, pp. 93–133.

Case 121

Clinical Presentation

74-year-old woman presenting with a long history of flank pain. Left uretero-pelvic junction (UPJ) obstruction was diagnosed with retrograde ureterography. Intravenous pyelography and ultrasound showed mild to moderate hydronephrosis. There was a question as to the functional significance of the left UPJ obstruction.

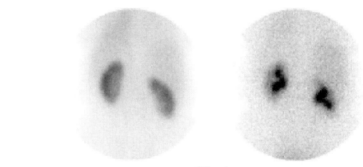

Fig. A

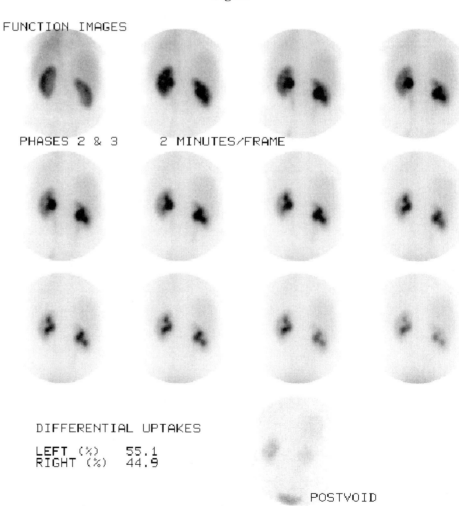

FUNCTION IMAGES

PHASES 2 & 3   2 MINUTES/FRAME

DIFFERENTIAL UPTAKES

LEFT (%)   55.1
RIGHT (%) 44.9

POSTVOID

Fig. B

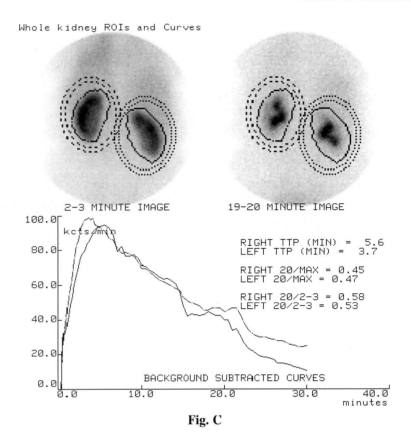

Whole kidney ROIs and Curves

2-3 MINUTE IMAGE   19-20 MINUTE IMAGE

RIGHT TTP (MIN) = 5.6
LEFT TTP (MIN) = 3.7

RIGHT 20/MAX = 0.45
LEFT 20/MAX = 0.47

RIGHT 20/2-3 = 0.58
LEFT 20/2-3 = 0.53

BACKGROUND SUBTRACTED CURVES

Fig. C

Technique

- 10 mCi technetium-99m-mercaptoacetyltriglycine (MAG-3) intravenously.
- Administer 20 mg furosemide intravenously at 20 minutes post tracer injection.
- Use low-energy all-purpose collimator.
- Energy window 20% centered at 140 keV.
- Imaging time is a dynamic sequence: 24 frames at 2 sec/frame; 16 frames at 15 sec/frame; 60 frames at 30 sec/frame.

Image Interpretation

Images from the functional phase (Fig. A) show the right kidney to be slightly smaller than the left kidney, mild cortical thinning on both sides, and prominent intrarenal and extrarenal collecting systems bilaterally. There is clear spontaneous drainage on both sides (Fig. B). Split function analysis shows the following:

	Left	Right
Split function analysis (%)	55	45
Residual cortical activity at 20 minutes	47	45

Total function, expressed as effective renal plasma flow (ERPF), is 204 mL/min (100% of expected for age, gender, and body surface area). The functional curves (Fig. C) confirm the impression from the functional images that there is spontaneous, albeit delayed, drainage from both kidneys. The delayed drainage is reflected in the elevated residual cortical activity at 20 minutes (RCA 20). There is a prompt, symmetrical response to furosemide within 1 minute after furosemide injection, demonstrating no evidence of obstruction. There is mild to moderate slightly asymmetrical dilatation of the collecting systems and mild bilateral hydronephrosis.

Differential Diagnosis

- Non-obstructed, dilated renal pelves.

Diagnosis and Clinical Follow-up

Mild bilateral intermittent UPJ obstruction was the final diagnosis. The mild symptoms and findings described previously were reassuring. No intervention was undertaken.

Discussion

As a rule of thumb, the pelvis emptying half-time after furosemide (time it takes for the pelvis to empty half its tracer activity) should be less than 10 minutes. If emptying half-time is 10 to 20 minutes, mild obstruction or dilatation, or both, is suggested. If the emptying half-time is more than 20 minutes, it is consistent with moderate- to high-grade or total obstruction. When response to furosemide is evaluated, kidney function must be taken into consideration. With diminished renal function, a less vigorous response to diuretics should be expected.

Suggested Readings

Conway JJ. "Well-tempered" diuresis renography: Its historical development, physiological and technical pitfalls, and standardized technique protocol. *Semin Nucl Med* 22:74–84, 1992.

Yung BCK, Sostre S, Gearhart JP. Normalized clearance-to-uptake slope ratio: A method to minimize false-positive diuretic renograms. *J Nucl Med* 34:762–768, 1993.

Case 122

Clinical Presentation

81-year-old woman with a history of renal stones and chronic flank pain presenting with accentuation of pain and hematuria. Intravenous pyelography and retrograde ureterography had previously demonstrated right-sided hydronephrosis. Two months before, the patient underwent laser lithotripsy, stone extraction, and stenting. The patency of the stent and split renal function have been questioned.

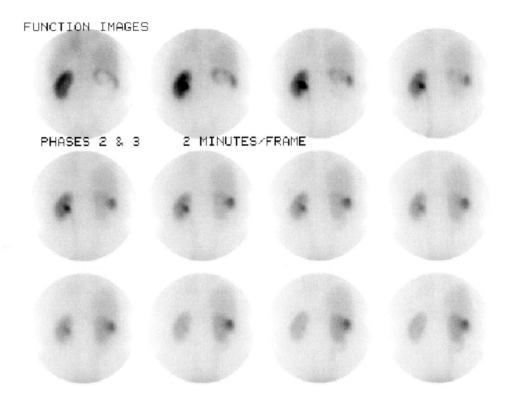

FUNCTION IMAGES

PHASES 2 & 3   2 MINUTES/FRAME

DIFFERENTIAL UPTAKES

LEFT (%)   82.7
RIGHT (%)   17.3

Fig. A

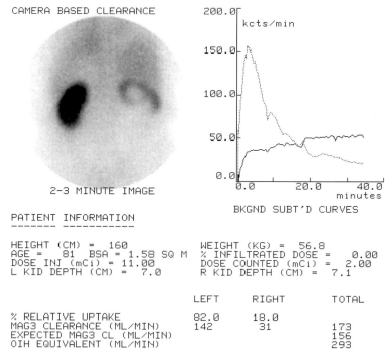

CAMERA BASED CLEARANCE

2-3 MINUTE IMAGE

BKGND SUBT'D CURVES

PATIENT INFORMATION
------- -----------

HEIGHT (CM) =   160   WEIGHT (KG) =   56.8
AGE =   81 BSA = 1.58 SQ M   % INFILTRATED DOSE =   0.00
DOSE INJ (mCi) = 11.00   DOSE COUNTED (mCi) =   2.00
L KID DEPTH (CM) = 7.0   R KID DEPTH (CM) =   7.1

	LEFT	RIGHT	TOTAL
% RELATIVE UPTAKE	82.0	18.0	
MAG3 CLEARANCE (ML/MIN)	142	31	173
EXPECTED MAG3 CL (ML/MIN)			156
OIH EQUIVALENT (ML/MIN)			293

Fig. B

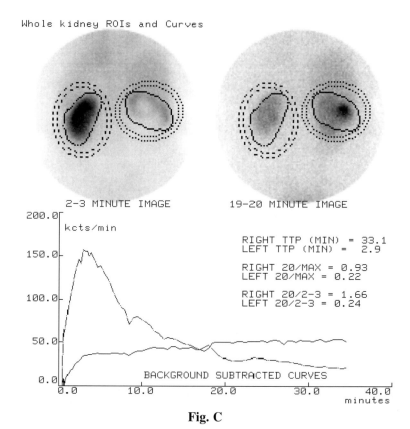

Whole kidney ROIs and Curves

2-3 MINUTE IMAGE   19-20 MINUTE IMAGE

BACKGROUND SUBTRACTED CURVES

RIGHT TTP (MIN) = 33.1
LEFT TTP (MIN) = 2.9

RIGHT 20/MAX = 0.93
LEFT 20/MAX = 0.22

RIGHT 20/2-3 = 1.66
LEFT 20/2-3 = 0.24

Fig. C

PEARLS/PITFALLS

- When obstruction of the renal collecting system is suspected, functional curves from each pelvis should always be reviewed. Because the pelvis of each kidney might be visualized at different times, careful frame by frame inspection of the study will identify when each pelvis is optimally visualized. The ROI can then be drawn using the most appropriate frames.

- When high-grade obstruction leads to marked reduction in function, the functional curve often has very low amplitude when it is compared with the curve from a well-functioning contralateral kidney. If the kidney curves are displayed simultaneously (Figs. B and C, upper right quadrant), the scaling will be to the curve with the highest count rate. The low count curve has low amplitude with little detail (Fig. B). By displaying and scaling the curves individually, the details are more apparent.

- The decision to give furosemide often has to be made quickly, while images are being acquired and the renal pelvis is full. The images must therefore be monitored as they are acquired.

- Because dehydration may lead to delayed elimination from the parenchyma and from the collecting system, patients should always be hydrated before radionuclide renography. Eating and drinking as usual on the day of the study is permitted, with an additional intake of 500 to 750 mL of water (10 mL/kg) encouraged in the hour before imaging.

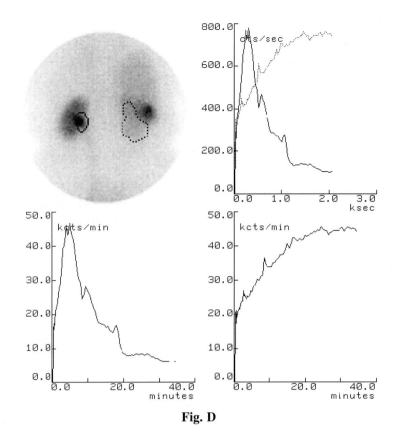

Fig. D

Technique

- 10 mCi technetium-99m mercaptoacetyltriglycine (MAG-3) intravenously.
- 20 mg furosemide intravenously at 20 minutes post tracer injection.
- Use low-energy all-purpose collimator.
- Energy window 20% centered at 140 keV.
- Imaging time is a dynamic sequence: 24 frames at 2 sec/frame; 16 frames at 15 sec/frame; 60 frames at 30 sec/frame.

Image Interpretation

Images from the functional phase (Fig. A) show a tilted right kidney with high-grade cortical thinning. The right kidney function is markedly reduced at 18% of total (Fig. B). The right collecting system is therefore not well visualized. In the late images (last three images in the lower row of Fig. A), however, a markedly dilated pelvis is evident. The functional whole kidney curves (Fig. C) show left sided continuous tracer accumulation up to 40 minutes post injection with no detectable effect of furosemide (given at about 20 minutes).

The left kidney is normal in size with homogeneous parenchymal distribution of tracer (Fig. A). The intrarenal and extrarenal collecting system appears normal, and the functional curves (Fig. C) confirm the impression of normal function and drainage. Left and right renal pelves were defined with a region of interest (ROI) by using the dynamic images where they were seen best (Fig. D, upper left quadrant). Time activity curves (TACs) for the ROIs were generated (Fig. D, upper right quadrant). The TAC for the left pelvis is displayed alone in the lower left quadrant and for the right pelvis in the lower right quadrant. The right pelvis curve demonstrates continuous accumulation of tracer (climbing curve) with no spontaneous decrease and no response to furosemide. These findings are diagnostic for high-grade or total obstruction. The amount of cortical thinning implies a long-standing process.

Notice the intrarenal accumulation laterally in the lower pole of the right kidney. This likely represents a drainage problem from the calyx due to a regional intrarenal impediment such as a stone or tissue debris. The left pelvis curve has a normal appearance.

Differential Diagnosis

- Chronic, high-grade right renal collecting system obstruction
- Hydronephrosis in poorly functioning kidney (unresponsive to furosemide) without obstruction

Diagnosis and Clinical Follow-up

The diagnosis was chronic obstruction. Additional stones were removed, and ureteroplasty was performed.

Suggested Readings

Conway JJ. "Well-tempered" diuresis renography: Its historical development, physiological and technical pitfalls, and standardized technique protocol. *Semin Nucl Med* 22:74–84, 1992.

Yung BCK, Sostre S, Gearhart JP. Normalized clearance-to-uptake slope ratio: A method to minimize false-positive diuretic renograms. *J Nucl Med* 34:762–768, 1993.

Case 123

Clinical Presentation

42-year-old woman presenting with hypertension that recently had become refractory to medication. Blood pressure was 200–220/110–120 mmHg. There was no current treatment with angiotensin-converting enzyme (ACE) inhibitors. The referring physicians were concerned that the hypertension might be secondary to renal artery stenosis (RAS).

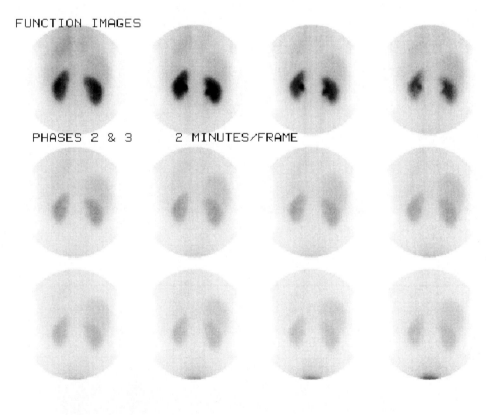

FUNCTION IMAGES

PHASES 2 & 3   2 MINUTES/FRAME

DIFFERENTIAL UPTAKES

LEFT (%)   49.2
RIGHT (%)   50.8

Fig. A—Baseline

Technique

- 6 and 12 mCi technetium-99m mercaptoacetyltriglycine (MAG-3) administered intravenously at 8 AM (baseline) and 3 PM (1 hour after 50 mg captopril orally).
- Hydration (500 to 700 mL water orally) was performed 1 hour before the test.
- If captopril is administered, blood pressure should be obtained 60, 30, and 0 minutes prior to imaging.
- Use a low-energy, general-purpose collimator.
- Energy window 20% centered at 140 keV.
- Imaging time is a dynamic sequence: 24 frames at 2 sec/frame; 16 frames at 15 sec/frame; 60 frames at 30 sec/frame.

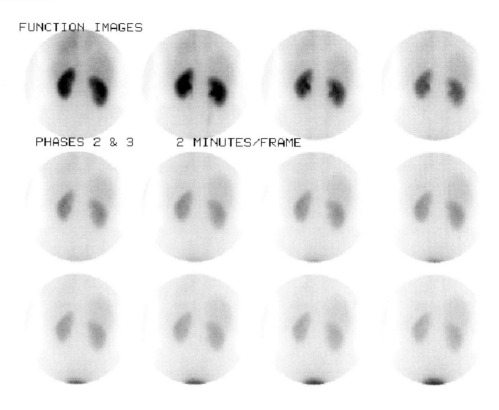

FUNCTION IMAGES

PHASES 2 & 3   2 MINUTES/FRAME

DIFFERENTIAL UPTAKES

LEFT (%)   50.5
RIGHT (%)   49.5

Fig. B—Captopril

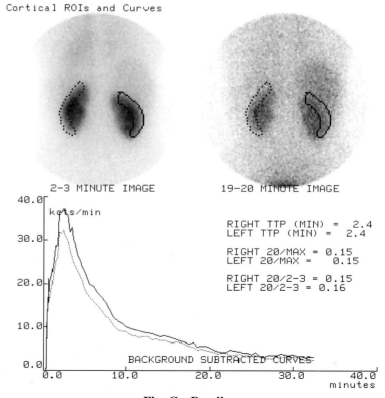

Cortical ROIs and Curves

2-3 MINUTE IMAGE   19-20 MINUTE IMAGE

RIGHT TTP (MIN) =   2.4
LEFT TTP (MIN) =   2.4

RIGHT 20/MAX = 0.15
LEFT 20/MAX =   0.15

RIGHT 20/2-3 = 0.15
LEFT 20/2-3 = 0.16

BACKGROUND SUBTRACTED CURVES

Fig. C—Baseline

Cortical ROIs and Curves

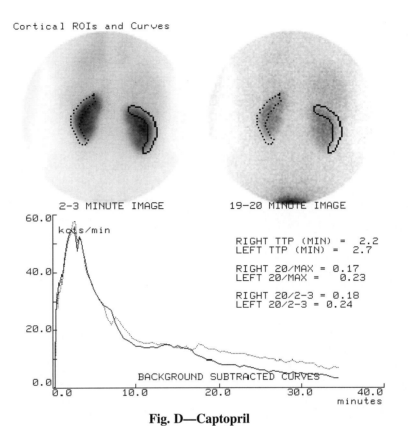

2-3 MINUTE IMAGE   19-20 MINUTE IMAGE

60.0 kcts/min

RIGHT TTP (MIN) = 2.2
LEFT TTP (MIN) = 2.7

40.0

RIGHT 20/MAX = 0.17
LEFT 20/MAX = 0.23

RIGHT 20/2-3 = 0.18
LEFT 20/2-3 = 0.24

20.0

BACKGROUND SUBTRACTED CURVES

0.0

0.0   10.0   20.0   30.0   40.0
                                minutes

Fig. D—Captopril

CAMERA BASED CLEARANCE

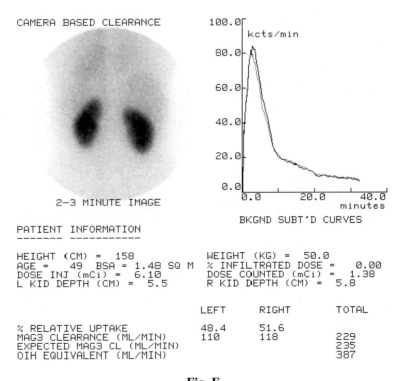

100.0 kcts/min

80.0

60.0

40.0

20.0

0.0

0.0   20.0   40.0
                minutes

2-3 MINUTE IMAGE

BKGND SUBT'D CURVES

PATIENT INFORMATION
‾‾‾‾‾‾‾ ‾‾‾‾‾‾‾‾‾‾‾

HEIGHT (CM) = 158   WEIGHT (KG) = 50.0
AGE =   49 BSA = 1.48 SQ M % INFILTRATED DOSE =   0.00
DOSE INJ (mCi) = 6.10   DOSE COUNTED (mCi) = 1.38
L KID DEPTH (CM) = 5.5   R KID DEPTH (CM) = 5.8

	LEFT	RIGHT	TOTAL
% RELATIVE UPTAKE	48.4	51.6	
MAG3 CLEARANCE (ML/MIN)	110	118	229
EXPECTED MAG3 CL (ML/MIN)			235
OIH EQUIVALENT (ML/MIN)			387

Fig. E

PEARLS/PITFALLS

- The captopril challenge study should, as a general rule, be performed first. If normal (as in this case), then there is no need for a baseline study.

- In certain clinical environments and for certain patients, a 1-day protocol in which the baseline study is done in the morning and the captopril study is done 5 to 6 hours later may be arranged for patient convenience.

- Standard hydration of all patients and for both studies is important to avoid false-positives, especially when using tubular agents in which the cortical retention is a major diagnostic variable.

- Crushing the captopril tablet will improve absorption of the medication. Inadequate absorption has been reported as a problem in some studies, leading to false-negative results.

- A fall in systemic systolic pressure to below 80 mmHg, for whatever reason, will compromise kidney function. Blood pressure must be monitored during the captopril challenge, and the pressure at the time of the study must be recorded. Captopril rarely causes a dramatic decrease in blood pressure because the action is primarily on the efferent arterioles. Vasovagal reactions, volume depletion, and so on are much more common reasons for a severe drop in blood pressure. *(continued)*

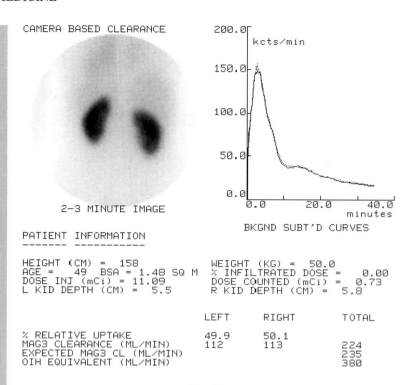

CAMERA BASED CLEARANCE

2-3 MINUTE IMAGE

BKGND SUBT'D CURVES

PATIENT INFORMATION
------- -----------

HEIGHT (CM) =   158   WEIGHT (KG) =   50.0
AGE =   49   BSA = 1.48 SQ M   % INFILTRATED DOSE =   0.00
DOSE INJ (mCi) = 11.09   DOSE COUNTED (mCi) =   0.73
L KID DEPTH (CM) =   5.5   R KID DEPTH (CM) =   5.8

	LEFT	RIGHT	TOTAL
% RELATIVE UPTAKE	49.9	50.1	
MAG3 CLEARANCE (ML/MIN)	112	113	224
EXPECTED MAG3 CL (ML/MIN)			235
OIH EQUIVALENT (ML/MIN)			380

Fig. F

Image Interpretation

Images from the functional phase of the baseline study (Fig. A) and during captopril challenge (Fig. B), displayed at 2 minutes per frame, starting at 1 minute post injection, show equal-sized kidneys with homogeneous parenchymal distribution and no collecting system abnormalities. Split function, time to maximum, and residual cortical activity at 20 minutes (RCA 20) are shown for baseline (Fig. C) and captopril (Fig. D) in the following table:

Baseline	Left	Right	Captopril	Left	Right
Split function (%)	49	51	Split function (%)	50	50
Time to max (min)			Time to max (min)		
(normal < 5 min)	2.4	2.4	(normal < 5 min)	2.7	2.2
RCA 20			RCA 20		
(normal < 30%)	15%	15%	(normal < 30%)	23%	17%

Although the RCA 20 is higher during the captopril portion of the test than it is at baseline, it is still within normal limits (normal retention < 30%). An increase of 10% or more, into or within the abnormal range, is considered significant.

There is therefore no evidence of functionally significant RAS or renovascular hypertension (RVH). The total function, expressed as effective renal plasma flow (ERPF), is normal at baseline (Fig. E), 229 mL/min, and during captopril challenge (Fig. F), 224 mL/min; the expected MAG-3 clearance for a woman this age, weight, and height is 235 mL/min.

(continued) ACE inhibitor therapy should be withheld 48 to 72 hours prior to the study. If this is clinically impossible or considered risky, one can withhold the evening dose the day before the study and the morning dose on the day of the study. Use the 1-day protocol (baseline first), and administer the morning dose or 1.5 times the morning dose as the challenge dose. The accuracy of this variant of the test is probably diminished, but the test is still useful (estimated decrease in sensitivity and specificity from high 80% to mid-70%).

- Both filtered agents and tubular agents can be used. The tubular agents are probably more reliable because of a better target to background ratio allowing for functional curves with less noise.

- The dose of technetium-99m used for captopril studies varies among the centers performing the studies from 4 mCi to 12 mCi.

- Some centers find it necessary to have the patients take nothing by mouth after midnight. The assumption is that food might interfere with captopril absorption.

Differential Diagnosis

- Normal study
- False negative study because of inadequate absorption of captopril

Diagnosis and Clinical Follow-up

The clinical suspicion for RAS was low to moderate. With this negative study, the post-test probability of functional RAS or RVH is very low (less than 5 to 10%). The patient's final diagnosis was essential hypertension.

Discussion

The reproducibility of modern camera-based methods for assessment of renal function is very good. In this patient, ERPF is almost the same in both the first and the second studies. A reproducibility of ± 5 to 10% is common.

The first-generation software for calculating glomerular filtration rate (GFR) and ERPF (Gates' method and Schlegel's method, respectively) was introduced in the mid-1980s. Improved versions were reported in 1989 to 1990, and third-generation software for calculation of ERPF with MAG-3 was released recently. Improvement in background subtraction, attenuation correction based on computed tomography–determined kidney depth, and measurement of injected dose are the most significant enhancements.

Kidney function is commonly assessed by calculating clearance, defined as the virtual volume plasma cleared per minute:

$$Clearance = \frac{Uc \times Uv}{Pc}$$

where Uc is urine concentration of a given substance, Uv is urine volume per unit time, and Pc is the plasma concentration of the substance. If the principle is applied to a filtered agent such as DTPA (or less accurately creatinine, which is filtered, secreted, and reabsorbed), the calculation provides GFR. If the principle is applied to tubular agents such as hippuran or MAG-3, then the effective renal plasma flow is generated.

Suggested Readings

Davidson R, Wilcox CS. Diagnostic usefulness of renal scanning after angiotensin converting enzyme inhibitors. *Hypertension* 18:299–303, 1991.

Dondi M, Fanti S, DeFabritis A, et al. Prognostic value of captopril renal scintigraphy in renovascular hypertension. *J Nucl Med* 33:2040–2044, 1992.

Erbsloh-Moller B, Dumas A, Roth D, et al. Furosemide-131-I-hippuran renography after angiotensin-converting enzyme inhibition for the diagnosis of renovascular hypertension. *Am J Med* 90:23–29, 1991.

Nally JV Jr, Black HRS. State-of-the-art review: Captopril renography—pathophysiological considerations and clinical observations. *Semin Nucl Med* 22:85–97, 1992.

Setaro JF, Saddler MC, Chen CC, et al. Simplified captopril renography in diagnosis and treatment of renal artery stenosis. *Hypertension* 18:289–298, 1991.

Case 124

Clinical Presentation

67-year-old man presenting with diabetes mellitus and hypertension that recently had become refractory. Blood pressure had been in the range of 180–220/90–110 mmHg. There was no ongoing treatment with angiotensin-converting enzyme (ACE) inhibitors.

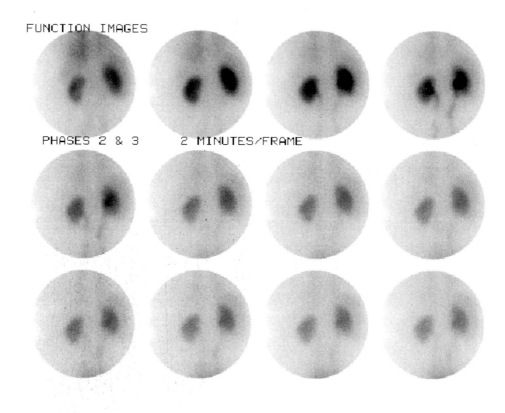

FUNCTION IMAGES

PHASES 2 & 3   2 MINUTES/FRAME

DIFFERENTIAL UPTAKES
LEFT (%)   42.2
RIGHT (%)   57.8

Fig. A—Baseline

Technique

- 6 mCi and 12 mCi technetium-99m mercaptoacetyltriglycine (MAG-3) administered intravenously at 8 AM (baseline) and 3 PM (1 hour after 50 mg captopril).
- Blood pressure 60, 30, and 0 minutes before the test: 180/100, 140/90, 130/90.
- Use a low-energy, general-purpose collimator.
- Energy window 20% centered at 140 keV.
- Imaging time is a dynamic sequence: 24 frames at 2 sec/frame; 16 frames at 15 sec/frame; 60 frames at 30 sec/frame.

PEARLS/PITFALLS

- A standardized protocol should be strictly followed; there should be hydration during the hour before both baseline and captopril studies.

- Administer 25 to 50 mg captopril crushed (to ensure absorption) 1 hour prior to imaging.

- A small dose of furosemide (20 to 40 mg) just before or early into imaging can eliminate the possibility that tracer will hang up in the intrarenal collecting system, a potential source of a false-positive study results.

- Reduce the captopril dose in older patients with arteriosclerosis. These patients have more difficulty compensating by means of peripheral vasoconstriction.

- If blood pressure falls to < 90 mmHg, invalid data are likely. Stop the study and expand the blood volume. Elevate the extremities (legs contain about ½ L of blood) and give intravenous fluids.

FUNCTION IMAGES

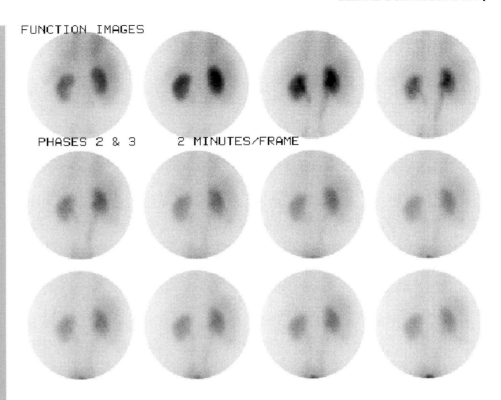

PHASES 2 & 3   2 MINUTES/FRAME

DIFFERENTIAL UPTAKES

LEFT (%)   47.3
RIGHT (%) 52.7

Fig. B—Captopril

Cortical ROIs and Curves

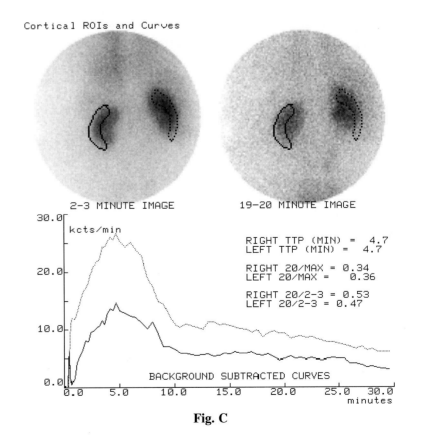

2-3 MINUTE IMAGE   19-20 MINUTE IMAGE

30.0
kcts/min

RIGHT TTP (MIN) = 4.7
LEFT TTP (MIN) = 4.7

20.0

RIGHT 20/MAX = 0.34
LEFT 20/MAX = 0.36

RIGHT 20/2-3 = 0.53
LEFT 20/2-3 = 0.47

10.0

BACKGROUND SUBTRACTED CURVES

0.0
0.0   5.0   10.0   15.0   20.0   25.0   30.0
minutes

Fig. C

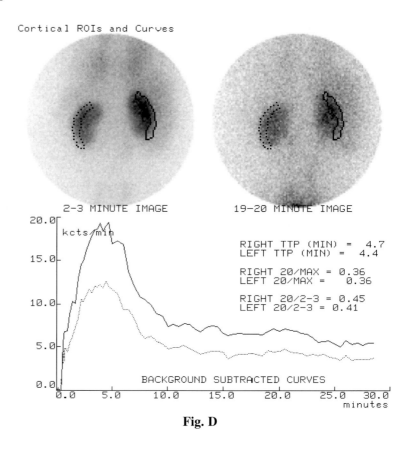

Fig. D

Image Interpretation

Images from the functional phase at baseline (Fig. A) and during captopril challenge (Fig. B) demonstrate the right kidney performing 58% of the total renal function and the left performing 42% at baseline, and 47% and 53% following captopril administration. Functional phase images during both baseline (Fig. A) and captopril challenge (Fig. B) show the left kidney to be slightly smaller than the right kidney. Homogeneous parenchymal distribution and normal collecting system were noted. Time to maximum and residual cortical activity at 20 minutes (RCA 20) are shown for baseline (Fig. C) and captopril (Fig. D) in the following table:

Baseline	Left	Right	Captopril	Left	Right
Time to max (min)	4.7	4.7	Time to max (min)	4.4	4.7
RCA 20	36%	34%	RCA 20	36%	36%

Thus, there is no change in time to maximum or cortical retention during captopril challenge compared with baseline. Functionally significant renal artery stenosis (RAS) or renovascular hypertension (RVH) is therefore very unlikely. At baseline the total function, expressed as effective renal plasma flow (ERPF), was moderately reduced at 131 mL/min (55% of expected considering age, gender, and body surface area). Time to maximum is just below the upper limit of normal, and cortical retention is just above upper limit of normal.

Differential Diagnosis

- Renal parenchymal disease
- False negative study because of inadequate absorption of captopril

Diagnosis and Clinical Follow-up

The diagnosis is not consistent with RAS and more suggestive of an intrarenal etiology. The pretest clinical suspicion of RAS or RVH was moderate. Serum creatinine was slightly elevated at the time of the study and increased gradually over the next 6 months. The elevated blood pressure did not increase further after adjustment of antihypertensives.

Discussion

The captopril study is clearly negative for RAS or RVH. There is clear evidence of abnormal function, however. The tracer is homogeneously distributed throughout the parenchyma, and there are no drainage abnormalities suggestive of postrenal problems. Diffuse intrarenal (also called medical or parenchymal) disease is therefore the most likely pathogenesis. The patient has long-standing (albeit well-controlled) diabetes. Diabetic nephropathy is first in a long list of diseases leading to kidney failure.

Suggested Readings

Davidson R, Wilcox CS. Diagnostic usefulness of renal scanning after angiotensin converting enzyme inhibitors. *Hypertension* 18:299–303, 1991.

Dondi M, Fanti S, DeFabritis A, et al. Prognostic value of captopril renal scintigraphy in renovascular hypertension. *J Nucl Med* 33:2040–2044, 1992.

Erbsloh-Moller B, Dumas A, Roth D, et al. Furosemide-131-I-hippuran renography after angiotensin-converting enzyme inhibition for the diagnosis of renovascular hypertension. *Am J Med* 90:23–29, 1991.

Nally JV Jr, Black HRS. State-of-the-art review: Captopril renography—pathophysiological considerations and clinical observations. *Semin Nucl Med* 22:85–97, 1992.

Setaro JF, Saddler MC, Chen CC, et al. Simplified captopril renography in diagnosis and treatment of renal artery stenosis. *Hypertension* 18:289–298, 1991.

Case 125

Clinical Presentation

65-year-old woman presenting with a history of peripheral vascular disease and hypertension. Over the last year her blood pressure has been increasingly difficult to control. She is now on three antihypertensives in high doses.

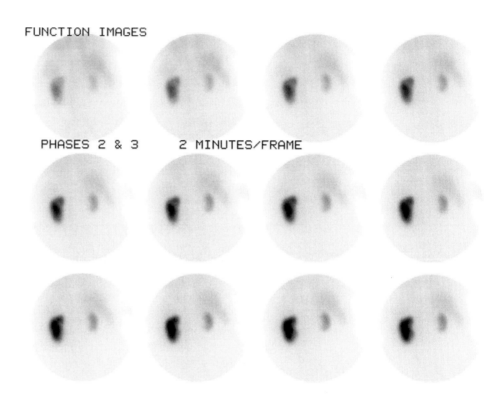

FUNCTION IMAGES

PHASES 2 & 3   2 MINUTES/FRAME

DIFFERENTIAL UPTAKES

LEFT (%)   89.4
RIGHT (%)   10.6

Fig. A—Captopril

Technique

- 8 mCi technetium-99m mercaptoacetyltriglycine (MAG-3) administered intra-venously 1 hour after 50 mg captopril (Figs. A–D).
- Baseline study done 5 days later (Figs. E–H).
- Hydration should be done prior to imaging for both studies.
- Blood pressure measurements taken 60, 30, and 0 minutes before the acquisition of captopril images were: 170/90 mmHg, 170/85 mmHg, and 160/65 mmHg, respectively for this patient.
- Use a low-energy, general-purpose collimator.
- Energy window 20% centered at 140 keV.
- Imaging time is dynamic sequence: 24 frames at 2 sec/frame; 16 frames at 15 sec/frame; 60 frames at 30 sec/frame.

PEARLS/PITFALLS

- Each kidney serves as its own control, such that each kidney is compared with itself at baseline. The change in each kidney, baseline versus captopril, permits the detection of bilateral RAS and RVH. The method also applies to patients with only one kidney.

- A change in cortical retention of more than 10% between captopril and baseline and a change in time to maximum of more than 2 minutes are considered significant changes using tubular agents.

- The curves of renal collecting system obstruction and RAS during captopril administration are similar and can be easily confused.

- Kidneys with very low function are always difficult to evaluate. Such kidneys may have RAS but too little function to generate a measurable response to captopril.

- RAS should always be considered a possibility in small kidneys with poor function.

- Equivocal results (intermediate probability for RAS/ev4) in the form of a partial response to captopril are not uncommon in patients with reduced renal function.

- Most centers recommend cessation of ACE inhibitors 24 to 72 hours before the test.

- Some centers reduce or stop diuretics 24 to 48 hours prior to the study.

- Intravenous ACE inhibitors are advocated by some to ensure effective and quick blockade. Severe hypotension may occur with this protocol, a significant risk in elderly patients.

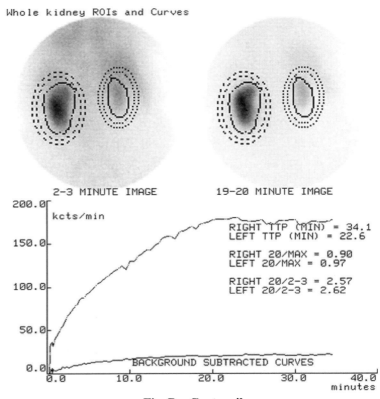

Fig. B—Captopril

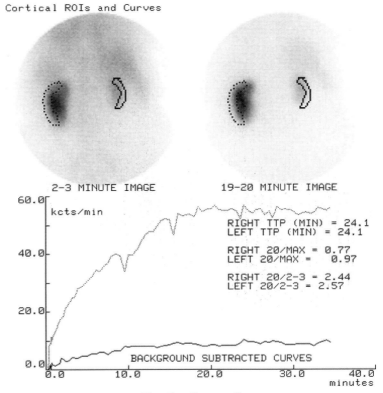

Fig. C—Captopril

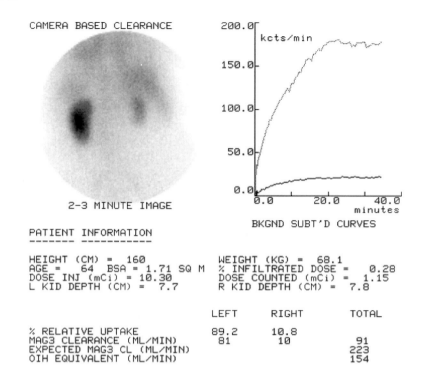

CAMERA BASED CLEARANCE

200.0 kcts/min

150.0

100.0

50.0

0.0

0.0   20.0   40.0
                minutes

2-3 MINUTE IMAGE

BKGND SUBT'D CURVES

PATIENT INFORMATION

HEIGHT (CM) =   160   WEIGHT (KG) =   68.1
AGE =   64 BSA = 1.71 SQ M % INFILTRATED DOSE =   0.28
DOSE INJ (mCi) = 10.30   DOSE COUNTED (mCi) =   1.15
L KID DEPTH (CM) = 7.7   R KID DEPTH (CM) =   7.8

	LEFT	RIGHT	TOTAL
% RELATIVE UPTAKE	89.2	10.8	
MAG3 CLEARANCE (ML/MIN)	81	10	91
EXPECTED MAG3 CL (ML/MIN)			223
OIH EQUIVALENT (ML/MIN)			154

Fig. D—Captopril

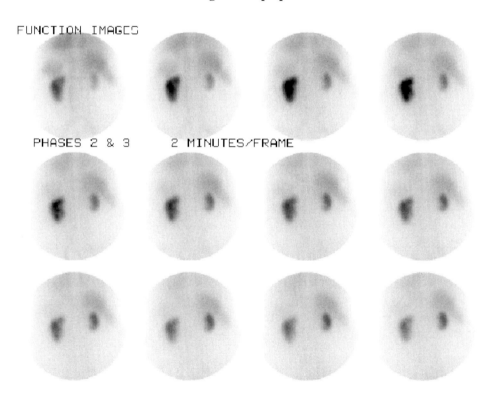

FUNCTION IMAGES

PHASES 2 & 3   2 MINUTES/FRAME

DIFFERENTIAL UPTAKES

LEFT (%)   89.6
RIGHT (%) 10.4

Fig. E—Baseline

Whole kidney ROIs and Curves

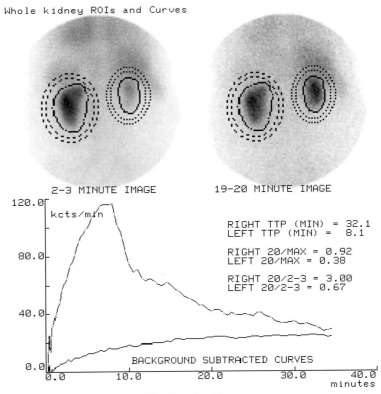

Fig. F—Baseline

Cortical ROIs and Curves

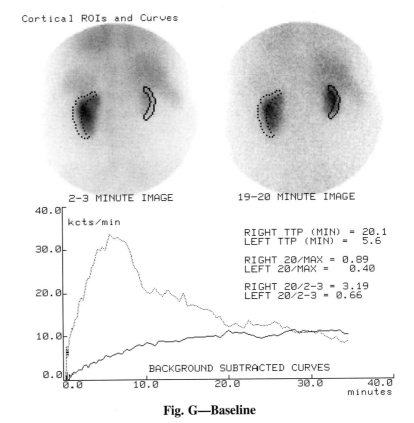

Fig. G—Baseline

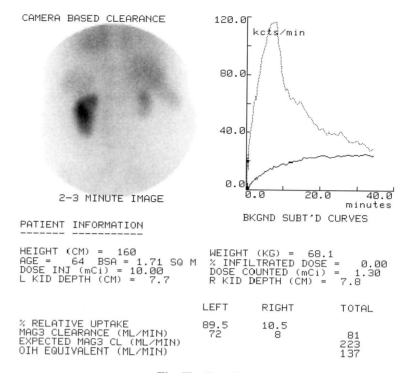

CAMERA BASED CLEARANCE

2-3 MINUTE IMAGE

BKGND SUBT'D CURVES

PATIENT INFORMATION
------- -----------

HEIGHT (CM) =   160   WEIGHT (KG) =   68.1
AGE =   64 BSA = 1.71 SQ M % INFILTRATED DOSE =   0.00
DOSE INJ (mCi) = 10.00   DOSE COUNTED (mCi) =   1.30
L KID DEPTH (CM) =   7.7   R KID DEPTH (CM) =   7.8

	LEFT	RIGHT	TOTAL
% RELATIVE UPTAKE	89.5	10.5	
MAG3 CLEARANCE (ML/MIN)	72	8	
EXPECTED MAG3 CL (ML/MIN)			81
OIH EQUIVALENT (ML/MIN)			223
			137

Fig. H—Baseline

Image Interpretation

Functional images from the captopril study (Fig. A) show that the left kidney is of normal size with inhomogeneous parenchymal distribution in the form of reduced tracer in the upper third. The renal collecting system is not visualized. The right kidney appears very small but with homogeneously distributed functioning parenchyma is present. No collecting system details were identifiable.

The functional whole kidney and cortex curves (Figs. B and C) are very abnormal. The left kidney curves are of continuous accumulation type; the right kidney curves have very low amplitude and appear flat. Total function is markedly reduced, MAG-3 clearance is 91 mL/min (Fig. D) (34% of expected).

Captopril	Left	Right
Split function (%)	89	11
Residual cortical activity at 20 min	>90	90
Time to peak (min)	23	>30

Functional images of the left kidney in baseline study (Fig. E) are similar to the images with captopril, but the collecting system is now visualized (from frame 4 forward). The functional whole kidney and cortex curves (Figs. F and G) for the left kidney now show a distinct peak and clearcut elimination.

The right kidney curves are very similar to the curves seen during captopril challenge. Total function is markedly reduced (Fig. H); MAG-3 clearance is 81 mL/min.

Baseline	Left	Right
Split function (%)	90	10
Residual cortical activity at 20 min	38	92
Time to peak (min)	8.1	>30

The marked increase in time to maximum and increase in cortical retention during captopril challenge compared with baseline are diagnostic for functionally significant renal artery stenosis (RAS) or renovascular hypertension (RVH) on the left side.

The atrophic right kidney with no appreciable change in time to maximum or cortical retention could represent end-stage RAS, but several other conditions could also lead to this pattern.

Differential Diagnosis

- Left renal artery stenosis with atrophic right kidney
- Bilateral renal artery stenosis

Diagnosis and Clinical Follow-up

Renal angiography was performed shortly after the second renogram, revealing (1) occluded right main renal artery and (2) 70% stenosis proximally in the left renal artery. Successful left renal artery angioplasty was performed. The blood pressure was subsequently responsive to a single drug regimen.

Discussion

When a functionally significant RAS develops, it leads to reduced filtration pressure that activates the intrarenal renin-angiotensin-aldosterone system locally. This activation constricts the efferent arterioles, ensuring a sufficient filtration pressure at the expense of flow and increase in systemic pressure. Angiotensin-converting enzyme (ACE) inhibitors block this defense and preservation mechanism, resulting in loss of filtration pressure. A drop in filtration means reduction in ultrafiltrate volume and decrease or cessation of luminal transport of tubular secreted agents resulting in retention.

Anatomical RAS is fairly common in the general population and equally common in individuals with or without hypertension (well-documented in autopsy and angiographic studies). Correction of a stenosis results in improvement of hypertension in only a small fraction of patients with hypertension and RAS. Arteriosclerotic stenosis is in the majority of patients secondary to the hypertension which accelerates development of arteriosclerosis. Hypertension *caused* by renal artery stenosis, on the other hand, is much more responsive to renal artery dilatation. A positive captopril study indicates functionally significant RAS and RVH and predicts positive response to renal artery dilatation or surgical intervention. Although angiography is the gold standard for diagnosis of anatomical RAS, the captopril renogram complements angiography by providing information about the physiological significance of the RAS.

Suggested Readings

Davidson R, Wilcox CS. Diagnostic usefulness of renal scanning after angiotensin converting enzyme inhibitors. *Hypertension* 18:299–303, 1991.

Dondi M, Fanti S, DeFabritiis A, et al. Prognostic value of captopril renal scintigraphy in renovascular hypertension. *J Nucl Med* 33:2040–2044, 1992.

Erbsloh-Moller B, Dumas A, Roth D, et al. Furosemide-131-I-hippuran renography after angiotensin-converting enzyme inhibition for the diagnosis of renovascular hypertension. *Am J Med* 90:23–29, 1991.

Nally JV Jr, Black HRS. State-of-the-art review: Captopril renography—pathophysiological considerations and clinical observations. *Semin Nucl Med* 22:85–97, 1992.

Setaro JF, Saddler MC, Chen CC, et al. Simplified captopril renography in diagnosis and treatment of renal artery stenosis. *Hypertension* 18:289–298, 1991.

Section IX

Biliary Scintigraphy

Case 126

Clinical Presentation

45-year-old man presenting with right upper quadrant pain.

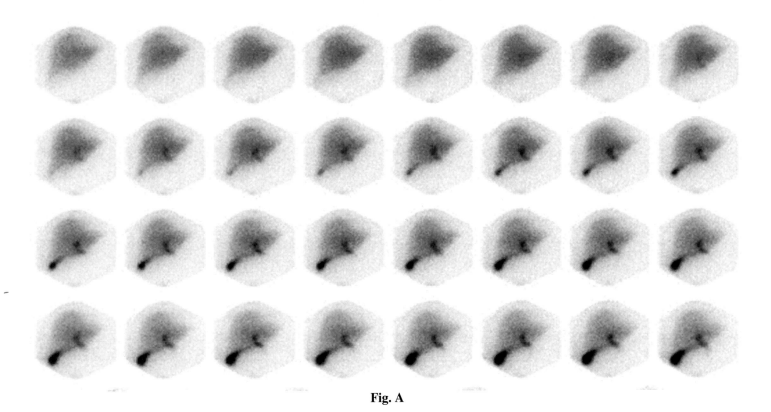

Fig. A

Technique

- Patient should take nothing by mouth for more than 4 hours and less than 24 hours prior to the test.
- Immediately following injection of 1.5 mCi technetium-99m–labeled diisopropyl-iminodiacetic acid (DISIDA) the patient should be positioned supine beneath the gamma camera.
- Continuous image acquisition in a 64 × 64 matrix is divided into 1-minute frames.
- Images (Fig. A) obtained in the left anterior oblique (LAO) projection with a slant-hole collimator.
- Delayed static images are acquired as necessary.

Image Interpretation

Images show rapid tracer uptake into the liver and subsequent excretion into the biliary tract and small bowel (Figs. A, B). The gallbladder is seen within 10 minutes.

PEARLS/PITFALLS

- Clearance of tracer from the cardiac blood pool found on top of the left lobe of the liver is a good indicator of hepatocellular function. Delayed blood pool clearance may indicate that hepatocellular dysfunction is responsible for lack of gallbladder visualization.

- Small bowel collection of tracer in the region of the gallbladder may be confused with collection in the gallbladder but can be cleared by instructing the patient to drink a small amount of water. The water usually empties quickly from the stomach and will wash away any tracer in the small bowel without stimulating cholecystokinin release.

- Look for signs of bowel obstruction, biliary reflux into the stomach, defects in the liver (metastases), and other serendipitous findings.

- Focal tracer uptake in the region of the gallbladder that increases and decreases over time is very unlikely to be in the gallbladder. The gallbladder should not contract unless stimulated by cholecystokinin.

- The caliber of the biliary ducts is not a parameter that can be accurately determined with biliary scintigraphy. Intense concentration of tracer in a duct of normal caliber can demonstrate "blooming" (through narrow angle scatter), which makes the duct look larger than it is. Figure C shows an image with two sections of intravenous tubing of identical diameter. One section (bottom) has approximately 10 times the concentration of activity as the *(continued)*

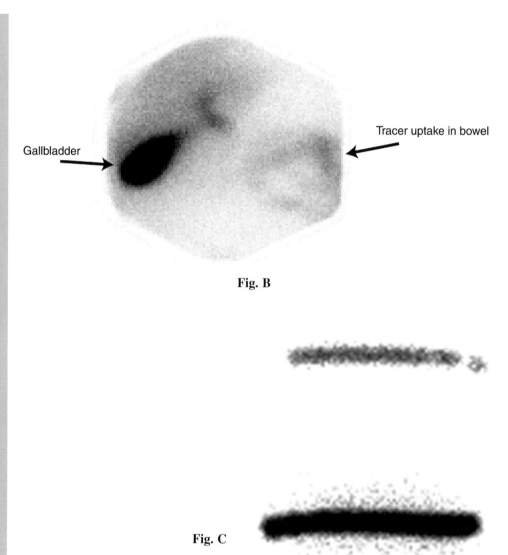

Gallbladder

Tracer uptake in bowel

Fig. B

Fig. C

Differential Diagnosis

- Normal study
- False-negative secondary to tracer in duodenum overlying gallbladder fossa (although this would be expected to vary over time):
  Bile leak into gallbladder fossa
  Acalculous cholecystitis
  Choledochal cyst overlying gallbladder fossa

Diagnosis and Clinical Follow-up

Patient was diagnosed as having peptic ulcer disease. No evidence of biliary disease was noted.

Discussion

The biliary imaging study is a very sensitive, specific test for cystic duct obstruction in patients with acute onset of right upper quadrant pain. The study has decreased in popularity in recent years, however, because of more conservative

(continued) other (top) and therefore appears to be of greater diameter.

- Time between the last meal and imaging can be as little as 2 hours, but the specificity of the test may be diminished if imaging is done less than 4 hours after a meal.

management of biliary tract obstruction and the increased use of more readily available imaging modalities such as ultrasound or computed tomography (CT) and magnetic resonance imaging (MRI). The anatomical imaging tests provide information about not only the liver and biliary tract but also the adjacent structures in the abdomen, making the anatomical imaging tests better suited for screening of abdominal pain. The scintigraphic study, on the other hand, provides information only about the liver and biliary tract, making it less valuable as a screening test. The study is therefore used more often in patients with equivocal findings on other tests. Often the patients have been in the hospital for a period of time and may have taken nothing by mouth for more than 24 hours, making interpretation of the biliary study more difficult.

The normal sequence of appearance of the tracer in the biliary collecting system and gastrointestinal tract has been debated. Some believe that the tracer should normally appear in the gallbladder before it appears in the small bowel. Others believe that the small bowel may be seen before the gallbladder in patients who have eaten recently or who have been fasting for several hours.

Suggested Readings

Hulse PA, Nicholson DA. Investigation of biliary obstruction. *Br J Hosp Med* 52:103–107, 1994.

Kim OH, Chung HJ, Choi BG. Imaging of the choledochal cyst. *Radiographics* 15:69–88, 1995.

Negrin JA, Zanzi I, Margouleff D. Hepatobiliary scintigraphy after biliary tract surgery. *Semin Nucl Med* 25:28–35, 1995.

Saini S. Imaging of the hepatobiliary tract. *N Engl J Med* 336:1889–1894, 1997.

Singer AJ, McCracken G, Henry MC, et al. Correlation among clinical, laboratory, and hepatobiliary scanning findings in patients with suspected acute cholecystitis. *Ann Emerg Med* 28:267–272, 1996.

Weissmann HS, Badia J, Sugarman LA, et al. Spectrum of 99m-Tc-IDA cholescintigraphic patterns in acute cholecystitis. *Radiology* 138:167–175, 1981.

Weissmann HS, Sugarman LA, Frank MS, et al. Serendipity in technetium-99m dimethyl iminodiacetic acid cholescintigraphy: Diagnosis of nonbiliary disorders in suspected acute cholecystitis. *Radiology* 135:449–454, 1980.

Weltman DI, Zeman RK. Acute diseases of the gallbladder and biliary ducts. *Radiol Clin North Am* 32:933–950, 1994.

Case 127

Clinical Presentation

71-year-old man presenting with a history of abdominal and chest pain. Ultrasound was normal. Myocardial infarction was ruled out.

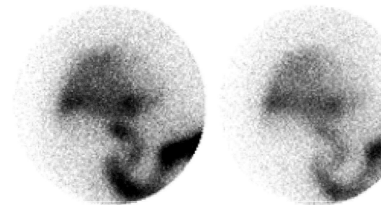

Fig. A

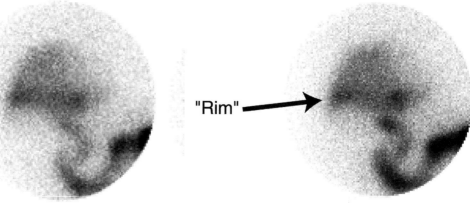

"Rim"

Fig. B

Technique

- Patient should take nothing by mouth for more than 4 hours and less than 24 hours prior to the test.
- Immediately following injection of 1.5 mCi technetium-99m–labeled diisopropyl-iminodiacetic acid (DISIDA) the patient should be positioned supine beneath the gamma camera.
- Continuous image acquisition in a 64 × 64 matrix is divided into 1-minute frames.
- Images obtained in left anterior oblique (LAO) projection with a slant-hole collimator.
- Delayed static images are acquired as necessary.

Image Interpretation

Serial 1-minute images (not shown) showed prompt uptake of the tracer by the hepatocytes. Images at 60 minutes (Fig. A, left) and 75 minutes (Fig. A, right) show tracer in liver and small bowel and a band of tracer ("rim sign") around the region of the gallbladder bed (Fig. B).

Differential Diagnosis

- Acute cholecystitis
- Gallbladder perforation
- Gangrenous cholecystitis
- Locally dilated biliary collecting system

Diagnosis and Clinical Follow-up

At surgery the patient had a gangrenous gallbladder removed.

PEARLS/PITFALLS

- The rim sign may be related to hyperperfusion. Flow images obtained during tracer injection may provide additional information about local inflammatory changes.

- The rim sign is nonspecific and may be caused by other structures such as a prominent porta hepatis.

Discussion

The rim sign is a nonspecific sign on biliary imaging that suggests gangrenous cholecystitis. When the finding is noted during biliary imaging, the referring physician should be contacted immediately because the condition may warrant more immediate attention.

Suggested Readings

Aburano T, Yokoyama K, Taniguchi M, et al. Diagnostic values of gallbladder hyperperfusion and the rim sign in radionuclide angiography and hepatobiliary imaging. *Gastrointest Radiol* 15:229–232, 1990.

Bohdiewicz PJ. The diagnostic value of grading hyperperfusion and the rim sign in cholescintigraphy. *Clin Nucl Med* 18:867–871, 1993.

Brachman MB, Goodman MD, Waxman AD. The rim sign in acute cholecystitis. Comparison of radionuclide, surgical, and pathologic findings. *Clin Nucl Med* 18:863–866, 1993.

Meekin GK, Ziessman HA, Klappenbach RS. Prognostic value and pathophysiologic significance of the rim sign in cholescintigraphy. *J Nucl Med* 28:1679–1682, 1987.

Oates E, Selland DL, Chin CT, et al. Gallbladder nonvisualization with pericholecystic rim sign: morphine-augmentation optimizes diagnosis of acute cholecystitis. *J Nucl Med* 37:267–269, 1996.

Case 128

Clinical Presentation

23-year-old woman presenting with a history of several weeks of intermittent abdominal and right upper quadrant pain.

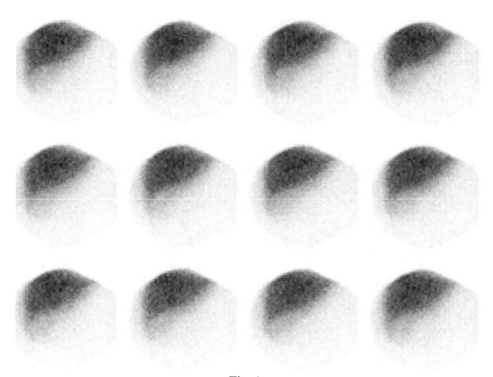

Fig. A

Technique

- Patient should take nothing by mouth for more than 4 hours and less than 24 hours prior to the test.
- Immediately following injection of 1.5 mCi technetium-99m–labeled diisopropyl-iminodiacetic acid (DISIDA) the patient should be positioned supine beneath the gamma camera.
- Continuous image acquisition in a 64 × 64 matrix is divided into 1-minute frames.
- Images obtained in the left anterior oblique (LAO) projection with a slant-hole collimator.
- Delayed static images are acquired as necessary.

Image Interpretation

Images in Figure A are samples of the 1-minute frames obtained during imaging. The patient was imaged continuously for 90 minutes without change in the distribution of tracer. These images show rapid uptake of tracer and homogeneous distribution of tracer throughout the hepatic parenchyma. No tracer movement into the biliary collecting system or bowel was noted during imaging.

Differential Diagnosis

- Choledocholithiasis
- Other causes of complete duct obstruction:
  Carcinoma of the distal biliary tract
  Metastatic disease
  External compression of the common bile duct
- Drug cholestasis
- Hepatitis
- Biliary atresia

Diagnosis and Clinical Follow-up

Common bile duct obstruction was the diagnosis. Endoscopic retrograde cholangiopancreatography (ERCP) demonstrated an edematous, inflamed Oddi's sphincter. Laparotomy revealed two impacted gallstones at Oddi's sphincter.

Discussion

This study demonstrates the typical appearance of complete common bile duct obstruction. Tracer uptake in the liver is normal because hepatocytes are functioning normally, but the obstruction in the biliary collecting system causes intrahepatic cholestasis.

Suggested Readings

Donohoe KJ, Woolfenden JM, Stemmer JL. Biliary imaging suggesting common duct obstruction in acute viral hepatitis. Case report. *Clin Nucl Med* 12:711–712, 1987.

Weissmann HS, Badia J, Sugarman LA, et al. Spectrum of 99m-Tc-IDA cholescintigraphic patterns in acute cholecystitis. *Radiology* 138:167–175, 1981.

Weltman DI, Zeman RK. Acute diseases of the gallbladder and biliary ducts. *Radiol Clin North Am* 32:933–950, 1994.

Case 129

Clinical Presentation

63-year-old man presenting with epigastric distress and a history of recent chole-cystectomy.

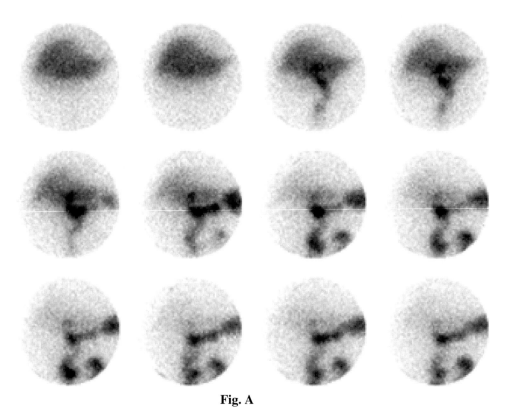

Fig. A

Technique

- Patient should take nothing by mouth for more than 4 hours and less than 24 hours prior to the test.
- Immediately following injection of 1.5 mCi technetium-99m–labeled diisopropyl-iminodiacetic acid (DISIDA) the patient should be positioned supine beneath the gamma camera.
- Continuous image acquisition in a 64 × 64 matrix is divided into 1-minute frames.
- Images obtained in the left anterior oblique (LAO) projection with a slant-hole collimator.
- Delayed static images are acquired as necessary.

Image Interpretation

Selected 1-minute images (Fig. A) obtained for 1 hour show uptake and excretion of tracer into the bowel. Reflux of tracer into the stomach (Fig. B, *arrow*) is noted following appearance of tracer activity in the bowel.

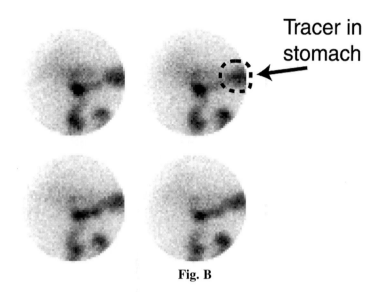

Tracer in stomach

Fig. B

Differential Diagnosis

- Normal variant
- Bile gastritis
- Superimposition of distal duodenum over stomach
- Biliary leak (from biliary tract or bowel perforation)

Diagnosis and Clinical Follow-up

The images demonstrate bile reflux into the stomach. No further workup of the reflux was obtained.

Discussion

Reflux of bile into the stomach can cause a gastritis that may be important in the diagnosis of epigastric discomfort. When bile reflux is noted on the biliary imaging study, it should be mentioned in the study report.

Suggested Reading

Weissmann HS, Sugarman LA, Frank MS, et al. Serendipity in technetium-99m dimethyl iminodiacetic acid cholescintigraphy: Diagnosis of nonbiliary disorders in suspected acute cholecystitis. *Radiology* 135:449–454, 1980.

Case 130

Clinical Presentation

55-year-old man with a history of intravenous drug abuse presenting with malaise and jaundice.

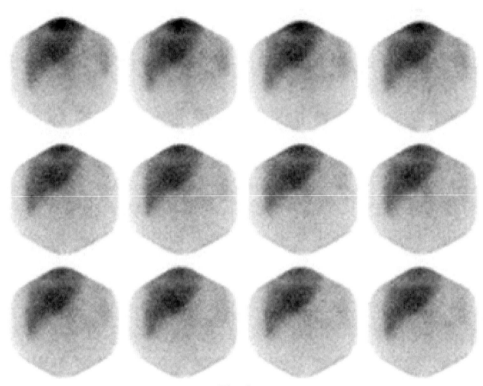

Fig. A

Technique

- Patient should take nothing by mouth for more than 4 hours and less than 24 hours prior to the test.
- Immediately following injection of 1.5 mCi technetium-99m–labeled diisopropyl-iminodiacetic acid (DISIDA) the patient should be positioned supine beneath the gamma camera.
- Continuous image acquisition in a 64 × 64 matrix is divided into 1-minute frames.
- Images obtained in left anterior oblique (LAO) projection with a slant-hole collimator.
- Delayed static images are acquired as necessary.

Image Interpretation

Figure A shows tracer uptake in the liver but also demonstrates tracer in the kidneys and persistent tracer activity in the blood pool (Fig. B). The delayed image obtained at 90 minutes shows persistent blood pool activity, but some activity is

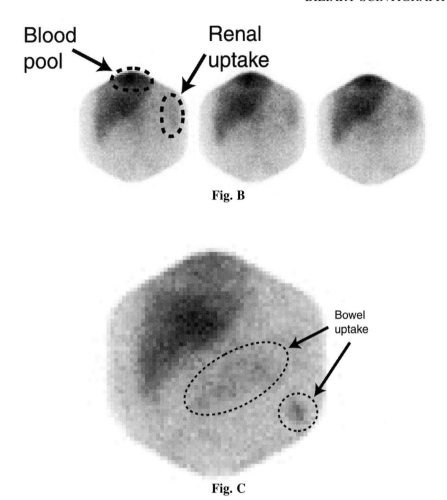

Fig. B

Fig. C

noted in the bowel (Fig. C). The bowel activity was confirmed on cinematic display, which showed the tracer moving in a pattern consistent with small bowel.

Differential Diagnosis

• Choledocholithiasis
• Other causes of complete duct obstruction:
  Carcinoma of the distal biliary tract
  Metastatic disease
  External compression of the common bile duct
• Drug cholestasis
• Hepatitis
• Biliary atresia

Diagnosis and Clinical Follow-up

Patient was diagnosed as having viral hepatitis. No evidence of biliary obstruction was noted on further workup.

Discussion

Because the cardiac blood pool is usually just above the left lobe of the liver, it can easily be monitored for the clearance of tracer from the blood pool. Delayed clearance also causes poor resolution of the liver contour and persistent diffuse background tracer activity. Although the kidneys are a secondary route of tracer excretion, they are posterior structures and therefore not seen very well on anterior views.

Suggested Readings

Aburano T, Yokoyama K, Shuke N, et al. 99mTc colloid and 99mTc IDA imagings in diffuse hepatic disease. *J Clin Gastroenterol* 17:321–326, 1993.

Kim EE, Moon TY, Delpassand ES, Podoloff DA, Haynie TP. Nuclear hepatobiliary imaging. *Radiol Clin North Am* 31:923–933, 1993.

Case 131

Clinical Presentation

83-year-old man with a cholecystostomy tube becoming febrile postoperatively.

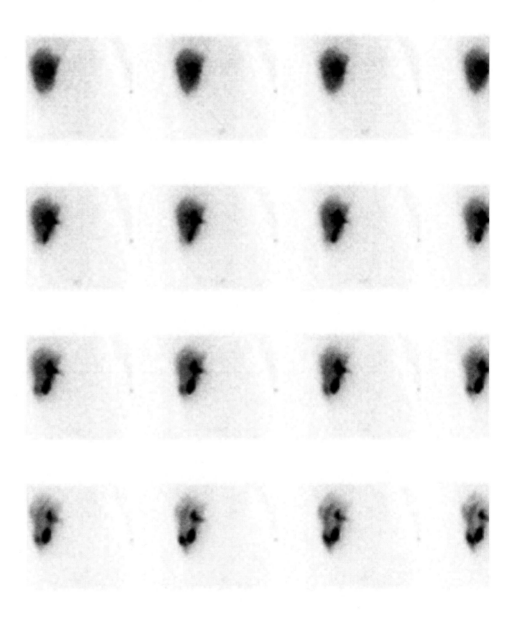

Fig. A

Technique

- Patient should take nothing by mouth for more than 4 hours and less than 24 hours prior to the test.

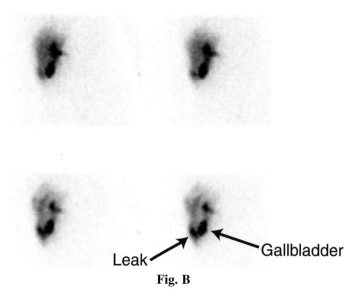

Fig. B

- Immediately following injection of 1.5 mCi technetium–99m–labeled diisopropyl-iminodiacetic acid (DISIDA) the patient should be positioned supine beneath the gamma camera.
- Continuous image acquisition in a 64×64 matrix is divided in 1-minute frames.
- Images obtained in left anterior oblique (LAO) projection with a slant-hole collimator.
- Delayed static images are acquired as necessary.

Image Interpretation

Selected 1-minute dynamic images (Fig. A) show prompt tracer uptake by the liver and subsequent appearance in the gallbladder. A second focus of accumulation is noted lateral to the gallbladder.

Differential Diagnosis

- Biliary tract leak
- Duodenal perforation
- Duodenal obstruction (rare)
- Metastatic hepatoma (very rare)

Diagnosis and Clinical Follow-up

The fluid accumulation lateral to the gallbladder is consistent with a bile leak (Fig. B). Computed tomography (CT) scan showed perihepatic fluid accumulation. Percutaneous drainage revealed the fluid to be bile.

Discussion

The biliary imaging study is an excellent test for demonstrating bile leak. In postoperative patients with perihepatic fluid accumulation, there may be a question not only as to the source of the fluid but also, more importantly, if the fluid is still accumulating. The biliary imaging study is the gold standard for demonstrating active bile leak.

PEARLS/PITFALLS

- If the leak is slow, delayed images may be necessary.

- If imaging is halted too early, a focal leak in the region of the gallbladder or bowel may be mistaken for expected excretion into normal structures. Continued imaging may be needed to show that local accumulation does not demonstrate the contour of normal structures.

Suggested Readings

Goletti O, Boni G, Lippolis PV, et al. Scintigraphic evaluation of biliary leakage following laparoscopic cholecystectomy. *Surg Laparosc Endosc* 3:286–289, 1993.

Kurzawinski TR, Selves L, Farouk M, et al. Prospective study of hepatobiliary scintigraphy and endoscopic cholangiography for the detection of early biliary complications after orthotopic liver transplantation. *Br J Surg* 84:620–623, 1997.

Peters JH, Ollila D, Nichols KE, et al. Diagnosis and management of bile leaks following laparoscopic cholecystectomy. *Surg Laparosc Endosc* 4:163–170, 1994.

Case 132

Clinical Presentation

71-year-old man with pancreatic cancer presenting with right upper quadrant pain. The patient was given narcotic analgesia before biliary scintigraphy was started.

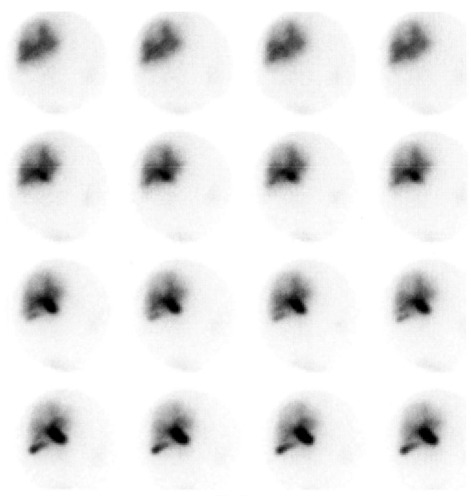

Fig. A

Technique

- Patient should take nothing by mouth for more than 4 hours and less than 24 hours prior to the test.
- Immediately following injection of 1.5 mCi technetium-99m–labeled diisopropyl-iminodiacetic acid (DISIDA) the patient should be positioned supine beneath the gamma camera.
- Continuous image acquisition in a 64 × 64 matrix is divided in 1-minute frames.

- Images obtained in left anterior oblique (LAO) projection with a slant-hole collimator.
- Delayed static images are acquired as necessary.

Image Interpretation

Selected 1-minute images (Fig. A) immediately after tracer injection demonstrate irregular tracer uptake in the liver. The defects noted in the liver correspond to lesions noted on computed tomography (CT) scan. The gallbladder was visualized, but no activity was noted in the bowel at 1 hour. The lack of small bowel visualization may be secondary to contraction of Oddi's sphincter caused by narcotics. A prominent hepatic duct is noted. This may be secondary to pooling of tracer in a normal caliber duct, however, and is not necessarily a sign of a dilated or obstructed duct.

Differential Diagnosis

- Hemangioma
- Hepatic cyst
- Metastasis
- Abscess
- Hepatoma

Diagnosis and Clinical Follow-up

Biopsy demonstrated that the liver defects seen on the biliary study were secondary to pancreatic cancer metastases.

Discussion

Biliary imaging studies may provide information about causes of right upper quadrant abdominal pain other than cholecystitis. Early images demonstrating tracer uptake in the liver can demonstrate not only diffuse hepatocellular dysfunction but also focal abnormalities in the liver. Intrahepatic lesions may also cause regional obstruction of bile flow. This may be demonstrated by delayed emptying or lack of tracer emptying from one or more hepatic segments. If complete cholestasis is present in the obstructed segment, visualization of tracer in a dilated biliary tree is unlikely.

Suggested Readings

Kinnard MF, Alavi A, Rubin RA, Lichtenstein GR. Nuclear imaging of solid hepatic masses. *Semin Roentgenol* 30:375–395, 1995.

Salvatori M. Imaging of hepatic focal lesions by nuclear medicine. *J Surg Oncol* 3(suppl):189–191, 1993.

Section X

Lymphoscintigraphy

Case 133

Clinical Presentation

50-year-old woman presenting with a history of breast cancer and status post-left breast lumpectomy, axillary lymph node dissection, and radiation. She was complaining of progressive ipsilateral arm and forearm swelling. Doppler studies were normal. She was referred for lymphoscintigraphy (LS) to evaluate lymphatic drainage.

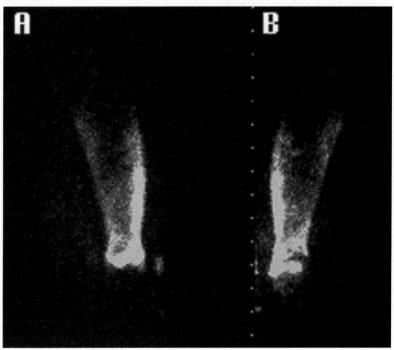

Figs. A, B

PEARLS/PITFALLS

- To maintain sterile conditions, two tuberculin syringes (one per injection site) are prepared equipped with a 26-gauge needle. Fifty μL of air are withdrawn followed by 50 μL of the FSC preparation. The small amount of volume minimizes the pain or burning sensation that may be felt during the intradermal injection, and the air pushes all the volume in, preventing loss of tracer in the tip of the syringe or within the needle. *(continued)*

Technique

- Radiopharmaceutical is filtered (0.22 μm) technetium-99m sulfur colloid (FSC) (Hung et al, 1995) at a concentration of 10 mCi (370 MBq)/mL and 0.5 mCi (18.5 MBq)/injection site.
- Administer two 0.05-cc intradermal injections of technetium Tc-99m FSC in the dorsum (as opposed to the web space) of the hand using sterile techniques. Injection of the contralateral extremity is sometimes used to provide a comparison. Patient is then asked to exercise the hand and arm to aid lymphatic drainage from the injection site.
- Static images of the forearm, arm, and shoulder are acquired for 15 minutes each, leaving the injection sites just outside the field of view. Images are obtained over the first 90 minutes post-injection or until lymph vessels and nodal groups are visualized. Delayed views (2 to 3 hours post injection) are also obtained to assess for dermal backflow or "cutaneous flare."

- *(continued)* Delayed views are essential in the evaluation of lymphedema because it takes longer for the superficial lymphatic vessels to fill in.

- There are several degrees of severity of lymphedema. Early changes include tortuosity and collateralization of lymphatic vessels, followed by focal flare, usually located in the elbow region. With increasing lymphedema, the cutaneous flare extends over the extremity, and there is decreased or nonvisualization of deep lymphatic vessels and lymph node groups.

- It is important to use sterile technique during the injection because lymphedematous areas are extremely sensitive to infection, which should be avoided since it is a confounding factor leading to potential worsening of lymphedema. Development of cellulitis may quickly lead to systemic infection, and aggressive intravenous antibiotherapy with hospital stay is usually needed.

- Assessment of lymphedema via LS may not be current practice in many nuclear medicine practices. However, development of new reconstructive and plastic surgical techniques as well as new drugs may lead to alleviation of lymphedema. LS allows for evaluation of lymph vessel patency and the severity of lymphedema, which may help identify which patient would benefit from such treatment.

Image Interpretation

Anterior (Fig. A) and posterior (Fig. B) delayed views of the left arm are shown. The hand is out of the field of view at the lower end of the field of view. The images demonstrate nonvisualization of deep lymphatic vessels and diffuse dermal backflow or cutaneous flare extending from the wrist up to the elbow region. Two faint brachial nodes are seen on the anterior view in the distal aspect of the arm.

Differential Diagnosis

- Lymphedema
- Cellulitis
- Edema secondary to vascular etiology

Diagnosis and Clinical Follow-up

Findings were consistent with lymphedema and severe functional impairment of lymphatic drainage from the left upper extremity.

Discussion

Radionuclide LS is a physiological, noninvasive technique that can be easily performed and readily repeated. This diagnostic tool provides unique functional information on lymphatic channels and nodes. Since it does not require direct intralymphatic administration, it can be applied in diverse clinical situations and in anatomic sites that may not be accessible to contrast lymphangiography. It is based on the principle that radiolabeled colloid or macromolecules of appropriate size and properties introduced into appropriate tissue planes are transported into lymphatic channels and drain into lymphatic nodes. This allows anatomical and functional visualization of the lymphatic system under normal and abnormal conditions (Ege, 1996). It has also been useful in assessing lymphatic drainage before and after reconstructive and plastic surgery (Slavin et al, 1997, and 1999).

A typical normal upper extremity LS will show rapid migration from the injection sites into the ulnar or radial vessels, or both, as well as a few main channels over the posterior wrist and forearm within a few minutes post-injection. The radiocolloid will then transit medially through the antecubital fossa to a brachial vessel in the medial upper arm into the axillary lymph node basin. Besides axillary nodes, epitrochlear and brachial nodes can also be visualized.

Suggested Readings

Browse NL. The diagnosis and management of primary lymphedema. *J Vasc Surg* 3:181, 1986.

Ege GN. Lymphoscintigraphy in oncology. In: *Nuclear Medicine,* Henkin RE, Boles MA, Dillehay GL, et al, eds. St. Louis, MO: Mosby-Year Book, Inc., 1996:1504–1523.

Gloviczki P, Calcagno D, Schirger A, et al. Noninvasive evaluation of the swollen extremity: Experiences with 190 lymphoscintigraphy examinations. *J Vasc Surg* 9:683–689, 1989.

Golueke PJ, Montgomery RA, Minken SL, Perler BA, Williams GM. Lymphoscintigraphy to confirm the clinical diagnosis of lymphedema. *J Vasc Surg* 10:306–312, 1989.

Hung JC, Wiseman GA, Wahner HW, et al. Filtered technetium-99m-sulfur colloid evaluated for lymphoscintigraphy. *J Nucl Med* 36:1895–1901, 1995.

Slavin SA, Upton J, Kaplan WD, Van den Abbeele AD. An investigation of lymphatic function following free tissue transfer. *Plast Reconstr Surg* 99:730–741, 1997.

Slavin SA, Van den Abbeele AD, Losken A, Swartz MA, Jain RK. Return of lymphatic function after flop transfer for acute lymphedema. *Annals of Surg* 229:421–427, 1999.

Ter SE, Alavi A, Kim CK, Merli G. Lymphoscintigraphy. A reliable test for the diagnosis of lymphedema. *Clin Nucl Med* 18:646–654, 1993.

Vendrell-Torne E, Setoain-Quinquer J, Domenech-Torne FM. Study of normal lymphatic drainage using radioactive isotopes. *J Nucl Med* 13:801–805, 1972.

Case 134

Clinical Presentation

42-year-old woman presenting with a history of pelvic surgery 2.5 years ago. There has been gradual onset of left extremity edema without a venous explanation. Lymphatic drainage is to be evaluated.

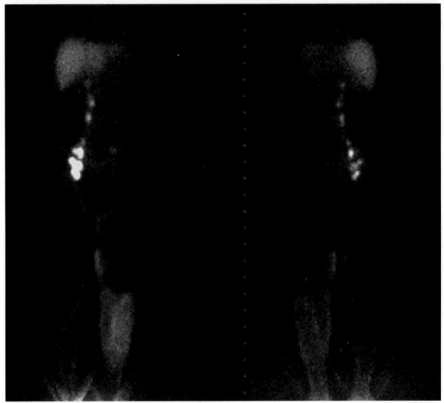

Figs. A, B

Technique

- Filtered (0.22 μm) technetium-99m sulfur colloid (FSC) (Hung et al, 1995) at a concentration of 10 mCi (370 MBq)/mL and 0.5 mCi (18.5 MBq)/injection site.
- Administer two 0.05-cc intradermal injections of technetium-99m FSC in the dorsum (as opposed to the web space) of each foot using sterile technique. Injection of the contralateral extremity is used to provide a comparison. Patient is then asked to go up and down a flight of stairs to aid lymphatic drainage from the injection site.
- Successive anterior and posterior whole body images are acquired at 8 cm/min up to the level of the chest, leaving the injection sites out of the field of view. Images are obtained over the first 90 minutes post-injection until lymph vessels and nodal groups are visualized up to the cisterna chyli and until the liver is visualized. Delayed views (2 to 3 hours post-injection) are also ob-

tained to assess for dermal backflow or "cutaneous flare." These are important in the diagnosis of lymphedema, which may not be evident on the earlier set of images.

- The end point of an exam occurs when the clinical question is answered.

Image Interpretation

Delayed anterior (Fig. A) and posterior (Fig. B) whole body views show a normal right lower extremity lymphoscintigraphy (LS) with visualization of deep lymphatic vessels along the right lower extremity, followed by filling of right inguinal and iliac nodes and progression of tracer into the right paraaortic nodal chain up to the level of the cisterna chyli. The liver is also visualized.

There is only faint visualization of deep lymphatic vessels in the left lower extremity and diffuse cutaneous flare from the knee to the ankle. Two areas of more focal flare are also seen in the medial aspect of the left thigh. There is only faint visualization of an inguinal lymph node and no further progression of activity beyond the inguinal region. The posterior view shows a popliteal lymph node.

Differential Diagnosis

- Low plasma osmotic pressure
- Obstruction of venous return
- Obstruction of lymphatic return

Diagnosis and Clinical Follow-up

Findings were consistent with severe functional impairment of lymphatic drainage from the left lower extremity and lymphedema in the lower portion of the extremity with progression into the thigh.

Discussion

A normal study, as demonstrated in the right lower extremity in this case, should demonstrate the major lymph vessels along the entire extremity and lymph node groups in the inguinal, iliac, and para-aortic regions up to the cisterna chyli. Occasionally, popliteal lymph nodes are seen. From the cisterna chyli, lymph drains into the thoracic duct and into the left subclavian vein. Visualization of the liver, therefore, confirms patent communication between the lymphatic and the venous systems.

Generally, extremity edema has three main etiologies: low plasma osmotic pressure (usually seen in cases of kidney or liver failure but also seen associated with inflammation and associated increased vascular permeability), obstruction of venous return (with etiologies ranging from heart failure to venous thrombus), and obstruction of lymphatic return. Some of the more commonly encountered causes of impaired lymphatic return include congenital deficiency of lymphatic vessels, luminal obstruction by lymphadenopathy (because of tumor or infection), compression of the lymphatic vessel lumen via fibrosis (secondary to radiation therapy) or edema (often venous in etiology) in the surrounding tissues, and node dissection associated with radiation therapy (frequently observed in patients with breast cancer or pelvic cancers).

A study of 17 patients (20 extremities) referred for lymphedema resulted in 8 true-positive, 9 true-negative, 0 false-positive, and 3 false-negative extremity im-

• *(continued)* LS is the diagnostic study of choice to evaluate lymphedema. Whereas conventional lymphangiography better demonstrates lymph vessel morphology, LS can readily demonstrate the presence of lymphedema, the location of major nodal groups, and the lymphatic drainage patterns at a lower price and with less radiation exposure to the patient. Also, lymphangiography is technically more difficult to perform, provides little functional information, and may have significant side effects (including local tissue necrosis, contrast reaction, and exacerbation of lymphedema).

ages; the 3 false-negatives were not imaged within the first hour, decreasing the sensitivity for detecting subtle pedal lymphedema and crossover filling of major lymph nodes (Ter Se et al, 1993). Another study of 115 patients (190 extremities) referred for the evaluation of extremity edema showed LS to be 92% sensitive and 100% specific for the diagnosis of lymphedema (Gloviczki et al, 1989).

Suggested Readings

Browse NL. The diagnosis and management of primary lymphedema. *J Vasc Surg* 3:181, 1986.

Ege GN. Lymphoscintigraphy in oncology. In: Henkin RE, Boles MA, Dillehay GL, et al, eds. *Nuclear Medicine,* St. Louis, MO: Mosby-Year Book, Inc., 1996, pp 1504–1523.

Gloviczki P, Calcagno D, Schirger A, et al. Noninvasive evaluation of the swollen extremity: Experiences with 190 lymphoscintigraphy examinations. *J Vasc Surg* 9:683–689, 1989.

Golueke PJ, Montgomery RA, Minken SL, Perler BA, Williams GM. Lymphoscintigraphy to confirm the clinical diagnosis of lymphedema. *J Vasc Surg* 10:306–312, 1989.

Hung JC, Wiseman GA, Wahner HW, et al. Filtered technetium-99m-sulfur colloid evaluated for lymphoscintigraphy. *J Nucl Med* 36:1895–1901, 1995.

Slavin SA, Upton J, Kaplan WD, Van den Abbeele AD. An investigation of lymphatic function following free tissue transfer. *Plast Reconstr Surg* 99:730–741, 1997.

Ter SE, Alavi A, Kim CK, Merli G. Lymphoscintigraphy. A reliable test for the diagnosis of lymphedema. *Clin Nucl Med* 18:646–654, 1993.

Vendrell-Torne E, Setoain-Quinquer J, Domenech-Torne FM. Study of normal lymphatic drainage using radioactive isotopes. *J Nucl Med* 13:801–805, 1972.

Case 135

Clinical Presentation

38-year-old woman presenting 2 weeks after excisional biopsy of a level III melanoma on her right flank. She had no palpable nodal disease and was scheduled for wide local excision the day of this study.

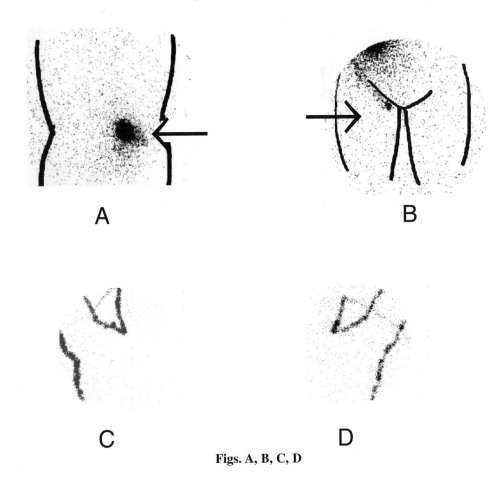

Figs. A, B, C, D

Technique

- 2 to 4 doses of 100 to 200 μCi technetium-99m filtered (0.22-μm filter) sulfur colloid diluted in a volume of 0.1 to 0.2 cc. One–cubic centimeter syringes with 25-gauge needles are recommended. Approximately 0.1 cc of air drawn behind the nuclide solution will ensure that the dose is emptied from the syringe during injection.
- For injection it is helpful to bend the needle to a 45-degree angle using the loosened cap as a sterile tool. Use of standard sterile betadine followed by alcohol prep is recommended.
- Draping the field will reduce the chance of skin contamination.
- Use a high-resolution collimator.
- Energy window 20% centered on 140 keV.
- Imaging time is 60 seconds per view.

375

PEARLS/PITFALLS

- Additional views (lateral and oblique) of a sentinel node to determine depth will aid in intraoperative localization. These extra views are strongly recommended for axillary nodes. Single photon emission computed tomography (particularly the cinematic projections) can also aid in more definitive localization.

- Poor progression of nuclide beyond the injection site can be due to an inadvertent subcutaneous injection; a repeat injection is recommended if a small tense wheal is not evident. The covering epidermis on the palms and soles is relatively thick and requires a deeper injection.

- Delayed imaging (at 2 to 4) hours has been recommended to increase the intraoperative target to background count ratios.

- Contamination of the skin or clothing can cause false-positive results. Great care should be taken to avoid contamination; draping the field with an opening only for the injection site should be considered.

- Although sentinel node lymphoscintigraphy is becoming well-established for use in cases of malignant melanoma, there is ongoing research into the use of this technique for breast cancer lesions. The technique for breast cancer is more difficult because injection around the primary lesion may require the use of ultrasonography if the lesion is not palpable. Interpretation can be more difficult because the fainter draining nodes may be obscured by a proximal injection site. Clinical trials are currently in progress to evaluate the usefulness of this method in patients with breast cancer.

- For imaging have the patient in position (the position planned for the surgical procedure is preferred) prior to injection. Following the preceding preparatory guidelines, administer 2 to 4 intradermal injections close to and surrounding the site of the original lesion. Obtain immediate 60-second static (or dynamic) images of the injection site. Shield the injection site or remove from field on future images for improved visualization of tracer movement. Obtain sequential 60-second acquisitions (or a dynamic study over the first 30 minutes followed by static views), repositioning the patient, if needed, to follow visualized lymph channels. Carefully mark skin location of sentinel node(s) (using radioactive marker to direct marking position in two planes). Adequate images can usually be obtained within 30 minutes to 1 hour after injection; a delayed image at 2 to 4 hours will show all nodal draining basins, however. This delay will also result in increased target to background ratio at the time of surgery.

Image Interpretation

Figure A is a posterior abdominal view obtained immediately after injection showing confluence of injection sites. The patient received a total of four injections because the first two injections were not clearly intradermal. Figure B is an image obtained 10 minutes after injection and shows intense increased uptake in a single groin node medially. Right and left anterior axillary views (Figs. C and D, respectively) acquired at 18 and 20 minutes post injection are negative (rough outlines of the arm and neck were drawn with a radioactive marker).

Differential Diagnosis

- Sentinel lymph node
- Skin contamination
- Tortuous lymphatic channel with transient "hang-up" of nuclide
- Secondary lymph node

Diagnosis and Clinical Follow-up

Pathological examination of this inguinal node was negative for melanoma.

Discussion

Malignant melanoma is a cancerous transformation of melatonin cells. The extent of disease is categorized according to the thickness of the primary lesion and the presence of lymph node or distant metastases. The spread of melanoma cells occurs via lymphatics (more common) and hematogenous routes. The surgical management of the primary lesion is wide local dermal excision. A radical lymph node dissection is indicated for palpable nodes. Elective lymph node dissection is only indicated in cases in which the primary lesions are 1 to 4 mm thick and there is no clinical evidence of metastases. The overall benefit of elective lymph node dissection is controversial and under investigation.

Lymphoscintigraphy is important because lymph drainage patterns are quite variable, particularly for head, neck, and truncal lesions. For all nodal groups, identification and biopsy of the primary draining node (sentinel node) can preempt further exploration if the sentinal node is negative for tumor. Use of an intraoperative gamma probe is useful for localization of radioactive nodes during surgery.

Suggested Readings

Albertini JJ, Cruse CW, Rapaport D, et al. Intraoperative radiolymphoscintigraphy improves sentinel lymph node identification for patients with melanoma. *Ann Surg* 223:217–224, 1996.

Krag DN, Meijer SJ, Weaver DL, et al. Minimal access surgery for staging of malignant melanoma. *Arch Surg* 130:654–660, 1995.

Krag D, Weaver D, Ashikaga T, et al. The sentinel node in breast cancer—a multicenter validation study. *N Engl J Med* 339:941–946, 1998.

Morton DL, Duan-Ren, Wong JH, et al. Technical details of intraoperative lymphatic mapping for early stage melanoma. *Arch Surg* 127:392–399, 1992.

O'Brien CJ, Uren RF, Thompson JF, et al. Prediction of potential metastatic sites in cutaneous head and neck melanoma using lymphoscintigraphy. *Am J Surg* 170:461–466, 1995.

Case 136

Clinical Presentation

36-year-old man presenting 18 months after noticing a change in the appearance of a mole on his back. An excisional biopsy performed 3 weeks prior to presentation showed a 1.04-mm level III malignant melanoma.

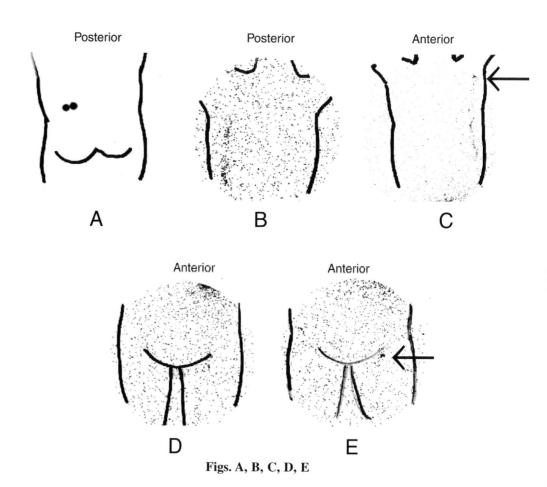

Figs. A, B, C, D, E

Technique

- 2 to 4 doses of 100 to 200 µCi technetium-99m filtered (0.22-µm filter) sulfur colloid diluted in a volume of 0.1 to 0.2 cc. One–cubic centimeter syringes with 25-gauge needles are recommended. Approximately 0.1 cc of air drawn behind the nuclide solution will ensure that the dose is emptied from the syringe during injection.
- For injection it is helpful to bend the needle to a 45-degree angle using the loosened cap as a sterile tool. Use of standard sterile betadine followed by alcohol prep is recommended.
- Draping the field will reduce the chance of skin contamination.
- High-resolution collimator.
- Energy window 20% centered on 140 keV.
- Imaging time is 60 seconds per view.

PEARLS/PITFALLS

- •Rapid imaging under direct supervision is important for the successful use of this technique. Nodes can appear at several locations within minutes of each other. Careful skin marking and conscientious communication of findings to the surgeon are very important.

- Cleaning up any contaminated area will help decrease confusion for the surgeon using the radiation probe during surgery.

- Covering the injection site with a 4 cm × 4 cm gauze pad while removing the needle will decrease the chances of tracer spraying or leaking out of the injection site to contaminate the surrounding area.

- The importance of tracer uptake in nodes distal to the first visualized node has been debated. Some surgeons pursue any nodes with radiotracer; some are primarily interested in the first node visualized in any single nodal group.

- For imaging have the patient in position (the position planned for the surgical procedure is preferred) prior to injection. Following the preceding preparatory guidelines, administer 2 to 4 subdermal injections close to and surrounding the site of the original lesion. Obtain immediate 60-second static (or dynamic) images of the injection site. Shield the injection site or remove from field on future images for improved visualization of tracer movement. Obtain sequential 60-second acquisitions (or a dynamic study over the first 30 minutes followed by static views), repositioning the patient, if needed, to follow visualized lymph channels. Carefully mark skin location of sentinel node(s) (using radioactive marker to direct marking position in two planes). Adequate images can usually be obtained within 30 minutes to 1 hour after injection; a delayed image at 2 to 4 hours will show all nodal draining basins, however. This delay will also result in increased target to background ratio at the time of surgery.

Image Interpretation

Figure A is a posterior abdominal view obtained immediately after injection showing the two sites of intradermal injection over the left flank. Eight minutes after injection, anterior views of the trunk (Fig. B) demonstrated a prominent lymph channel on the left ascending to the left axilla. Fourteen minutes after injection an axillary node was seen on the anterior chest view (Fig. C). Eighteen minutes after injection faint uptake was seen in a left groin node (Fig. D). Fifteen minutes later this node was more prominent (Fig. E).

Differential Diagnosis

- Sentinel lymph node
- Skin contamination
- Tortuous lymphatic channel with transient "hang-up" of nuclide
- Secondary lymph node

Diagnosis and Clinical Follow-up

Pathological examination of the axillary and inguinal nodes showed no evidence of lymphatic spread of disease.

Discussion

This case is an example of the unpredictability of lymph drainage patterns, particularly in the trunk at approximately the level of the umbilicus and any midline location in the back or the anterior chest and abdomen. Lymph drainage patterns are quite variable in the head and neck as well. There are two sentinel nodes in this case: one in the ipsilateral axilla and one in the groin. Drainage to two or more lymph node beds is observed in approximately 60% of cases; drainage to three or more nodal groups occurs in 10% of cases. Lymphoscintigraphy can identify sentinel nodes in a number of distant nodal beds.

Suggested Readings

McCarthy WH, Shaw HM, Cascinelli N, et al. Elective lymph node dissection for melanoma: Two perspectives. *World J Surg* 16:203–213, 1992.

Slingluff CL, Stidman KR, Ricci WM, Stanley WE, Seigler HG. Surgical management of regional lymph nodes in patients with melanoma. *Ann Surg* 219:120–130, 1994.

Uren RF, Howman-Giles RB, Shaw HM, Thompson JF, McCarthy WH. Lymphoscintigraphy in high-risk melanoma of the trunk: Predicting draining node groups, defining lymphatic channels and locating the sentinel node. *J Nucl Med* 34:1435–1450, 1993.

Uren RF, Howman-Giles RB, Thompson JF, et al. Mammary lymphoscintigraphy in breast cancer. *J Nucl Med* 36:1775–1780, 1995.

Wells KE, Cruse CW, Daniels S, et al. The use of lymphoscintigraphy in melanoma of the head and neck. *Plast Reconstr Surg* 93:757–761, 1994.

Section XI

Central Nervous System Scintigraphy

Case 137

Clinical Presentation

62-year-old woman presenting with increasing short-term memory loss over the past 3 years. A radionuclide brain perfusion single photon emission computed tomography (SPECT) study was ordered to evalute the perfusion pattern.

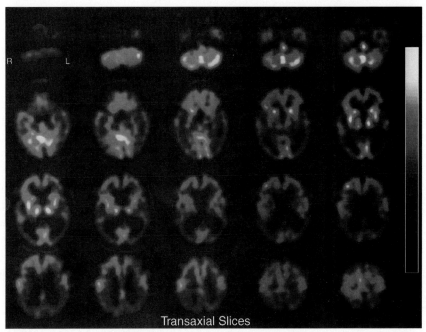

Fig. A (see Color Plate 11, page IV)

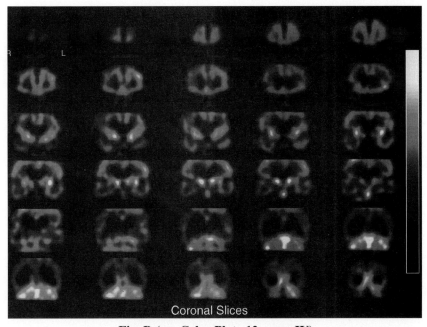

Fig. B (see Color Plate 12, page IV)

- Sulci, gyri, and ventricles tend to appear larger in older patients because of atrophy. This is a common finding.

- Temporal lobe perfusion defects can be missed on axial images. Coronal slices are useful for the evaluation of the temporal lobes.

- Brain perfusion scans are normalized to the cerebellum. Any visible defect below 60% of cerebellar activity (blue area in the color scale) noted over a span of two adjacent slices should be considered abnormal.

- It is normal to observe a few small perfusion defects in healthy subjects because of sulci and wide gyri.

- Consider Pick's disease or dementia of the frontal type if there is involvement of frontal and occasionally temporal lobes.

- While evaluating disease progress by comparing with previous studies, be aware of the differences in the perfusion patterns between HMPAO and ECD studies because their normal distribution varies. Always check for image orientation (left and right sides of the patient) before correlating with magnetic resonance, computed tomography, or other SPECT studies because protocols used for image processing may differ.
(continued)

Technique

- 20 mCi of technetium-99m-labeled-hexamethyl propylene amine oxime (HMPAO) (or ECD) injected intravenously.
- Energy window 10% centered over the 140-keV peak.
- Imaging time: 20 to 30 minutes after injection (1 hour if using ECD).
- Acquisition protocol is 30 minutes using an annular SPECT system, 360 degrees, 120 images, 15 sec/image, matrix size 128 × 128, 1 byte per pixel.
- Patient should be supine, with the head slightly elevated and eyes closed. Patient's head should be as close to the camera as possible and strapped tightly with a nonattenuating object such as Velcro, rubber, or elastic to avoid head motion.
- Environment should be a quiet room with lights dimmed (avoid disturbances and noise).
- Patient's head should be in the center of the axis of rotation. Adjust head position so that the area of interest lies in the center.

Image Interpretation

The axial (Fig. A) and coronal (Fig. B) views display a global reduction in the radiotracer uptake with increased background activity (notice the halo around the brain representing scalp uptake). Lateral frontal perfusion defects are seen on the left side. Marked reduction in the perfusion to the temporal lobes (medial, lateral, and inferior aspects) is seen bilaterally in the axial and coronal slices. The left side is more affected than the right side is. Marked reduction in the perfusion to the entire parietal cortex is noted bilaterally. Symmetrical radiotracer uptake is visible in the basal ganglia and thalami.

Differential Diagnosis

- Alzheimer's disease
- Parkinson's disease
- Multi-infarct dementia

Diagnosis and Clinical Follow-up

There are bilateral temporoparietal perfusion defects, left more than right, in a pattern consistent with Alzheimer's disease.

Discussion

As with positron emission tomography (PET) imaging, perfusion abnormalities detected with SPECT imaging in patients with Alzheimer's disease correlate with the severity of the disease. Early in the disease the defects can be asymmetrical and of variable intensity. As the disease progresses, the defects become more prominent, with relative sparing of the basal ganglia and cerebellum.

If Parkinson's disease is excluded, the probability of Alzheimer's disease is more than 90% with bilateral temporal or parietal, or both, perfusion defects. This pattern is seen in 65% of patients with Alzheimer's.

• *(continued)* Patient motion as well as tilted axis can be misrepresented as perfusion defects in different views. Always correlate the asymmetry with the slice above and below and also with corresponding views in other planes.

• The reported accuracy of SPECT in early Alzheimer's disease has varied over a wide range. Recent data, however, suggest a high accuracy even in very mild disease.

Suggested Readings

Holman BL, Chandak PK, Garada BM. Atlas of Brain Perfusion SPECT. Available: http://www.med.harvard.edu/BWHRad/BrainSPECT/

Holman BL, Johnson KA, Garada B, Carvalho PA, Satlin A. The scintigraphic appearance of Alzheimer's disease: A prospective study using technetium 99m-HMPAO SPECT. *J Nucl Med* 33:181–185, 1992.

Case 138

Clinical Presentation

34-year-old woman with intractable complex partial seizures since the age of 22 admitted for the evaluation of the seizure focus. Depth electrode placement showed spike activity in the frontal and temporal lobes.

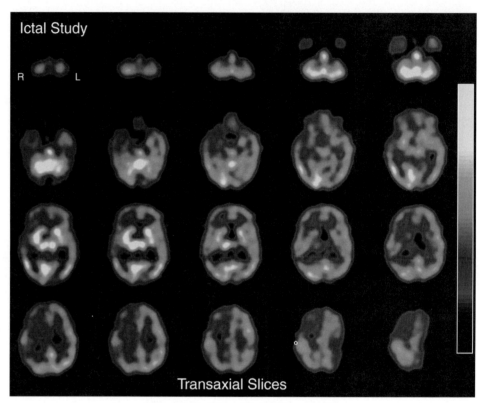

Fig. A (see Color Plate 13, page V)

Technique

- 20 mCi of technetium-99m hexamethyl propylene amine oxime (HMPAO) (or ECD) injected intravenously.
- Energy window is 10% centered over the 140 keV peak.
- Imaging time is 20 to 30 minutes after injection (1 hour if using ECD).
- Acquisition protocol is 30 minutes using an annular single photon emission computed tomography (SPECT) system, 360 degrees, 120 images, 15 sec/image. Matrix size is 128 × 128, 1 byte per pixel.
- Patient is supine, with the head slightly elevated and eyes closed. Patient's head is as close to the camera as possible and strapped tightly

PEARLS/PITFALLS

- There are some important differences between HMPAO and ECD. Although both agents are blood flow tracers, ECD may be a less effective flow tracer at high flows and may reflect metabolism in addition to flow.

- Magnetic resonance imaging (MRI) and MRI/SPECT image fusion are useful for the exact anatomic location of the seizure focus.

- While evaluating disease progress by comparing with previous studies, be aware of the differences in the perfusion patterns between HMPAO and ECD studies.

- Always check for image orientation (left and right sides) before correlating with MRI, CT, or other SPECT studies because protocols used for image processing may differ.

- Patient motion as well as tilting of the head can be misrepresented as severe perfusion defects in different views. Always correlate the asymmetry with the slice above and below and also with corresponding views in other planes.

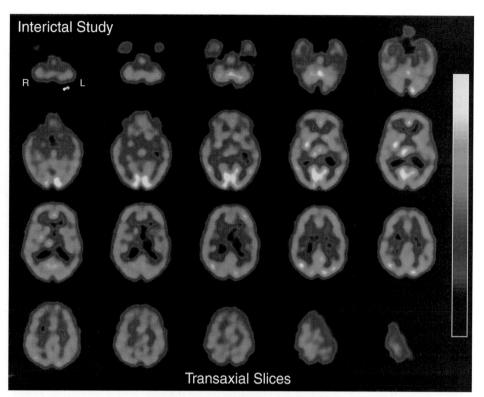

Fig. B (see Color Plate 14, page V)

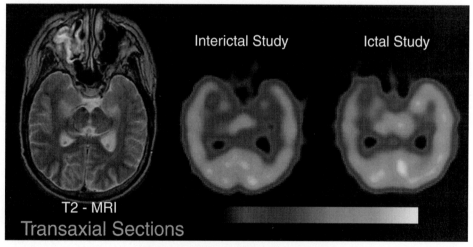

Fig. C (see Color Plate 15, page VI)

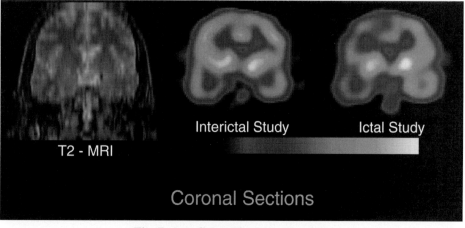

Fig. D (see Color Plate 16, page VI)

with a nonattenuating object, such as Velcro, rubber, or elastic to avoid head motion.
- Lights are dimmed and the room is quiet (avoid disturbances and noise).
- Seizure induced by voice activation. Preferably, for ictal imaging, the patient is injected during (have an intravenous line ready) or immediately following the seizure.

Image Interpretation

The ictal perfusion study (Fig. A) demonstrates marked hyperperfusion in the left superior temporal lobe, moderate hyperperfusion in the left hemisphere, and relative hypoperfusion in the right hemisphere and the temporal lobe. The interictal (baseline) study (Fig. B) shows areas of relative hypoperfusion in the temporal lobes bilaterally. Hypoperfusion is also noted in the left thalamus and basal ganglia.

Differential Diagnosis

- Epileptic focus
- Encephalitis
- Tumor
- Luxury perfusion
- Focal sensory or motor stimulation at the time of imaging
- Hallucinations secondary to dementia or schizophrenia

Diagnosis and Clinical Follow-up

The diagnosis was hyperperfusion in the left superior temporal lobe consistent with seizure focus.

Suggested Reading

Holman BL, Chandak PK, Garada BM. *Atlas of Brain Perfusion SPECT.* Available: http://www.med.harvard.edu/BWHRad/BrainSPECT/

Case 139

Clinical Presentation

25-year-old woman in otherwise good health presenting with several episodes of severe headaches. Magnetic resonance imaging (MRI) demonstrated a small area of enhancement in the right thalamus and stereotactic biopsy confirmed the diagnosis of grade III astrocytoma. An ^{18}F-fludeoxyglucose (^{18}FDG) positron emission tomography (PET) study was performed to define the metabolic extent of the lesion, determine if additional lesions were present, and serve as a baseline for monitoring the effect of radiation therapy.

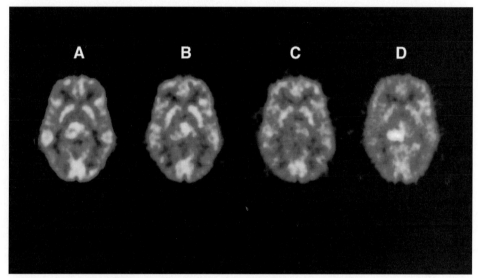

Figs. A, B, C, D (see Color Plate 17, page VI)

Technique

- Patient should take nothing by mouth for 12 hours before radiopharmaceutical administration. Switch all glucose-containing intravenous solution to normal saline on the day before imaging.
- 10 mCi of ^{18}FDG administered intravenously 45 minutes prior to image acquisition.

- Since the rate of [18]FDG accumulation and the time at which plateau concentrations are achieved vary with tumor type, the choice of the delay between injection and imaging is critical.

- Patients must fast, and all intravenous solutions containing glucose must be stopped for at least 4 hours before injection of [18]FDG. It is important to determine that all intravenous drugs (antibiotics, chemotherapy agents) administered before and during the study do not contain glucose.

- Because of the high target to background ratios in many tumors, comparisons with transmission images and color displays are extremely useful for defining tumor margins precisely.

- When the DUR method is used to evaluate the effects of chemotherapy or radiation therapy, it is essential that imaging always be performed at the same time after [18]FDG injection.

- If a patient eats within 4 hours before an [18]FDG PET or single photon emission computed tomography (SPECT) and the examination cannot be rescheduled, the dose of [18]FDG should be increased and the injection delayed as long as possible.

- Dose infiltration can seriously confound quantification of [18]FDG images by the DUR (SUV) method. Infiltrations should be noted in the patient's record.

- Because of its relatively low resolution, [18]FDG SPECT may not be useful for diagnosis and staging of brain tumors.

- Imaging device: whole-body PET camera with in-plane and axial resolutions of 5.0 mm full width half maximum (FWHM), 9.5-cm field of view, 15 contiguous slices of 6.5-mm separation and sensitivity of approximately 5,000 cps/μCi.
- Image acquisition performed as 10-minute acquisitions in two bed positions.
- Transmission measurements use analytic attenuation correction.
- Image reconstruction: conventional filtered back-projection algorithm to an in-plane resolution of 7-mm FWHM. All projection data are corrected for nonuniformity of detector response, dead time, random coincidences, attenuation, and scattered radiation.

Image Interpretation

Prior to therapy, the transaxial [18]FDG PET image of the brain demonstrated an intense focus of increased accumulation in the anterior aspect of the right thalamus (Fig. A). The location of this lesion corresponded well with the area of enhancement on MRI. Midway in a course of radiation therapy, the degree and extent of the hypermetabolic focus decreased (Fig. B). In the study performed after completion of therapy (Fig. C), further regression of the tumor was evident. However, 6 months after completion of therapy, the PET study revealed intense focal hypermetabolism in the posterior aspect of the right thalamus (Fig. D).

Diagnosis and Clinical Follow-up

After radiation therapy, the patient's symptoms decreased significantly. However, 6 months later, at the time of the fourth study, symptoms started to recur and the patient died several weeks later.

Discussion

Compared with conventional single photon radionuclide procedures, PET has several advantages: (1) resolution and sensitivity are considerably higher; (2) implementation of corrections for photon attenuation and scatter are straightforward; (3) the images are quantitative; (4) a variety of radiopharmaceuticals that do not have single photon analogues are available; (5) the short physical half-lives of many of the radiopharmaceuticals facilitate repetitive studies.

Currently, numerous PET radiopharmaceuticals are available for tumor detection and therapeutic monitoring, including [15]O water, [15]O butanol and ^{13}N ammonia for measuring perfusion, [18]FDG for studying glucose metabolism, [11]C- methionine and ^{18}F-tyrosine for evaluating amino acid transport and protein synthesis, ^{11}C-thymidine for studying cell proliferation, and numerous [11]C- and ^{18}F-labeled receptor ligands. However, despite this plurality of tracers, FDG has become the "work horse" of clinical PET. In fact, [18]FDG and clinical PET are nearly synonymous. The central role of [18]FDG is based on both fundamental aspects of tissue metabolism and practical considerations. On the theoretical side, it is well-established that rapidly dividing tumor cells have accelerated glucose use under anaerobic conditions. Explanations for this phenomenon (Pasteur effect) include both increased hexokinase activity in tumor cells and increased concentrations of glucose transport proteins. On the practical side, there are at least three reasons for the prominent status of [18]FDG: (1) current synthetic methods for preparing [18]FDG yield sufficient quantities of tracer for numerous studies; (2) compared with other PET radiopharmaceuticals, the fact that [18]FDG is a "trapped tracer" greatly simplifies imaging procedures; (3) because ^{18}F has a relatively long half-life (110 min) compared with other PET agents, regional distribution facilities can supply imaging centers without on-site cyclotrons.

Although histology is a reliable and standardized method for classifying brain tumors, it cannot fully explain their clinical behavior and in some cases [18]FDG-PET imaging can be more helpful. The most extensive study of [18]FDG-PET imaging of brain tumors was reported by DiChiro (1987). In this investigation of 100 consecutive patients, differences in glucose metabolism between high- and low-grade lesions were shown to be highly significant. DiChiro examined the PET images of patients with high-grade gliomas (grades III and IV), for which histological criteria could not define a subset with a better prognosis than the others. With PET, patient survival could be predicted by the ratio of [18]FDG accumulation in tumor versus normal tissue. Patients with a high ratio had a median survival of 5 months, whereas patients with a lower ratio had a median survival of 19 months. Although all these tumors were histologically malignant, [18]FDG-PET could discriminate rapidly progressing tumors from those with a more prolonged course. Multiple studies have shown similar results. Also, tumors that are initially hypometabolic (i.e., low grade) frequently develop areas of increased metabolism at the time of malignant degeneration, and this change in character can be easily detected by PET.

In addition to assessing degree of malignancy and providing initial prognostic information, [18]FDG-PET can also provide helpful information during and after brain tumor therapy. In the early days after surgical resection of a tumor, anatomic imaging often demonstrates contrast enhancement at the surgical margin. Although this may indicate residual tumor, it can also be caused by surgical manipulation of normal tissue. Anatomic imaging cannot discriminate between these two possibilities but [18]FDG-PET can. Perhaps the most important application of PET in the clinical management of brain tumors is the differentiation of tumor recurrence from radiation necrosis. Radiation therapy to the brain may cause dramatic tissue necrosis that is indistinguishable from tumor recurrence by anatomic imaging. [18]FDG-PET can reliably discriminate between recurrent tumor, which has increased [18]FDG uptake, and necrotic, edematous tissue, which has reduced [18]FDG uptake.

Suggested Readings

Alavi JB, Alavi A, Chawluk J, et al. Positron emission tomography in patients with glioma. A predictor of prognosis. *Cancer* 1988;62:1074–1078.

Di Chiro G. Positron emission tomography using (^{18}F) fluorodeoxyglucose in brain tumors. A powerful diagnostic and prognostic tool. *Invest Radiol* 1987;22:360–371.

Di Chiro G, Oldfield E, Wright DC, et al. Cerebral necrosis after radiotherapy and/or intraarterial chemotherapy for brain tumors: PET and neuropathologic studies. *AJR Am J Roentgenol* 1988;150:189–197.

Doyle WK, Budinger TF, Valk PE, et al. Differentiation of cerebral radiation necrosis from tumor recurrence by [^{18}F]FDG and [82]Rb positron emission tomography. *J Comput Assist Tomogr* 1987;11:563–570.

Francavilla TL, Miletich RS, Di Chiro G, et al. Positron emission tomography in the detection of malignant degeneration of low-grade gliomas. *Neurosurgery* 1989;24:1–5.

Patronas NJ, Di Chiro G, Brooks RA, et al. Work in progress: [18F] fluorodeoxyglucose and positron emission tomography in the evaluation of radiation necrosis of the brain. *Radiology* 1982;144:885–889.

Patronas NJ, Di Chiro G, Kufta C, et al. Prediction of survival in glioma patients by means of positron emission tomography. *J Neurosurg* 1985;62;816–822.

Phelps ME, Huang SC, Hoffman EJ, et al. Tomographic measurements of local cerebral glucose metabolism in humans with (F-18)-2-fluoro-2-deoxy-D-glucose: Validation of method. Ann Neurol 1979;6:371–388.

Sokoloff L, Reivich M, Kennedy C, et al. The ^{14}C-deoxyglucose method for the measurement of local cerebral glucose utilization: Theory, procedure and normal values in the conscious and anesthetized albino rat. *J Neurochem* 1977;28:897–916.

Warburg O. On the origin of cancer cell. *Science* 1956;123:309–314.

Case 140

Clinical Presentation

49-year-old man diagnosed 10 months prior to the study with glioblastoma multiforme in the left posterior frontal parasagittal region. Surgical resection was performed, followed by 6 weeks of radiation therapy. He presented to the emergency room with sudden onset of right-sided weakness and numbness. Magnetic resonance imaging (MRI) showed a left posterior medial, frontal, and parietal mass and edema. A dual isotope brain scan was then ordered.

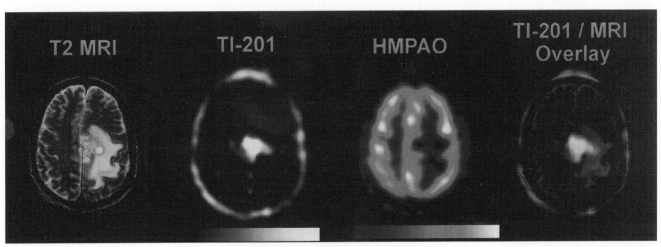

Fig. A (see Color Plate 18, page VI)

Technique

- 3 mCi thallium-201 thallous chloride injected intravenously. After the thallium-201 study was completed, 20 mCi of technetium-99m labeled hexamethyl propylene amine oxime (HMPAO) (or ECD) were then injected intravenously without moving the patient.
- Energy window for thallium-201 was 62 to 92 keV and for technetium-99m was 130 to 150 keV.
- Imaging time begins 20 to 30 minutes after each injection (1 hour after ECD).
- Acquisition protocol: 30 minutes per study using an annular single photon emission computed tomography (SPECT) system and without changing the patient's position between the acquisitions.

Image Interpretation

Thallium-201 SPECT demonstrated an abnormal area of increased thallium uptake involving the left medial temporoparietal region. No other areas of abnormal increased thallium accumulation were noted. HMPAO SPECT showed good overall uptake of the radiotracer with normal background activity and symmetrical radiotracer uptake in the basal ganglia and thalami (not seen here). Decreased radiotracer uptake was seen in the left medial temporoparietal cortex, indicating reduced perfusion. No other areas of abnormal increased or decreased radiotracer uptake were seen. On quantitative analysis, thallium uptake (lesion to contralateral scalp ratios) from three different suspicious areas—4.98, 4.87, and 6.05—were noted.

Differential Diagnosis

- The finding of increased thallium uptake and decreased perfusion is very specific for tumor recurrence. It is unlikely that any other lesion would cause these findings in a patient with a similar history.

Diagnosis and Clinical Follow-up

The HMPAO perfusion defect surrounding a focus of increased thallium uptake with a high lesion-to-scalp thallium uptake ratio indicates a high probability of solid tumor recurrence (low is ≤ 2.0 and high is ≥ 2.0).

Discussion

The dual isotope technique described here is used by neurosurgeons and neuro-oncologists not only to predict recurrence but also to assess residual disease following surgical resection, to evaluate response to therapy, and to differentiate radiation necrosis from recurrent disease. In a patient with a large abnormality on computed tomography (CT) or MRI, it also helps to guide the biopsy and minimize sampling error by directing the surgeon to the site of focal thallium uptake that most likely represents the site of recurrence.

Suggested Readings

Holman BL, Chandak PK, Garada BM. Atlas of Brain Perfusion SPECT. Available: http://www.med.harvard.edu/BWHRad/BrainSPECT/

Schwartz RB, Carvalho PA, Alexander E III, et al. Radiation necrosis vs high grade recurrent glioma: Differentiation using dual isotope SPECT with Tl and Tc-HMPAO. *Am J Neuroradiol* 12:1187–1192, 1991.

Case 141

Clinical Presentation

34-year-old woman presenting 2 weeks after a subarachnoid hemorrhage. Two hours prior to the study, she had a sudden deterioration in mental status and no clinical evidence of cerebral or brain stem function. The patient returned 17 hours later for a repeat study.

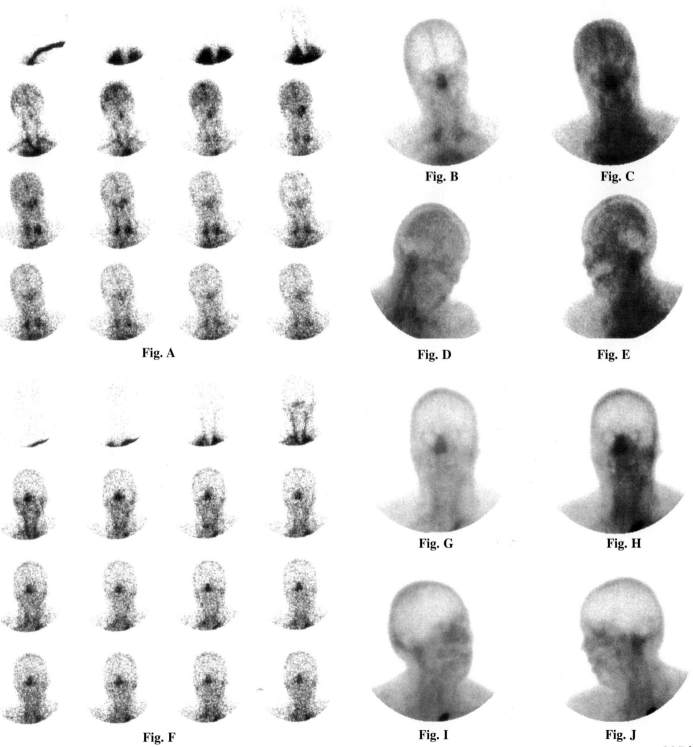

Fig. A

Fig. B

Fig. C

Fig. D

Fig. E

Fig. F

Fig. G

Fig. H

Fig. I

Fig. J

- A tourniquet wrapped tightly around the head above the eyes and ears can reduce overlying scalp activity.

- A systolic blood pressure less than 60 mmHg may invalidate the test.

- Imaging within several hours (we use 6 hours) of cessation of brain function can result in false-negative tests.

- Scalp and cerebral bleeding can lead to false-negative readings if not correlated to clinical and imaging findings.

- The clinical significance of small areas of residual cerebral blood flow seen on HMPAO static images in the absence of middle and anterior cerebral arterial blood flow is unknown, but it is conceivable that the legal significance may be more important.

Technique

- Flow: 20 mCi of technetium-99m–diethylenetriamine pentaacetic acid (DTPA) or 10 to 30 mCi of technetium-99m and hexamethyl propylene amine oxime (HMPAO) (volume less than 1 cc is preferable).
- For injection: rapid bolus of radiopharmaceutical followed by saline flush, central line access, is preferred.
- For statics: 10 mCi of HMPAO (total dose of HMPAO for flow and statics no greater than 30 mCi).
- Use a high-resolution collimator.
- Energy window 20% centered on 140 keV.
- Patient position: anterior with top of skull at the top of the field of view.
- Imaging time: 60-second dynamic at 1 sec/frame; for statics, 3 min/frame.

Image Interpretation

Figure A is the flow study compressed into 3-second frames. Carotid flow is normal bilaterally; middle and anterior cerebral flow are reduced. An immediate DTPA static image (Fig. B) demonstrates sagittal sinus uptake. Figures C, D, and E are the anterior, right lateral, and left lateral static images obtained 10 minutes after injection of 10 mCi of HMPAO. Cerebral uptake is reduced below the level expected but is present.

The patient returned to the department 17 hours later for a repeat brain flow scan. At that time, both carotid arteries were visualized, but there was no anterior or middle cerebral artery flow (Fig. F). The "hot nose" sign is noted (see Discussion). There was no uptake in the sagittal sinus on the immediate DTPA static image (Fig. G). HMPAO images (Figs. H, I, and J) showed no cerebral uptake.

Differential Diagnosis

(Second Set of Images)

- Brain death
- Poor tracer preparation resulting in lack of accumulation in central nervous system (may cause false-positive planar images but will not alter accuracy of flow images)
- Attenuation artifact, such as metallic skull implant or metal between head and camera

Diagnosis and Clinical Follow-up

The patient had no spontaneous respiration on the apnea test. She was declared brain dead immediately after the second study.

Discussion

Brain death is inevitably followed by cardiopulmonary death. Criteria for determination of brain death include absence of brain stem reflexes (gag, corneal, oculovestibular, and so on) and lack of spontaneous respiration with the apnea test. Confirmatory tests include an electroencephalogram or brain flow imaging, or both. Although contrast arteriography is widely available, many institutions rely on radionuclide angiography using technetium-99m–DTPA or glucoheptonate. Because these agents do not cross the blood-brain barrier, a single dynamic acquisition in the anterior projection is obtained. More recently, lipophilic radio-pharmaceuticals (such as HMPAO) have been used to assess cerebral flow and function. These agents do cross the blood-brain barrier and permit visualization of the brain in several projections.

Reservations about the use of HMPAO originated from concern about the labeling stability. A false-positive test because of free technetium-99m pertechnetate is, however, very unlikely, particularly with the newer stable radiopharmaceuticals. Although paper chromatography for in vitro quality control is recommended prior to use, this is not always feasible. Some authors assess labeling in vivo with images of the thyroid, lungs, and liver. Another acceptable precaution is to obtain a good quality flow study prior to static imaging (the carotid arteries should be distinctly visualized). Since HMPAO is often supplied in a volume that is too large for an ideal flow agent, a portion of the dose, or an additional DTPA dose, can be used for the flow injection.

The "hot nose sign" is not pathognomonic for cessation of brain flow. It is, however, frequently seen in cases of brain death. This finding has been attributed to external carotid collateral flow through the facial and ophthalmic arteries once internal carotid flow is interrupted by an elevated intracranial pressure. Similarly, what appears to be sagittal sinus visualization in the absence of arterial flow may represent increased blood supply to the falx from the external carotid system (e.g., anterior falcial arteries).

This case illustrates the importance of waiting for several hours to image after clinical evidence of brain death. Cerebral blood flow can be visualized in the time period in which the intracranial pressure has risen enough to affect brain stem function but is not yet elevated enough to interrupt internal carotid artery flow.

Suggested Readings

de la Riva A, Gonzalez FM, Llamas-Elvira JM, et al. Diagnosis of brain death: Superiority of perfusion studies with 99Tcm-HMPAO over conventional radionuclide cerebral angiography. *Br J Radiol* 65:289–294, 1992.

Grunwald F, Biersack HJ. In vivo quality control of technetium-99m-HMPAO. *J Nucl Med* 32:1316, 1991. Letter.

Larar GN, Nagel JS. Technetium-99m-HMPAO cerebral perfusion scintigraphy: considerations for timely brain death declaration. *J Nucl Med* 33:2209–2213, 1992.

Laurin NR, Driedger AA, Hurwitz GA, et al. Cerebral perfusion imaging with technetium-99m HM-PAO in brain death and severe central nervous system injury. *J Nucl Med* 30:1627–1635, 1989.

Lee VW, Hauck RM, Morrison MC, et al. Scintigraphic evaluation of brain death: Significance of sagittal sinus visualization. *J Nucl Med* 28:1279–1283, 1987.

Reid RH, Gulenchyn KY, Ballinger JR. Clinical use of technetium-99m HMPAO for determination of brain death. *J Nucl Med* 30:1621–1626, 1989.

Spieth ME, Ansari AN, Kawada TK, Kimura RL, Siegel ME. Direct comparison of Tc-99m DTPA and Tc-99m HMPAO for evaluating brain death. *Clin Nucl Med* 19:867–871, 1994.

Case 142

Clinical Presentation

70-year-old male presenting with a history of anterior cerebral artery aneurysm and with new onset of seizures. The patient was unresponsive.

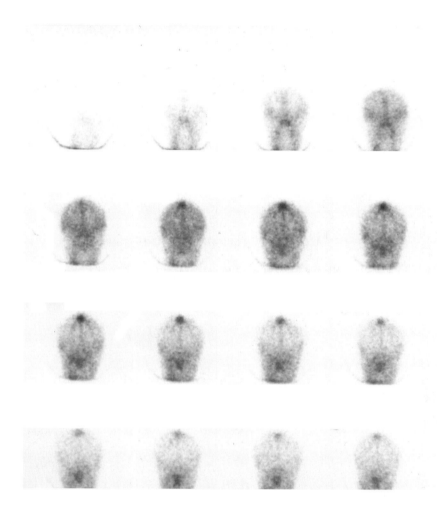

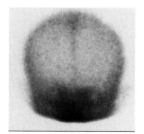

Fig. A

CENTRAL NERVOUS SYSTEM SCINTIGRAPHY

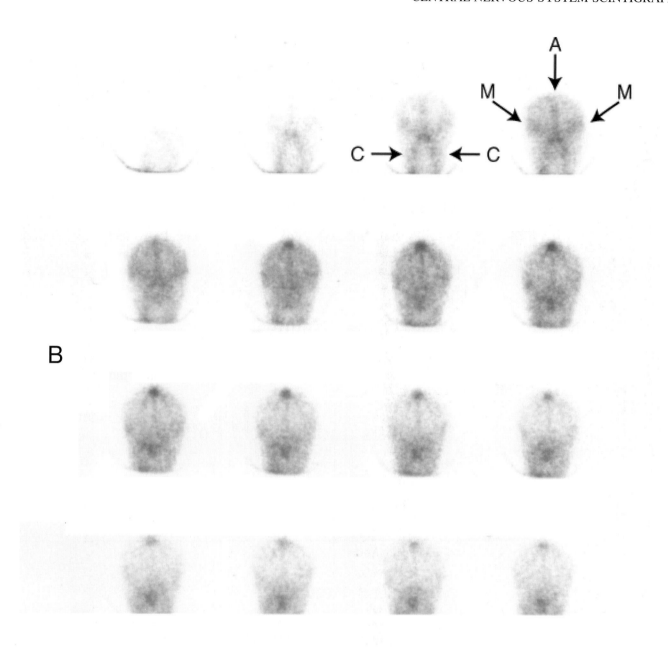

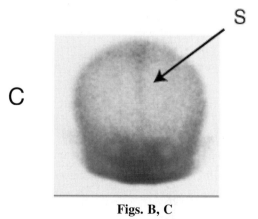

Figs. B, C

Technique

- 20 mCi of technetium-99m–diethylenetriamine pentaacetic acid (DTPA) as a rapid intravenous bolus.
- Use a high-resolution collimator.
- Energy window 20% centered on 140 keV.
- Patient position: anterior with top of skull at the top of the field of view.
- Imaging time: flow is 60-second dynamic at 1 sec/frame; for statics, 3 min/frame.

Image Interpretation

Figure A shows the DTPA flow study in sequential 3-second frames. The carotid (C), middle cerebral (M), and anterior cerebral (A) arteries are marked in Figure B. Note that the anterior cerebral vessels are seen as a single structure. Sagittal sinus filling (S) can be seen on the immediate static image (Fig. C).

Differential Diagnosis

- Normal brain blood flow
- False-negative because study was obtained too soon after the loss of cerebral function

Diagnosis and Clinical Follow-up

The diagnosis was normal brain blood flow.

Discussion

Compared with Case 141, the carotid, anterior, and middle cerebral arteries are clearly visualized.

Suggested Readings

de la Riva A, Gonzalez FM, Llamas-Elvira JM, et al. Diagnosis of brain death: Superiority of perfusion studies with 99Tcm-HMPAO over conventional radionuclide cerebral angiography. *Br J Radiol* 65:289–294, 1992.

Grunwald F, Biersack HJ. In vivo quality control of technetium-99m-HMPAO. *J Nucl Med* 32:1316, 1991. Letter.

Hansen AVE, Lavin PJM, Moody EB, Sandler MP. False-negative cerebral radionuclide flow study, in brain death, caused by a ventricular drain. *Clin Nucl Med* 18:502–505, 1992.

Larar GN, Nagel JS. Technetium-99m-HMPAO cerebral perfusion scintigraphy: Considerations for timely brain death declaration. *J Nucl Med* 33:2209–2213, 1992.

Laurin NR, Driedger AA, Hurwitz GA, et al. Cerebral perfusion imaging with technetium-99m HM-PAO in brain death and severe central nervous system injury. *J Nucl Med* 30:1627–1635, 1989.

Lee VW, Hauck RM, Morrison MC, et al. Scintigraphic evaluation of brain death: Significance of sagittal sinus visualization. *J Nucl Med* 28:1279–1283, 1987.

Reid RH, Gulenchyn KY, Ballinger JR. Clinical use of technetium-99m HMPAO for determination of brain death. *J Nucl Med* 30:1621–1626, 1989.

Speith M, Abella E, Sutter C, et al. Importance of the lateral view in the evaluation of suspected brain death. *Clin Nucl Med* 20:965–968, 1995.

Spieth ME, Ansari AN, Kawada TK, Kimura RL, Siegel ME. Direct comparison of Tc-99m DTPA and Tc-99m HMPAO for evaluating brain death. *Clin Nucl Med* 19:867–871, 1994.

Case 143

Clinical Presentation

35-year-old man presenting with mental status changes and suspected brain death following Lyme's disease.

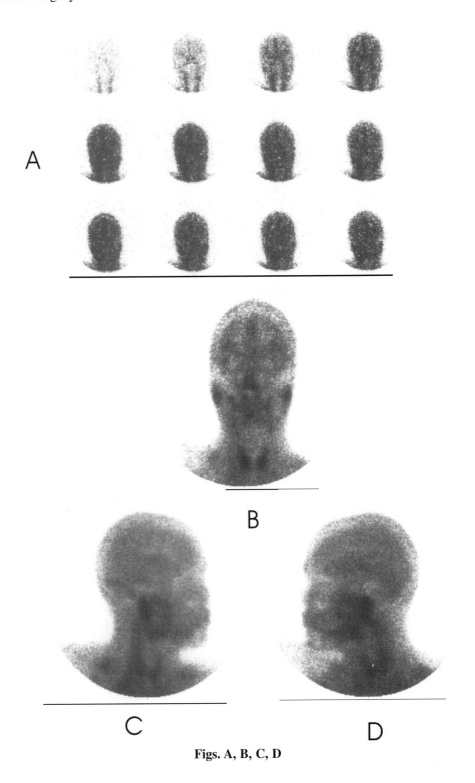

Figs. A, B, C, D

Technique

- 30 mCi technetium-99m–hexamethyl propylene amine oxime (HMPAO) as a rapid intravenous bolus.
- Use a high-resolution collimator.
- Energy window 20% centered on 140 keV.
- Patient position: anterior with top of skull at the top of the field of view.
- Imaging time: 60-second dynamic at 1 sec/frame; for statics, 3 min/frame.

Image Interpretation

Figure A shows the HMPAO flow study in sequential 3-second frames. The carotid, middle, and anterior cerebral arteries are visualized (see preceding DTPA case). Cerebral uptake is seen on the 15-min delayed anterior (Fig. B), right lateral (Fig. C), and left lateral (Fig. D) views. All structures are normal.

Differential Diagnosis

- Normal brain perfusion

Diagnosis and Clinical Follow-up

The diagnosis was normal brain perfusion.

Discussion

With HMPAO, the resolution of the vascular structures during flow imaging is reduced. This is due to higher background counts and a larger volume of injectate (resulting in a poorer bolus). The HMPAO flow study in this case is of a better quality because the flow study was done with a smaller volume of injectate (approximately 10 mCi), which improves the quality of the bolus and subsequent flow images.

Suggested Readings

de la Riva A, Gonzalez FM, Llamas-Elvira JM, et al. Diagnosis of brain death: Superiority of perfusion studies with 99Tcm-HMPAO over conventional radionuclide cerebral angiography. *Br J Radiol* 65:289–294, 1992.

Grunwald F, Biersack HJ. In vivo quality control of technetium-99m-HMPAO. *J Nucl Med* 32:1316, 1991. Letter.

Hansen AVE, Lavin PJM, Moody EB, Sandler MP. False-negative cerebral radionuclide flow study, in brain death, caused by a ventricular drain. *Clin Nucl Med* 18:502–505, 1992.

Larar GN, Nagel JS. Technetium-99m-HMPAO cerebral perfusion scintigraphy: Considerations for timely brain death declaration. *J Nucl Med* 33:2209–2213, 1992.

Laurin NR, Driedger AA, Hurwitz GA, et al. Cerebral perfusion imaging with technetium-99m HM-PAO in brain death and severe central nervous system injury. *J Nucl Med* 30:1627–1635, 1989.

Lee VW, Hauck RM, Morrison MC, et al. Scintigraphic evaluation of brain death: Significance of sagittal sinus visualization. *J Nucl Med* 28:1279–1283, 1987.

Reid RH, Gulenchyn KY, Ballinger JR. Clinical use of technetium-99m HMPAO for determination of brain death. *J Nucl Med* 30:1621–1626, 1989.

Speith M, Abella E, Sutter C, et al. Importance of the lateral view in the evaluation of suspected brain death. *Clin Nucl Med* 20:965–968, 1995.

Spieth ME, Ansari AN, Kawada TK, Kimura RL, Siegel ME. Direct comparison of Tc-99m DTPA and Tc-99m HMPAO for evaluating brain death. *Clin Nucl Med* 19:867–871, 1994.

Case 144

Clinical Presentation

48-year-old woman with subarachnoid hemorrhage presenting with decerebrate posturing to sternal rub, lower extremity withdrawal to pain, and absent brain stem reflexes (corneal, gag, oculocephalic). Her electroencephalogram (EEG) demonstrated no evidence of cerebral cortical activity.

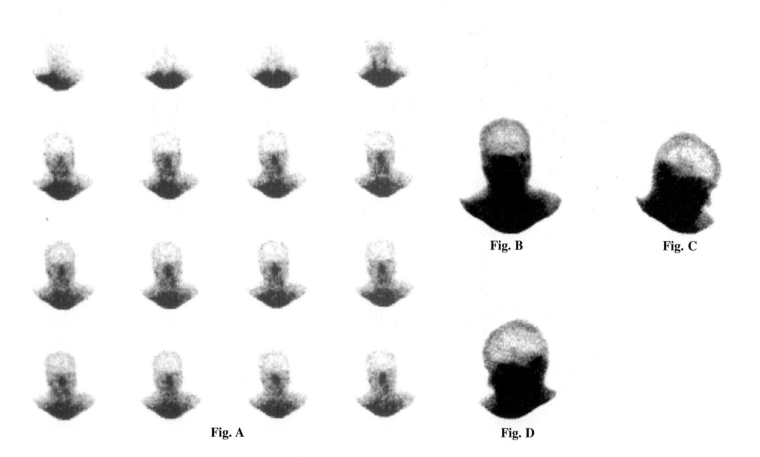

Fig. A

Fig. B

Fig. C

Fig. D

Technique

- 25 mCi of technetium-99m–hexamethyl propylene amine oxime (HMPAO) in 2 divided doses.
- Use a high-resolution collimator.
- Energy window 20% centered on 140 keV.
- Patient position: anterior with top of skull at the top of the field of view.
- Imaging time: 60-second dynamic at 1 sec/frame; for statics, 3 min/frame.

Image Interpretation

The cerebral flow study in Figure A demonstrates adequate carotid artery flow and no evidence of middle or anterior flow. The 15-minute delayed static images (Figs. B, C, and D) demonstrate uptake in the deep gray matter, seen best on the lateral views just above the intense activity at the base of the skull.

Differential Diagnosis

- Evolving brain death
- Bilateral subdural hematomas
- Faulty radiopharmaceutical preparation (would show normal flow phase of study, however)

Diagnosis and Clinical Follow-up

The subsequent apnea test demonstrated spontaneous breathing on withdrawal from assisted ventilation. The patient expired 5 hours later.

Discussion

This is an example of residual cerebral uptake of radionuclide in the absence of middle and anterior cerebral blood flow on the anterior flow images. The patient's clinical status was consistent with minimal residual cerebral function. The clinical significance of this finding is unclear because the patient progressed to complete brain death within several hours.

Suggested Readings

Hansen AVE, Lavin PJM, Moody EB, Sandler MP. False-negative cerebral radionuclide flow study, in brain death, caused by a ventricular drain. *Clin Nucl Med* 18:502–505, 1992.

Speith M, Abella E, Sutter C, et al. Importance of the lateral view in the evaluation of suspected brain death. *Clin Nucl Med* 20:965–968, 1995.

Section XII

Gastrointestinal Scintigraphy

Case 145

Clinical Presentation

A 30-year-old man volunteered for a gastric emptying study to establish normal values. There was no history of gastric complaints.

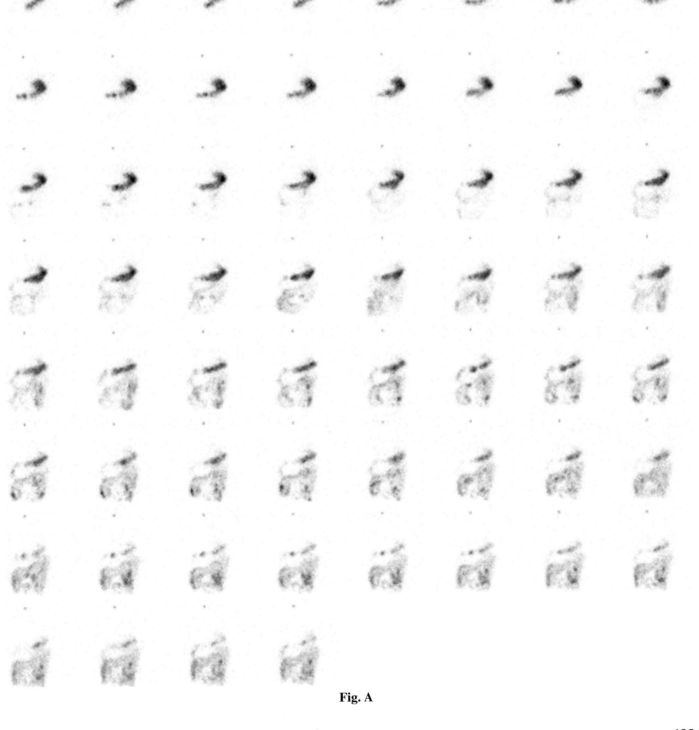

Fig. A

Technique

- 200 μCi technetium-99m–labeled sulfur colloid mixed with two scrambled whole eggs.
- Meal ingestion time less than 5 minutes.
- Subject placed supine between the heads of a dual-headed gamma camera.
- Anterior and posterior data collected continuously for 60 to 90 minutes and divided into 1-minute frames.
- Anterior, posterior, and geometric mean time-activity curves generated from the region of interest (ROI) drawn around the stomach (Fig. B).

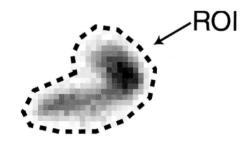

Fig. B

Image Interpretation

Images (Fig. A, only anterior images displayed here) and emptying curves (Fig. C) show prompt, smooth emptying of tracer from the stomach. The emptying curves show the gastric emptying half-time was approximately 30 minutes.

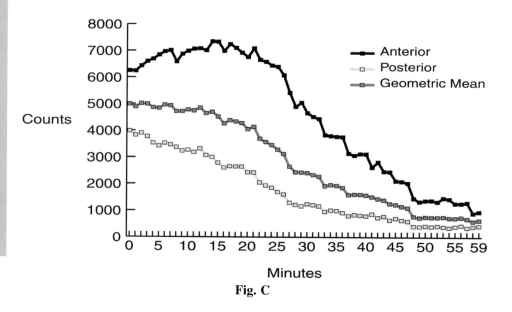

Fig. C

Differential Diagnosis

- Normal study

Diagnosis and Clinical Follow-up

The patient was a normal volunteer.

Discussion

The scintigraphic gastric emptying study is the most physiological of gastric motility studies. Unlike other examinations, it does not require invasive instrumentation and allows ingestion of a meal composed of familiar food.

There is considerable debate in the nuclear medicine community as to the optimal method to perform the study and analyze the results. Not debated, however, is the fact that the method used in any particular institution should have normal values established for the meal, imaging parameters, patient position, and environment. Meal composition, patient position, and ambient conditions can all affect gastric emptying rate. These parameters must be carefully reproduced to allow comparison of values from a specific patient to established normals or previous studies on the same patient.

Suggested Readings

O'Hara S. Pediatric gastrointestinal nuclear imaging. *Radiol Clin North Am* 34:845–862, 1996.

Parkman HP, Miller MA, Fisher RS. Role of nuclear medicine in evaluating patients with suspected gastrointestinal motility disorders. *Semin Nucl Med* 25:289–305, 1995.

Stacher G, Bergmann H. Scintigraphic quantitation of gastrointestinal motor activity and transport: Oesophagus and stomach. *Eur J Nucl Med* 19:815–823, 1992.

Case 146

Clinical Presentation

43-year-old woman presenting with insulin-dependent diabetes mellitus (IDDM) and bowel malrotation.

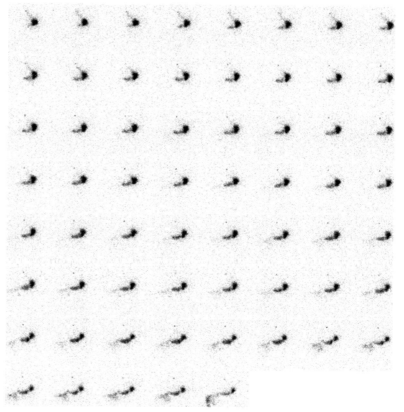

Fig. A

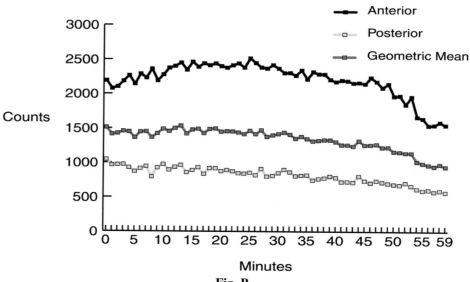

Minutes

Fig. B

- Patient symptoms during the gastric emptying study should be noted. If the emptying rate is normal but the patient complains of the usual symptoms following ingestion of the meal, the symptoms may not be related to gastric emptying disturbances.

- If the emptying curves are plotted directly from the counts in the region of interest, the emptying rate will be overestimated. Tracer activity must be corrected for decay of technetium-99m.

- Some centers will have the patient stand and walk around after 60 or 90 minutes if emptying is delayed. This may accelerate emptying, but an upright emptying rate should not be compared with the emptying rate while the patient is supine.

Technique

- 200 µCi technetium-99m–labeled sulfur colloid mixed with two scrambled whole eggs.
- Meal ingestion time less than 5 minutes.
- Subject placed supine between the heads of a dual-headed gamma camera.
- Anterior and posterior data collected continuously for 60 to 90 minutes and divided into 1-minute frames.
- Anterior, posterior, and geometric mean time-activity curves generated.

Image Interpretation

Images (Fig. A) and emptying curves (Fig. B) show poor emptying of tracer from the stomach. At 90 minutes, 65% of the initial radiolabeled meal remained in the stomach.

Differential Diagnosis

- Diabetic gastroparesis
- Hypomotility secondary to previous surgery
- Hypomotility secondary to medication
- Gastric outlet obstruction
- Hypothyroidism
- Muscular dystrophy
- Anxiety

Diagnosis and Clinical Follow-up

Findings consistent with delayed gastric emptying. No follow-up was available.

Discussion

As many as 30 to 50% of patients with diabetes can have delayed gastric emptying. Patients with the most severe upper gastrointestinal complaints are likely to have delayed gastric emptying, but the majority of patients with delayed emptying are asymptomatic. Abnormal emptying rates can influence blood glucose levels. Therefore, diagnosis and management of gastric emptying disturbances are important for control of diabetes.

Suggested Readings

Abrahamsson H. Gastrointestinal motility disorders in patients with diabetes mellitus. *J Intern Med* 237:403–409, 1995.

Farrell FJ, Keeffe EB. Diabetic gastroparesis. *Dig Dis* 13:291–300, 1995.

Samsom M, Smout AJ. Abnormal gastric and small intestinal motor function in diabetes mellitus. *Dig Dis* 15:263–274, 1997.

Case 147

Clinical Presentation

48-year-old obese female presenting with non–insulin-dependent diabetes.

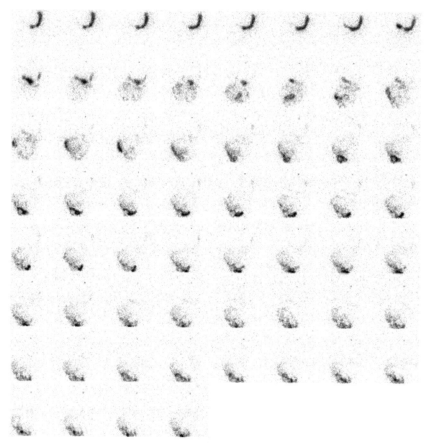

Fig. A

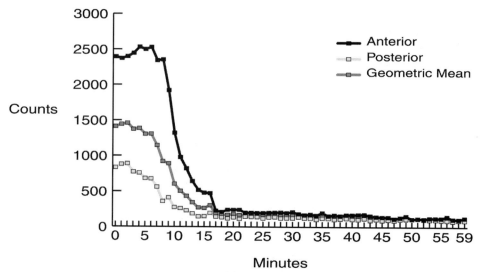

Fig. B

PEARLS/PITFALLS

- The patient should ingest the meal in the imaging room with the gamma camera set up and ready to go. The patient can then be put into position quickly, before appreciable emptying has occurred.

- If images are acquired only every 10 or 15 minutes in patients with rapid emptying, the emptying curve will demonstrate activity in the stomach at time zero, followed by nothing in the stomach on the second image.

Technique

- 200 μCi technetium-99m–labeled sulfur colloid mixed with two scrambled whole eggs.
- Meal ingestion time less than 5 minutes.
- Subject placed supine between the heads of a dual-headed gamma camera.
- Anterior and posterior data collected continuously for 60 to 90 minutes and divided into 1-minute frames.
- Anterior, posterior, and geometric mean time-activity curves generated.

Image Interpretation

Anterior images (Fig. A; posterior images not shown) and emptying curves (Fig. B) demonstrate rapid and complete emptying of tracer from the stomach.

Differential Diagnosis

- Hypermotility medication
- Dumping syndrome
- Hyperthyroidism
- Zollinger-Ellison syndrome

Diagnosis and Clinical Follow-up

Final diagnosis not known. No follow-up was available.

Discussion

Delayed emptying is the most commonly considered gastric motility abnormality in diabetic patients. Some patients, however, particularly those with type II diabetes, may demonstrate abnormally rapid emptying. Because some patients demonstrate rapid emptying, it is important that the patient ingest the meal within 10 minutes and get into position for imaging as soon as the test meal is finished.

Suggested Readings

Horowitz M, Wishart JM, Jones KL, et al. Gastric emptying in diabetes: An overview. *Diabet Med* 13:S16–S22, 1996.

Kong MF, Macdonald IA, Tattersall RB. Gastric emptying in diabetes. *Diabet Med* 13:112–119, 1996.

Smith U. Gastric emptying in type 2 diabetes: Quick or slow? *Diabet Med* 13:S31–S33, 1996.

Case 148

Clinical Presentation

44-year-old woman presenting with a history of chronic constipation. The patient had an "unusual episode" of diarrhea 24 hours following the first set of images and was therefore rescheduled to repeat the study several weeks later.

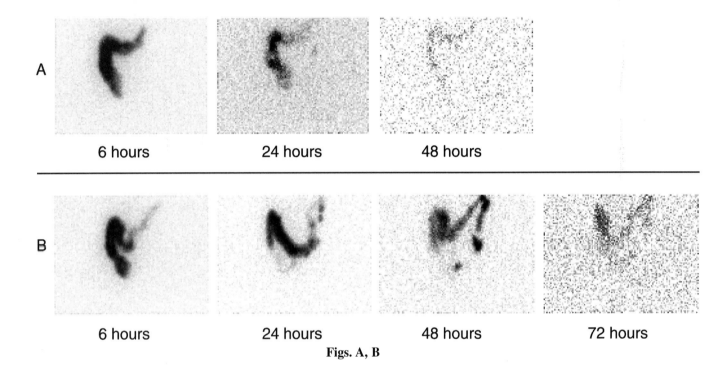

A

6 hours   24 hours   48 hours

B

6 hours   24 hours   48 hours   72 hours

Figs. A, B

Technique

- 100 μCi indium-111 DTPA orally in orange juice.
- Anterior and posterior images of the abdomen obtained at 6, 24, 48, and 72 hours.

Image Interpretation

The initial set of images (Fig. A) demonstrates tracer to the midtransverse colon. After an unusual episode of diarrhea, the diminished tracer could still be seen collecting just behind the midtransverse colon. A second study (Fig. B), done shortly thereafter, again shows tracer to the midtransverse colon on 6- and 24-hour images. At 48 hours, some tracer is seen to move beyond the transverse colon, but, as that is eliminated, most residual tracer is again seen predominately in the transverse colon on the 72-hour images.

Differential Diagnosis

Causes of functional obstruction (no anatomic lesion or stricture) include several neural lesions:

PEARLS/PITFALLS

- Geometric mean of the anterior and posterior counts that have been decay-corrected can provide information about total emptying of tracer from the bowel.

- The bowel can also be divided into various regions of interest so that a graph of tracer transit through each region is recorded. This provides more quantitative information than other methods of measuring bowel motility.

- Parasympathetic injury
- Multiple sclerosis
- Chaga's disease (damage to myenteric plexus)
- Hirschsprung's disease (usually diagnosed in infancy)
- Chronic idiopathic intestinal pseudo-obstruction
- Anticholinergic drugs

Diagnosis and Clinical Follow-up

After considering a partial bowel resection at the mid-colon, the patient elected to pursue less invasive therapy. She continues to have problems with constipation.

Discussion

Most anatomic causes of bowel obstruction (see Differential Diagnosis) should be ruled out with more anatomic studies before the colon transit scintigraphy study is obtained. Colon transit scintigraphy can help distinguish between generalized slow transit constipation and a lesion responsible for focal obstruction. The study is noninvasive, physiological, and simple to perform. Indium-111 DTPA is the preferred radiopharmaceutical because of the tracer half-life and dosimetry.

Suggested Readings

Mahendrarajah K, Van der Schaaf AA, Lovegrove FT, et al. Surgery for severe constipation: The use of radioisotope transit scan and barium evacuation proctography in patient selection. *Aust N Z J Surg* 64:183–186, 1994.

Maurer AH, Krevsky B. Whole-gut transit scintigraphy in the evaluation of small-bowel and colon transit disorders. *Semin Nucl Med* 25:326–338, 1995.

McLean R, Smart R, Barbagallo S, et al. Colon transit scintigraphy using oral indium-111-labeled DTPA. Can scan pattern predict final diagnosis? *Dig Dis Sci* 40:2660–2668, 1995.

Roberts JP, Newell MS, Deeks JJ, et al. Oral [111In]DTPA scintigraphic assessment of colonic transit in constipated subjects. *Dig Dis Sci* 38:1032–1039, 1993.

Smart RC, McLean RG, Gaston-Parry D, et al. Comparison of oral iodine-131-cellulose and indium-111-DTPA as tracers for colon transit scintigraphy: Analysis by colon activity profiles. *J Nucl Med* 32:1668–1674, 1991.

Case 149

Clinical Presentation

75-year-old man on Coumadin (warfarin sodium) for atrial fibrillation presenting with melena and anemia.

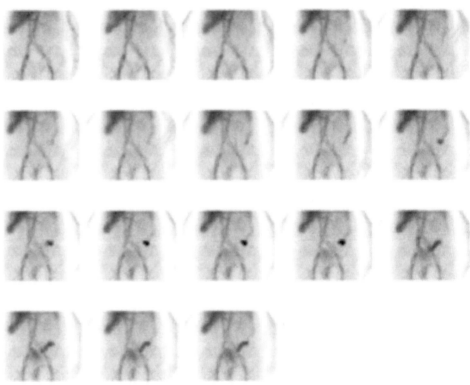

Fig. A

Technique

- See Case 50, for precautions related to labeling and injecting blood products.
- Label 3 mL autologous red blood cells with 20 to 25 mCi technetium-99m in vitro and inject intravenously.
- Patient positioned supine beneath a large field of view gamma camera.
- Anterior abdominal image data collected continuously and divided into 1-minute frames.
- Data collected for 60 to 90 minutes and displayed in cinematic format.

Image Interpretation

Serial anterior images of the abdomen (Fig. A) demonstrate a faint focus of activity in the region of the splenic flexure or upper portion of the descending colon that moves inferiorly toward the pelvis over several minutes.

- *(continued)* Bleeding sites should be followed for several minutes to most accurately determine their location.
- Poor labeling of the red blood cells can cause accumulation of pertechnetate in the gastric mucosa. This may be mistaken for gastritis or gastric bleeding.
- Excretion of the tracer in the urinary collecting system, particularly if there is hydronephrosis or hydroureter, can mimic hemorrhage.
- Genital blood pool can either mimic or hide rectal bleeding. A lateral view can distinguish the anterior genital activity from the posterior rectal accumulation of tracer.
- Retrograde movement of tracer can falsely suggest a more proximal bleeding site if continuous acquisition and cinematic display are not performed.
- Quantitative assessment of bleeding is difficult to do because of variables such as bowel motility, amount of tracer used, pooling of the blood within loops of bowel, and soft tissue attenuation.
- Delayed images may document the occurrence of interval bleeding between injection of tracer and the delayed image. It is not clear, however, that this information adds any more to patient management than observation of blood in the stool or other signs of bleeding. Normal bowel motility means the location of tracer on delayed images may have little to do with the original site of extravasation.

Differential Diagnosis

- Gastrointestinal bleeding in large bowel
- Atypical small bowel bleeding site
- Extraluminal bleeding site, collecting in the left abdomen

Diagnosis and Clinical Follow-up

The study was thought to represent a gastrointestinal bleed originating in the region of the splenic flexure of the colon. Colonoscopy revealed diverticula throughout the colon. No specific bleeding site was noted.

Discussion

Gastrointestinal bleeding scintigraphy is the most sensitive and specific test for the diagnosis of gastrointestinal bleeding. Bleeding rates of as little as 0.1 mL/min can be detected and localized to a general region of the bowel. The study can be used to document the occurrence and location of acute bleeding before the patient is taken to angiography. If the patient demonstrates bleeding soon after tracer injection, angiography is likely to be more helpful than if bleeding is less frequent.

The study is most often done with tracers that persist in the blood pool, such as labeled red blood cells, because many patients referred for the study have intermittent bleeding that may not be seen for more than 1 hour following tracer injection. Sulfur colloid, another tracer that is used occasionally, is cleared too rapidly from the blood to demonstrate anything but bleeding occurring within 10 to 15 minutes of tracer injection.

Suggested Readings

Emslie JT, Zarnegar K, Siegel ME, et al. Technetium-99m-labeled red blood cell scans in the investigation of gastrointestinal bleeding. *Dis Colon Rectum* 39:750–754, 1996.

Ng DA, Opelka FG, Beck DE, et al. Predictive value of technetium Tc 99m-labeled red blood cell scintigraphy for positive angiogram in massive lower gastrointestinal hemorrhage. *Dis Colon Rectum* 40:471–477, 1997.

Suzman MS, Talmor M, Jennis R, et al. Accurate localization and surgical management of active lower gastrointestinal hemorrhage with technetium-labeled erythrocyte scintigraphy. *Ann Surg* 224:29–36, 1996.

Case 150

Clinical Presentation

68-year-old man presenting with melena and falling hematocrit.

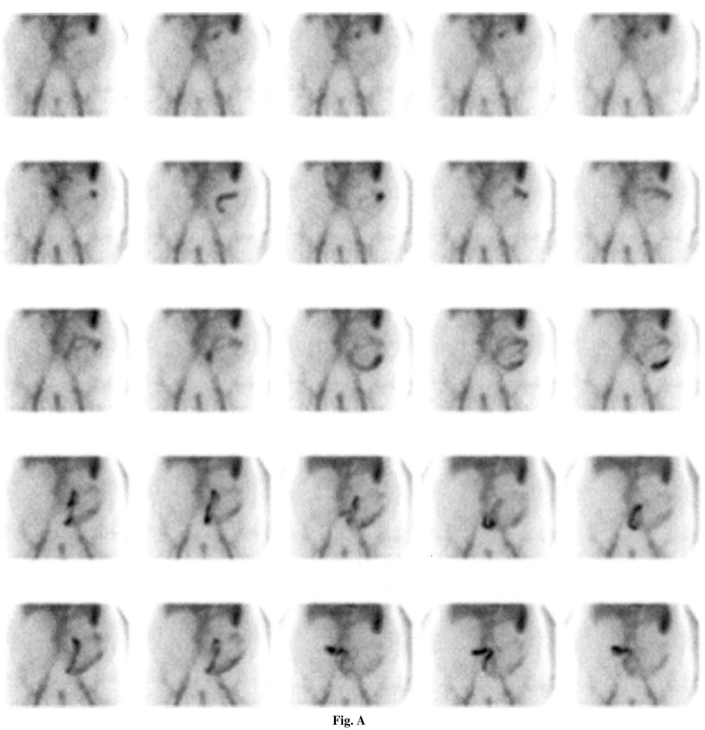

Fig. A

Technique

- See Cardiac functional imaging for precautions related to labeling and reinjecting blood products.
- 3 ml autologous red blood cells are labeled with 20–25 mCi Tc-99m in vitro and injected intravenously.
- Patient positioned supine beneath large field of view gamma camera.
- Anterior abdominal image data collected continuously and divided into one-minute frames.
- Data collected for 60 to 90 minutes and displayed in cinematic format.

Image Interpretation

Serial 1-minute anterior images over the abdomen (Fig. A) show tracer collection just at the upper edge of the field of view that moves inferiorly and outlines the "C loop" of the duodenum before it crosses midline to the left upper quadrant. The tracer then moves in a serpiginous pattern on the left side of the abdomen before crossing over to the right side of the abdomen. Later images taken after repositioning of the camera (not shown) demonstrate that the tracer accumulation is occurring just distal to the stomach.

Differential Diagnosis

- Upper small bowel bleeding
- Biliary tract hemorrhage
- Intraperitoneal bleeding (the pattern of tracer movement seen in this study would be very unlikely consistent with bleeding into any structure other than the bowel lumen)

Diagnosis and Clinical Follow-up

Endoscopy demonstrated a duodenal ulcer.

Discussion

Small bowel bleeding will follow a serpentine pattern of tracer movement much different than that seen with large bowel bleeding. If bleeding is intermittent, however, and bowel motility is diminished, focal accumulation of tracer that does not move can be very difficult to localize. Continued acquisition of images is needed in these patients because delayed static images will only identify the site of tracer accumulation at the time the image is acquired. This may have little to do with the site of origin.

Because the tracer collection began at the edge of the field of view, it was not clear whether the bleeding was coming from the duodenum or from above it. It is not uncommon that the gamma camera is repositioned to better observe a bleeding site. Careful review of the study during acquisition will allow repositioning of the gamma camera to best visualize the source of hemorrhage.

Suggested Readings

Dusold R, Burke K, Carpentier W, et al. The accuracy of technetium-99m-labeled red cell scintigraphy in localizing gastrointestinal bleeding. *Am J Gastroenterol* 89:345–348, 1994.

Lau WY, Yuen WK, Chu KW, et al. Obscure bleeding in the gastrointestinal tract originating in the small intestine. *Surg Gynecol Obstet* 174:119–124, 1992.

Case 151

Clinical Presentation

47-year-old man presenting with a history of elevated liver function tests.

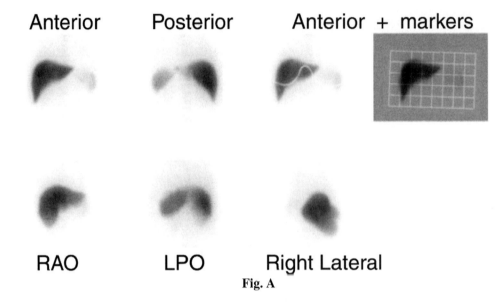

Anterior   Posterior   Anterior + markers

RAO   LPO   Right Lateral

Fig. A

Technique

- 3 mCi technetium-99m–labeled sulfur colloid injected intravenously.
- Planar images in anterior, posterior, anterior with markers, right anterior oblique, left posterior oblique, right lateral projections obtained at 15 minutes after tracer injection.

Image Interpretation

Images (Fig. A) show homogenous distribution of tracer and normal liver and spleen contour. A grid of 5-cm squares is superimposed on the first anterior view as a measurement reference. No colloid shift is noted.

Differential Diagnosis

- Normal liver and spleen scan
- Mild hepatocellular disease (liver and spleen scan not sensitive for mild hepatocellular disease)
- Focal lesion <1.5 cm (below resolution limits of imaging technique)

Diagnosis and Clinical Follow-up

Normal liver and spleen scan. The patient had mild elevation of liver function tests that resolved spontaneously.

PEARLS/PITFALLS

- Imaging with iminodiacetic acid (IDA) tracers should be considered for the evaluation of hepatocellular function.

- Liver and spleen scanning is used in some centers for the evaluation of liver function following liver transplant.

- Single photon emission computed tomography (SPECT) improves the sensitivity of the liver and spleen scan for the diagnosis of focal space-occupying lesions.

- Livers with acute hepatocellular dysfunction may demonstrate normal Kupfer cell function for a period of time before inflammation and decreased blood flow alter colloid uptake.

- The role of liver and spleen scanning in the routine diagnosis of hepatic masses or hepatocellular dysfunction is questioned. CT, ultrasound, and magnetic resonance imaging provide more sensitive and specific anatomic information.

Discussion

The liver and spleen scan demonstrates reticuloendothelial function in the liver, spleen, and bone marrow. The test was popular prior to computed tomography (CT) scanning and ultrasound for making the diagnosis of focal hepatic lesions and for demonstrating liver size and function. The study is not commonly used today because of poor specificity and sensitivity compared with anatomic imaging studies, particularly for focal lesions. Focal lesions smaller than 1.5 cm may be missed on liver and spleen scanning. When seen, focal hepatic or splenic defects may be caused by a variety of lesions, and further imaging is almost always necessary.

Liver and spleen scanning can be helpful in the workup of patients with elevated liver function tests. In these patients, the study is a simple, relatively inexpensive, noninvasive method to distinguish between diffuse and focal liver disease and to provide a rough estimate of hepatic function.

Suggested Readings

Klingensmith WC, Fritzberg AR, Zerbe GO, et al. Relative role of Tc-99m-diethyl-IDA and Tc-99m-sulfur colloid in the evaluation of liver function. *Clin Nucl Med* 5:341–346, 1980.

Shah AN, Dodson F, Fung J. Role of nuclear medicine in liver transplantation. *Semin Nucl Med* 25:36–48, 1995.

Case 152

Clinical Presentation

67-year-old woman presenting with a history of diabetes and gastrointestinal bleeding.

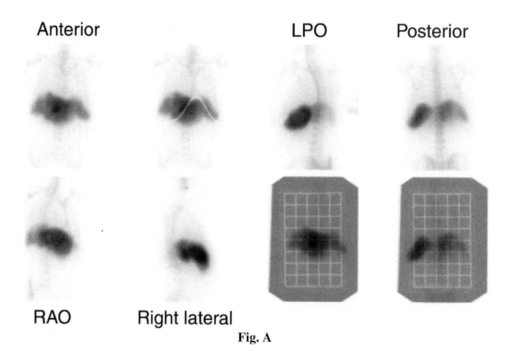

Anterior **LPO** **Posterior**

RAO **Right lateral**

Fig. A

Technique

- 3 mCi technetium-99m–labeled sulfur colloid injected intravenously.
- Planar images in anterior, posterior, anterior with markers, right anterior oblique, left posterior oblique, right lateral projections obtained at 15 minutes after tracer injection.

Image Interpretation

Planar images (Fig. A) demonstrate irregular, diminished uptake in a shrunken right hepatic lobe. The left lobe also shows some irregularity. Posterior images show more tracer uptake in the spleen than in the liver. Bone marrow uptake is also noted in most views.

Differential Diagnosis

- Hepatic cirrhosis
- Radiation port
- Partial liver resection (may help to explain the diminished size of the right lobe)
- Acute hepatitis (would explain poor hepatic uptake of tracer but not the diminished size of the right lobe)

Diagnosis and Clinical Follow-up

Biopsy revealed hepatic cirrhosis. The cause was unclear. The patient died within the year from esophageal variceal bleeding.

Discussion

Cirrhosis is a chronic process that leads to fibrotic scarring and subsequent diminished blood flow and function in the liver. The liver and spleen scan reflects these findings because the decreased hepatic blood flow and reticuloendothelial function result in decreased uptake of the colloid. The reticuloendothelial activity in the spleen and bone marrow become relatively more important, accumulating the tracer that would have otherwise been concentrated in the liver, which is also known as a "colloid shift."

The diminished uptake in the right lobe of the liver compared with the left lobe is not infrequently seen in patients with evolving cirrhosis. Some authors have suggested preferential "streaming" of the portal blood to the right lobe, delivering more toxins, such as ethanol, to this tissue, but this has not been clearly shown to occur. In advanced cirrhosis, both right and left lobes are commonly seen to be diminished in size and show poor tracer concentration.

Suggested Readings

Aburano T, Yokoyama K, Shuke N, et al. 99mTc colloid and 99mTc IDA imagings in diffuse hepatic disease. *J Clin Gastroenterol* 17:321–326, 1993.

Blomquist L, Wang Y, Kimiaei S, et al. Change in size, shape and radiocolloid uptake of the alcoholic liver during alcohol withdrawal, as demonstrated by single photon emission computed tomography. *J Hepatol* 21:417–423, 1994.

Rutland MD, Que L. Assessing diffuse liver disease with the hepatic uptake rate of 99mTc-colloids. *Nucl Med Commun* 16:26–30, 1995.

Section XIII

Vascular Scintigraphy

Case 153

Clinical Presentation

68-year-old woman presenting with breast cancer and indwelling left-sided central line (single lumen Port-a-Cath). There is poor blood return from the central line. The study is performed to rule out obstruction or thrombus.

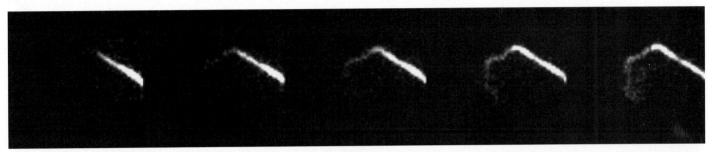

Fig. A

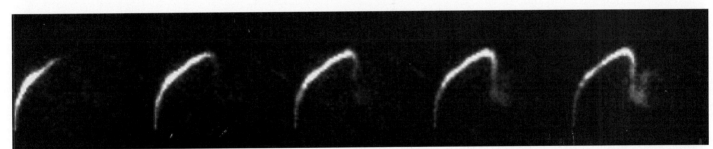

Fig. B

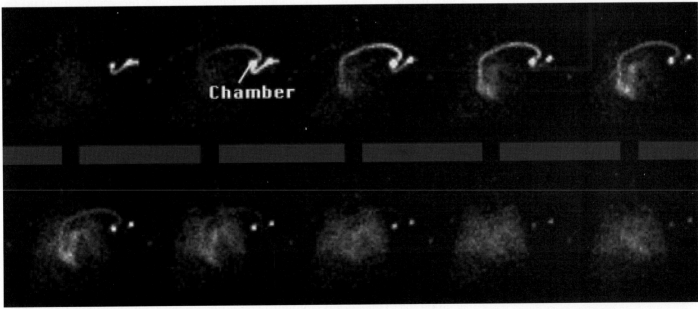

Fig. C

PEARLS/PITFALLS

- If the patient is scheduled for another nuclear medicine study, that radiopharmaceutical may be used for the flow study instead of technetium-99m pertechnetate. Also, because of the short acquisition time and the high count rate, these studies can be performed even if the patient has recently undergone another nuclear medicine study.

- It is important to inject not only the line but also the ipsilateral arm vein. The arm injection will allow detection of thrombus around the line that may be occluding the vessel lumen while the central line remains patent. If injections of the line and the ipsilateral arm vein fail to demonstrate the SVC, the contralateral arm vein should be injected to confirm SVC patency.

- Note the more oblique route taken by the left brachiocephalic vein compared with the right brachiocephalic vein.

- If activity does not clear from the chamber or increases over time, infiltration into the chest wall should be considered. This is why the injection of the line should always be the last one, because residual activity in the chest wall would prevent visualization of venous structures given the short acquisition time.

- If the patient is experiencing pain during the injection, the tracer may have infiltrated the chest wall or the tip of the catheter may have moved out of the SVC (for example, cephalad into the jugular vein, which may result in pain or unusual sensation in the neck upon injection). *(continued)*

Technique

- Potassium perchlorate (400 mg) is administered by mouth 15 minutes prior to the administration of technetium-99m pertechnetate to block thyroid uptake.
- Indwelling catheters with subcutaneous chambers (such as Port-a-Cath's) need to be accessed using sterile techniques.
- With the patient lying supine, butterfly needles connected to a three-way stopcock are connected to the accessed central line ports, and also placed into a vein in each upper extremity.
- Following placement of the lines, 1-mL syringes containing approximately 5 mCi of technetium-99m pertechnetate in a volume of 0.1 to 0.3 mL as well as 10-mL syringes containing 10 mL of normal saline are connected to each stopcock. The patient is placed under a large field of view gamma camera fitted with a low-energy, parallel hole, high-resolution collimator with a 20% energy window centered at 140 keV. The camera is positioned over the anterior chest and shoulders with the heart in the center of the field of view. The tracer is then administered as a bolus injection followed by a rapid infusion of a 10 mL flush of normal saline starting with the upper extremity ipsilateral to the central line, followed by the contralateral arm, and finally the central line in rapid sequence.
- Digital dynamic images are obtained in a 64×64 matrix at 1 frame a second for 120 seconds. At the completion of the study, the central line is flushed with 5 mL of heparin lock flush solution. Data are then reviewed in a cine format as well as 1 sec/frame digital images.

Image Interpretation

The injection into the left arm (Fig. A) shows normal transit of tracer into the left axillary, subclavian, and brachiocephalic veins into the superior vena cava (SVC) and cardiac chambers.

The flow study obtained following injection of the tracer into the right upper extremity (Fig. B) demonstrates normal flow of tracer through the right axillary, subclavian, and brachiocephalic veins into the SVC and cardiac chambers.

The injection through the port of the left-sided central line (Fig. C) shows activity flowing from the subcutaneous chamber through the central line into the SVC and the right cardiac chambers, followed by activity into the lungs and return to the left heart.

Diagnosis and Clinical Follow-up

The diagnosis was normal upper extremity venous flow and normal flow through the central line. The central line and upper extremity venous system are patent.

Discussion

Radionuclide venography provides a quick answer to the clinical question regarding patency of a vessel and that of the central line in which it lies. It is faster than conventional venography, is less expensive, and results in lower radiation exposure and lower procedural risks (such as reaction to iodinated contrast). A patent catheter, however, does not exclude venous thrombosis of the vein in which it lies (see Case 156). It is imperative to perform the injection into the ipsilateral arm in addition to the injection(s) into the central line because it may demonstrate thrombosis of that vessel as defined by abrupt stop of the tracer bolus or presence

- *(continued)* A patent central line does not imply patent vessels. Injection of the ipsilateral arm is essential to assess venous patency.

- If there is significant resistance to injection, the injection should be stopped. A forced injection into an obstructed system may result in disconnection of the syringe with the risk of contamination. It may also potentially cause dislodgment of a downstream thrombus, resulting in pulmonary embolism, or even line rupture.

- Radionuclide venography should not be performed to differentiate between extrinsic and intrinsic obstruction. Morphological modalities such as CT or MRI should be used for that purpose.

of collaterals or reflux into venous structures normally not visualized, or a combination of these.

It is important to keep in mind the normal more oblique route taken by the left brachiocephalic vein compared with the more vertical route taken by the right subclavian vein. If activity is seen transiting from the left subclavian vein in an horizontal fashion to the right side of the neck followed by filling of right-sided vessels, this may be due to total obstruction of the left brachiocephalic vein and transit to the right-sided vessels via collaterals such as the jugular arch.

Note that after the injection of the left-sided central line, the activity clears from the chamber, the line, and the vessels. The focus to the left of the chamber represents residual activity within a tubing connection that lies on the patient's chest.

Suggested Readings

Chasen MH, Charnsangavej C. Venous chest anatomy: Clinical implications. Categorical course in chest radiology. RSNA 1992;121–134.

Horattas MC, Wright DJ, Fenton AH, et al. Changing concepts of deep venous thrombosis of the upper extremity-report of a series of review of the literature. *Surgery* 1988;104:561–567.

Maxfield WS, Meckstroth GR. Technetium-99m superior vena cavography. *Radiology* 1969;92:913–917.

Miyamae T. Interpretation of Tc-99m superior vena cavograms and results of studies in 92 patients. *Radiology* 1973;108:339–352.

Muramatsu T, Miyame T, Dohi Y. Collateral pathways observed by radionuclide superior cavography in 70 patients with superior vena caval obstruction. *Clin Nucl Med* 1991;16:332–336.

Savolaine ER, Schlembach PJ. Scintigraphy compared to other imaging modalities in benign superior vena cava obstruction accompanying fibrosing mediastinitis. *Clin Imaging* 1989;13:234–238.

Case 154

Clinical Presentation

72-year-old man with a history of squamous cell cancer of the bladder, status post-chemotherapy, and removal of the central line now presenting with facial and neck swelling and prominent veins in the neck, upper chest, and upper abdomen. A flow study is requested to rule out superior vena cava (SVC) syndrome.

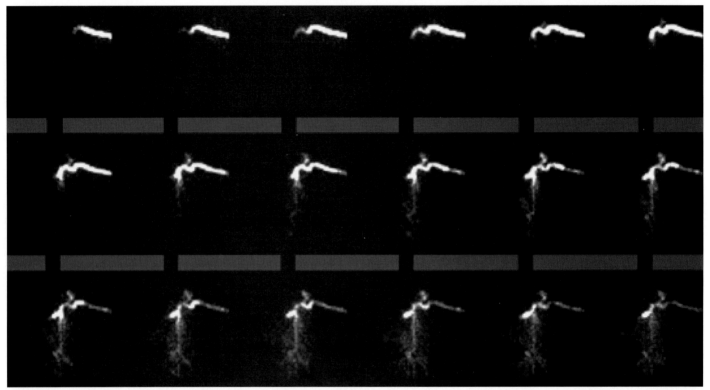

Fig. A

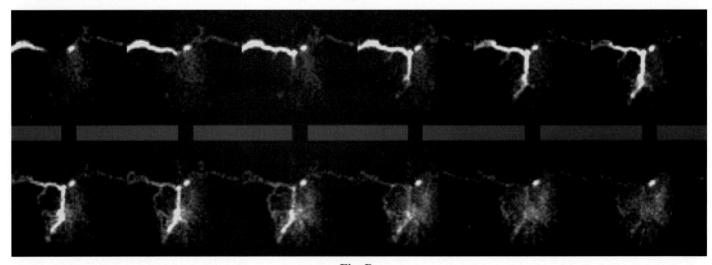

Fig. B

Technique

- Potassium perchlorate (400 mg) is administered by mouth 15 minutes prior to the administration of technetium-99m pertechnetate to block thyroid uptake.
- Indwelling catheters with subcutaneous chambers (such as Port-a-Cath's) need to be accessed using sterile techniques.
- With the patient lying supine, butterfly needles connected to a three-way stopcock are then connected to the accessed central line ports and also placed into a vein in each upper extremity.
- Following placement of the lines, 1-mL syringes containing approximately 5 mCi of technetium-99m pertechnetate in a volume of 0.1 to 0.3 mL as well as 10-mL syringes containing 10 mL of normal saline are connected to each stopcock. The patient is placed under a large field of view gamma camera fitted with a low-energy, parallel hole, high-resolution collimator with a 20% energy window centered at 140 keV. The camera is positioned over the anterior chest and shoulders with the heart in the center of the field of view. The tracer is then administered as a bolus injection followed by a rapid infusion of a 10 mL flush of normal saline starting with the upper extremity ipsilateral to the central line, followed by the contralateral arm, and finally the central line in rapid sequence.
- Digital dynamic images are obtained in a 64×64 matrix at 1 frame a second for 120 seconds. At the completion of the study, the central line is flushed with 5 mL of heparin lock flush solution. Data are then reviewed in a cine format as well as 1 sec/frame digital images.

Image Interpretation

Injection via the left upper extremity (Fig. A) shows flow of tracer through the axillary and subclavian veins followed by reflux into the left jugular vein and possible transit of activity into the left brachiocephalic vein. With continuous flushing, there is subsequent filling of a large number of collaterals extending from the chest into the abdomen. The SVC is not visualized.

Injection via the right upper extremity (Fig. B) demonstrates flow of tracer through the right axillary and subclavian veins followed by activity flowing into possibly the azygous vein as well as numerous collaterals in the chest wall connecting with intradiaphragmatic collateral vessels. The focal activity in the left mid-chest is residual tracer activity from the left arm injection. Again, the SVC is not visualized.

Differential Diagnosis

- Intrinsic causes: venous thrombi or emboli; tumors; foreign bodies
- Extrinsic causes: compression by masses; cicatrizing processes such as mediastinal fibrosis

Diagnosis and Clinical Follow-up

Findings are consistent with SVC obstruction and SVC syndrome. A follow-up chest computed tomography (CT) scan demonstrated a 4- $\times$ 5-cm soft-tissue mass in the superior mediastinum causing extrinsic compression of the SVC. The azygous vein appeared distended, and numerous collateral vessels were seen in the neck and anterior chest wall.

Discussion

Obstruction of the SVC is easily demonstrated by the flow study following injection in both upper extremities. Nonvisualization of the SVC following injection into one upper extremity does not imply SVC obstruction because it may be related to obstruction in ipsilateral vessels more distal to the SVC. This is why injection of the contralateral extremity should always be performed in this context, because it could demonstrate patency of the SVC. In the present case, both upper extremity injections failed to demonstrate the SVC and show a high degree of collateral formation, suggesting a high degree of obstruction.

Collateral flow patterns to the SVC include the paravertebral, azygous-hemiazygous, internal mammary, lateral thoracic, and anterior jugular venous systems, and some of these collateral systems were demonstrated in this patient.

Suggested Readings

Chasen MH, Charnsangavej C. Venous chest anatomy: Clinical implications. Categorical course in chest radiology. RSNA 1992;121–134.

Horattas MC, Wright DJ, Fenton AH, et al. Changing concepts of deep venous thrombosis of the upper extremity-report of a series and review of the literature. *Surgery* 1998;104:561–567.

Maxfield WS, Meckstroth GR. Technetium-99m superior vena cavography. *Radiology* 1969;92:913–917.

Miyamae T. Interpretation of Tc-99 superior vena cavograms and results of studies in 92 patients. *Radiology* 1973;108:339–352.

Muramatsu T, Miyame T, Dohi Y. Collateral pathways observed by radionuclide superior cavography in 70 patients with superior vena caval obstruction. *Clin Nucl Med* 1991;16:332–336.

Savolaine ER, Schlembach PJ. Scintigraphy compared to other imaging modalities in benign superior vena cava obstruction accompanying fibrosing mediastinitis. *Clin Imaging* 1989;13:234–238.

Case 155

Clinical Presentation

44-year-old patient with colon cancer who has been receiving chemotherapy through an indwelling central line. There is no problem injecting, but there is difficulty in withdrawing blood from the central line. A flow study is requested to assess patency of the central line.

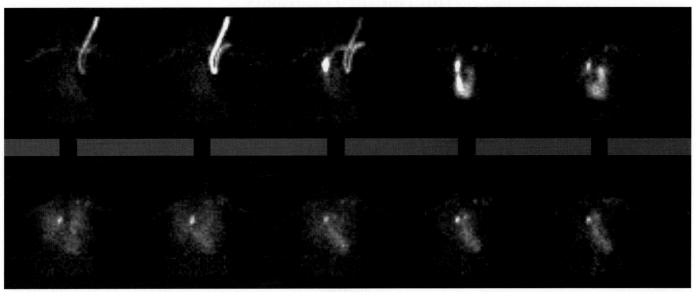

Fig. A

Technique

- Potassium perchlorate (400 mg) is administered by mouth. 15 minutes prior to the administration of technetium-99m pertechnetate to block thyroid uptake.
- Indwelling catheters with subcutaneous chambers (such as Port-a-Caths) need to be accessed using sterile techniques and special needles.
- With the patient lying supine, butterfly needles connected to a three-way stopcock are then connected to the accessed central line ports and also placed into a vein in each upper extremity.
- Following placement of the lines, 1-mL syringes containing approximately 5 mCi of technetium-99m pertechnetate in a volume of 0.1 to 0.3 mL as well as 10-mL syringes containing 10 mL of normal saline are connected to each stopcock. The patient is placed under a large field of view gamma camera fitted with a low-energy, parallel hole, high-resolution collimator with a 20% energy window centered at 140 keV. The camera is positioned over the anterior chest and shoulders with the heart in the center of the field of view. The tracer is then administered as a bolus injection followed by a rapid infusion of a 10 mL flush of normal saline starting with the upper extremity ipsilateral to the central line, followed by the contralateral arm, and finally the central line in rapid sequence.
- Digital dynamic images are obtained in a 64 × 64 matrix at 1 frame a second for 120 seconds. At the completion of the study, the central line is flushed with

5 mL of heparin lock flush solution. Data are then reviewed in a cine format as well as 1 sec/frame digital images.

Image Interpretation

Serial dynamic images (Fig. A) demonstrate normal transit of the tracer through the central line into the superior vena cava (SVC) and cardiac chambers. Following clearance of activity from the vessels and the cardiac chambers, there is, however, persistent tracer uptake in the region of the tip of the line despite continuous flushing. The venous blood flow through both upper extremities was normal (images not shown).

Differential Diagnosis

- Retention at the tip of the catheter
- Residual activity within overlying tubing or connections
- Residual activity in the vessel
- Residual activity within a collateral vessel

Diagnosis and Clinical Follow-up

The findings are suggestive of a "fibrin sheath" deposit at the tip of the catheter. The patient received urokinase, and blood return improved following urokinase therapy.

Discussion

Fibrin deposits are found around almost all indwelling catheters after 1 week. When this fibrin sheath extends over the tip of the line, it may result in difficulties in withdrawing blood because it can be pulled against or into the tip of the catheter during the drawing process. There is less of a problem injecting into those lines because these fibrin deposits form a loose mesh through which fluid can circulate.

This diagnosis is important to make because it requires "local" thrombolytic therapy, like urokinase, rather than systemic anticoagulative therapy with heparin.

Suggested Readings

Chasen MH, Charnsangavej C. Venous chest anatomy: clinical implications. Categorical course in chest radiology. RSNA 1992;121–134.

Horattas MC, Wright DJ, Fenton AH, et al. Changing concepts of deep venous thrombosis of the upper extremity-report of a series and review of the literature. *Surgery* 1988;104:561–567.

Maxfield WS, Meckstroth GR. Technetium-99m superior vena cavography. *Radiology* 1969;92:913–917.

Miyamae T. Interpretation of Tc-99m Superior vena cavograms and results of studies in 92 patients. *Radiology* 1973;108:339–352.

Muramatsu T, Miyame T, Dohi Y. Collateral pathways observed by radionuclide superior cavography in 70 patients with superior vena caval obstruction. *Clin Nucl Med* 1991;16:332–336.

Savolaine ER, Schlembach PJ. Scintigraphy compared to other imaging modalities in benign superior vena cava obstruction accompanying fibrosing mediastinitis. *Clin Imaging* 1989;13:234–238.

Case 156

Clinical Presentation

44-year-old woman with breast cancer who has been receiving chemotherapy through an indwelling right-sided central line recently complaining of right-sided upper extremity swelling.

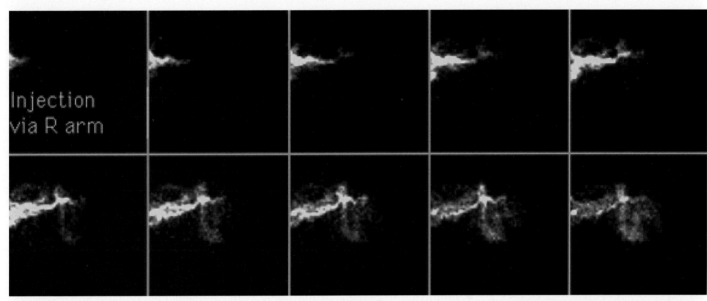

Fig. A

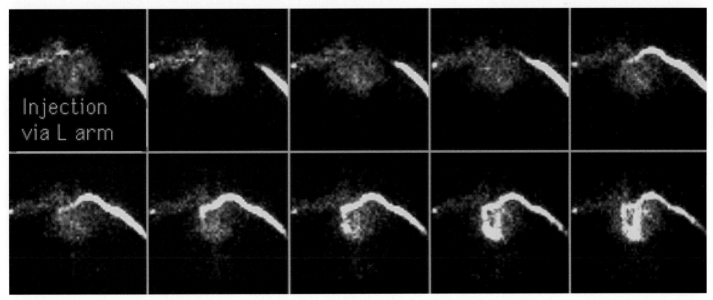

Fig. B

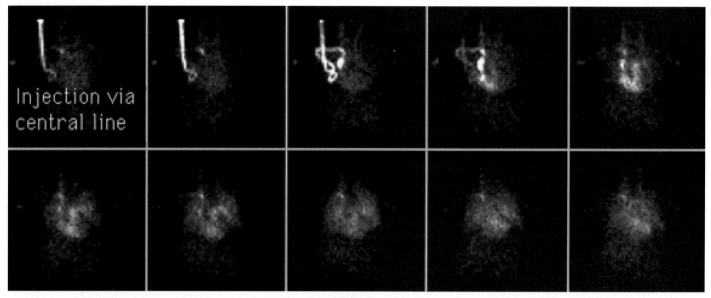

Fig. C

- Radionuclide venography may be performed in conjunction with other nuclear medicine studies.

- Careful attention should always be paid to the region of the tip of a central line. A persistent focus of tracer activity at this location suggests the presence of a fibrin mesh at the line tip. This could be the cause of a central line that flushes well but from which there is difficulty in withdrawing blood.

- Both upper extremities should always be imaged. If an abnormality is detected on one side, the contralateral study provides assessment of the superior vena cava. *(continued)*

Technique

- Potassium perchlorate (400 mg) is administered by mouth 15 minutes prior to the administration of technetium-99m pertechnetate to block thyroid uptake.

- Indwelling catheters with subcutaneous chambers (such as Port-a-Cath's) need to be accessed using sterile techniques.

- With the patient lying supine, butterfly needles connected to a three-way stopcock are then connected to the accessed central line ports and also placed into a vein in each upper extremity.

- Following placement of the lines, 1-mL syringes containing approximately 5 mCi of technetium-99m pertechnetate in a volume of 0.1 to 0.3 mL as well as 10-mL syringes containing 10 mL of normal saline are connected to each stopcock. The patient is placed under a large field of view gamma camera fitted with a low-energy, parallel hole, high-resolution collimator with a 20% energy window centered at 140 keV. The camera is positioned over the anterior chest and shoulders with the heart in the center of the field of view. The tracer is then administered as a bolus injection followed by a rapid infusion of a 10 mL flush of normal saline starting with the upper extremity ipsilateral to the central line, followed by the contralateral arm, and finally the central line in rapid sequence.

- Digital dynamic images are obtained in a 64×64 matrix at 1 frame a second for 120 seconds. At the completion of the study, the central line is flushed with 5 mL of heparin lock flush solution. Data are then reviewed in a cine format as well as 1 sec/frame digital images.

Image Interpretation

Injection via the right upper extremity (Fig. A) demonstrates filling of collateral vessels extending from the level of the right axillary vein, along the right brachiocephalic vein up to the right jugular vein. The right brachiocephalic vein and the SVC are not visualized. The activity progresses across the neck into another collateral (the jugular arch), and the cardiac chambers are filling in via the collaterals.

Injection via the left arm (Fig. B) shows normal progression of tracer

- *(continued)* The central line should be injected last after the arm veins. This is done in case there is extravasation from the line into the soft tissues of the thorax that could obscure subsequent imaging.

- The presence of a patent central line does not exclude the presence of a thrombus. Thrombus may form concentrically around a catheter without obstructing its lumen. The ipsilateral injection is essential in the evaluation of the patency of a central line.

- Radionuclide venography is not an effective means by which to distinguish intrinsic from extrinsic causes of venous stenosis or obstruction. If there is reason to suspect a nonthrombotic cause of obstruction, anatomic imaging such as a chest CT may be useful.

through the left axillary, subclavian, and brachiocephalic veins into the SVC, confirming patency of the SVC.

The last injection via the central line (Fig. C) shows normal progression of tracer through the line, the SVC, and cardiac chambers.

Differential Diagnosis

- Intrinsic causes: thrombi, emboli, tumors, webs, foreign bodies.
- Extrinsic causes: impression from masses or musculoskeletal structures; cicatrizing processes such as mediastinal fibrosis.

Diagnosis and Clinical Follow-up

The findings are consistent with a high-grade obstruction of the right subclavian vein possibly extending into the right axilla. Based on the clinical and scintigraphic findings, an upper extremity thrombus was diagnosed and the patient was placed on heparin.

Discussion

Radionuclide venography is a rapid and sensitive means to detect or exclude upper extremity thrombosis. It is also a useful means to assess for patency of central lines and an early way to detect the formation of a fibrin mesh at the tip of an indwelling line.

At our institution, the majority of patients who undergo this test have indwelling central lines and frequently an underlying malignancy. These factors predispose to thrombus formation.

The study in this patient demonstrated the fact that a patent central line does not exclude venous thrombus. Second, the contralateral arm injection was helpful in defining patency of the SVC when a high-grade obstruction was seen in the ipsilateral venous system, preventing definite visualization of the SVC from the right upper extremity injection because of collateral formation.

Although this patient's central line was patent, the vein in which it lay was totally obstructed based on the significant collateral formation demonstrated by the ipsilateral arm injection. The right subclavian and brachiocephalic veins as well as the SVC cannot be explicitly assessed on this study, because tracer was shunted to collateral vessels around the venous obstruction. The right brachiocephalic vein and the SVC could be involved with thrombus, or they could conceivably be patent. From the left-sided injection, we know that the superior vena cava in this patient was patent.

Suggested Readings

Fielding JR, Nagel JS, et al. Upper extremity DVT. Correlation of MR and nuclear medicine flow imaging. *Clin Imaging* 1997;21:260–263.

Kida T. Demonstration of collateral pathways in superior vena cava syndrome by means of radionuclide venography. *Clin Nucl Med* 1985;10:195–196.

Podoloff DA, et al. Evaluation of sensitivity and specificity of upper extremity radionuclide venography in cancer patients with indwelling central venous catheters. *Clin Nucl Med* 1992;17:457–462.

Van Houtte P, et al. Radionuclide venography in the evaluation of superior vena cava syndrome. *Clin Nucl Med* 1981;6:177–183.

Case 157

Clinical Presentation

67-year-old man presenting with abdominal pain. Computed tomography (CT) scan showed an appendiceal mass and a 2-cm lesion in the dome of the right lobe of the liver.

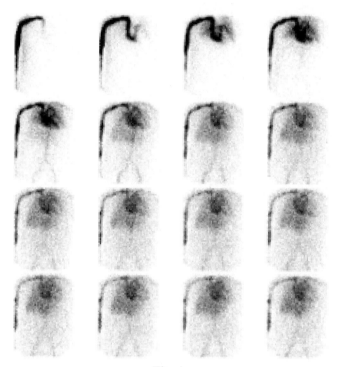

Fig. A

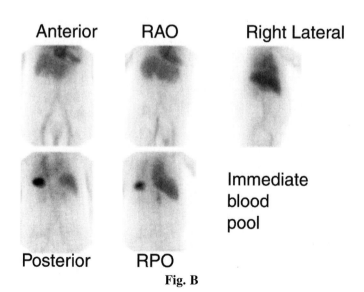

Anterior   RAO   Right Lateral

Posterior   RPO

Immediate blood pool

Fig. B

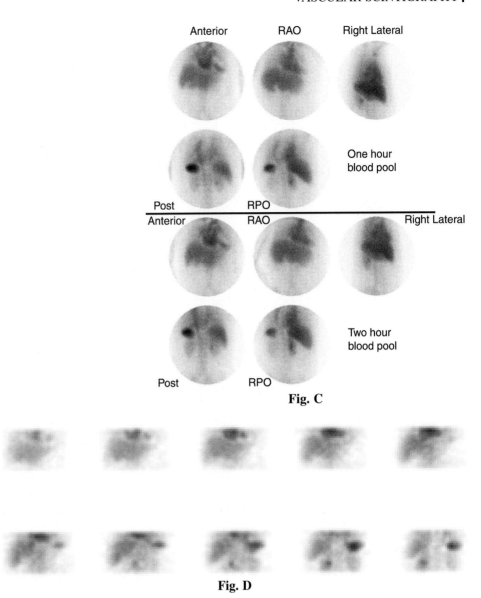

Fig. C

Fig. D

Technique

- 3 cc autologous red blood cells labeled in vitro with 25 mCi technetium-99m.
- Flow images obtained during tracer injection in a 64 × 64 matrix for 1.5 seconds per frame.
- Delayed images obtained in anterior, right anterior oblique, right lateral, posterior, and right posterior oblique views for 500,000 counts at 5 minutes after tracer injection, at 1 hour and at 2 hours.
- Use a low-energy, all-purpose collimator.

Image Interpretation

Selected flow images (Fig. A) show normal blood flow to the liver. Immediate (Fig. B), 1 hour–delayed, and 2 hour–delayed (Fig. C) planar images show a normal hepatic blood pool. Coronal reconstructions from single photon emission computed tomography (SPECT) acquisition also showed normal tracer distribution (Fig. D).

Differential Diagnosis

(False negative studies)

- Hemangioma too small for detection with gamma camera
- Thrombosed hemangioma
- Excessive patient motion during image acquisition

Diagnosis and Clinical Follow-up

The appendiceal mass noted on CT was felt to be an abscess. The 2-cm lesion in the right lobe of the liver was felt to be a hemangioma by CT criteria. The hemangioma was probably too small to be seen with blood pool imaging.

Discussion

The liver blood pool study is the gold standard for the diagnosis of hepatic hemangioma. Although characteristic findings on CT and magnetic resonance imaging (MRI) may obviate the need for a scintigraphic study in patients with low suspicion of metastatic disease, patients with atypical findings on CT and MRI are often referred for blood pool imaging.

Flow images are done to evaluate the lesion for signs of increased blood flow. Hemangiomas are characterized by areas of very sluggish blood flow through large, cavernous vascular channels. Increased blood flow to the lesion on flow images is not characteristic of hemangioma and should raise the possibility of metastatic disease or some other cause of increased blood flow. Delayed images demonstrate the distribution of the blood pool. The large blood pool and slow flow of cavernous hemangiomas will characteristically show an area of increased tracer activity that becomes more intense on delayed images.

The advantage of the scintigraphic study is the prolonged residence time of the tracer in the blood pool. This allows several hours for equilibration of the blood pool in patients with unusually sluggish flow through the hemangioma. CT contrast resides in the blood pool for only a very short time, often not long enough to allow equilibration with the blood pool of the hemangioma. Unfortunately, as was the case for this study, the sensitivity of the test decreases when the size of the lesion is less than 2 cm.

Suggested Readings

Achong DM, Oates E. Hepatic hemangioma in cirrhotics with portal hypertension: Evaluation with Tc-99m red blood cell SPECT. *Radiology* 191:115–117, 1994.

Bonanno N, Baldari S, Cerrito A, et al. Diagnosis of hepatic hemangiomas with 99mTc-labeled red blood cell scanning: Value of SPECT. *J Nucl Biol Med* 35:135–140, 1991.

Middleton ML. Scintigraphic evaluation of hepatic mass lesions: Emphasis on hemangioma detection. *Semin Nucl Med* 26:4–15, 1996.

Rubin RA, Lichtenstein GR. Scintigraphic evaluation of liver masses: Cavernous hepatic hemangioma. *J Nucl Med* 34:849–852, 1993.

Case 158

Clinical Presentation

33-year-old woman presenting with left upper quadrant pain. Ultrasound showed a hepatic lesion.

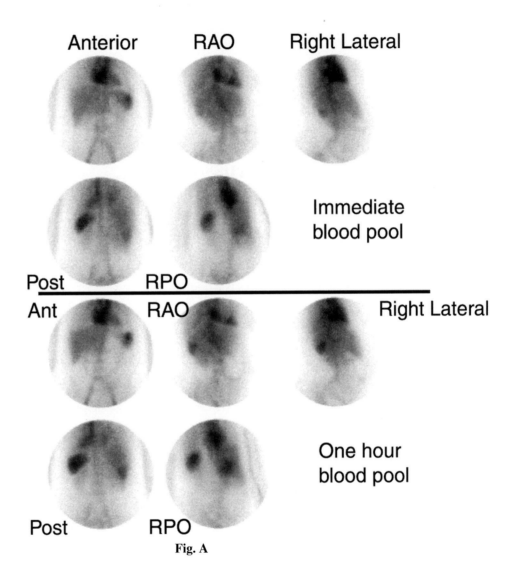

Anterior   RAO   Right Lateral

Immediate blood pool

Post   RPO

Ant   RAO   Right Lateral

One hour blood pool

Post   RPO

Fig. A

Technique

- 3 cc autologous red blood cells labeled in vitro with 25 mCi technetium-99m.
- Flow images obtained during tracer injection in a 64 × 64 matrix for 1.5 seconds per frame.
- Delayed images obtained in anterior, right anterior oblique, right lateral, posterior, and right posterior oblique views for 500,000 counts at 5 minutes after tracer injection and at 1 hour.
- Use a low-energy, all-purpose collimator.

Image Interpretation

Flow images (not shown) show no areas of abnormally increased flow. Immediate images show a faint area of increased tracer accumulation in the posterior portion of the right lobe of the liver. One hour–delayed images show more intense concentration of tracer in the same location (Fig. A).

Differential Diagnosis

- Cavernous hemangioma
- Hepatic angiosarcoma (rare)
- Hepatoma (rare)

Diagnosis and Clinical Follow-up

The findings are consistent with cavernous hemangioma. No further evidence of liver disease was noted.

Discussion

The flow images (not shown) were done in the posterior projection. This is because the liver lesion was noted to be posterior on ultrasound. The imaging study that initially discovered the lesion should always be reviewed before the scintigraphic study is performed.

The increasing tracer accumulation between the immediate and the first-hour images is a finding that is characteristic for hemangiomas. This is caused by slow flow of blood through the lesion, sometimes requiring more than 1 hour for the radiolabeled blood pool to equilibrate with that in the hemangioma.

Suggested Readings

Farlow DC, Chapman PR, Gruenewald SM, Antico VF, Farrell GC, Little JM. Investigation of focal hepatic lesions: is tomographic red blood cell imaging useful? *World J Surg* 1990; 14:463–467.

Kinnard MF, Alavi A, Rubin RA, Lichtenstein GR. Nuclear imaging of solid hepatic masses. *Semin Roentgenol* 1995; 30:375–395.

Rubin RA, Lichtenstein GR. Scintigraphic evaluation of liver masses: cavernous hepatic hemangioma [clinical conference] [see comments]. *J Nucl Med* 1993; 34:849–852.

Case 159

Clinical Presentation

41-year-old man presenting with right upper quadrant pain. Ultrasound showed lesions in the liver.

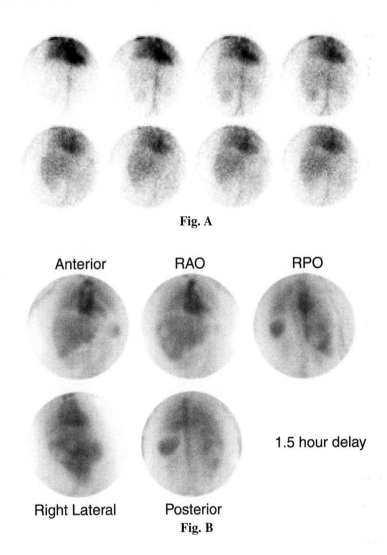

Fig. A

Anterior   RAO   RPO

1.5 hour delay

Right Lateral   Posterior

Fig. B

Technique

- 3 cc autologous red blood cells labeled with 25 mCi technetium-99m in vitro.
- Flow images should be obtained during tracer injection in a 64 × 64 matrix for 1.5 seconds per frame.
- Images obtained in anterior, right anterior oblique, right lateral, posterior, and right posterior oblique views for 500,000 counts each 5 minutes after tracer injection at 1 hour and 2 hours.
- Use a low-energy, all-purpose collimator.

Image Interpretation

Selected flow images (Fig. A) show no evidence of focally increased flow to the liver. There is some suggestion of decreased flow to the dome of the right lobe and irregularity in tracer distribution on the later flow images. Delayed images at 1.5 hours (Fig. B) show focal defects throughout the liver, particularly pronounced on the right lateral view.

Differential Diagnosis

- Neoplastic disease (primary and metastatic)
- Cyst
- Abscess

Diagnosis and Clinical Follow-up

Scan was read as not consistent with hemangioma. Biopsy demonstrated carcinoid metastases.

Discussion

Hepatic parenchymal defects that persist on delayed images are consistent with space-occupying lesions and are not consistent with hemangioma. Flow images may demonstrate focally increased flow in the presence of hepatocellular carcinoma, but the finding is not specific. Flow can also be increased in other neoplasms or arterioportal shunting.

Suggested Readings

Dwamena BA, Belcher KK, Dasika N, et al. Focal hyperemia on RBC blood-flow imaging. A scintigraphic marker of arterioportal venous shunting in hepatic cavernous hemangiomas? *Clin Nucl Med* 22:542–545, 1997.

Hobbs KE. Hepatic hemangiomas. *World J Surg* 14:468–471, 1990.

Intenzo C, Park C, Walker M, et al. Hepatic angiosarcoma mimicking cavernous hemangioma. *Clin Nucl Med* 20:375, 1995.

Middleton ML. Scintigraphic evaluation of hepatic mass lesions: Emphasis on hemangioma detection. *Semin Nucl Med* 26:4–15, 1996.

Rubin RA, Lichtenstein GR. Scintigraphic evaluation of liver masses: Cavernous hepatic hemangioma. *J Nucl Med* 34:849–852, 1993.

Shih WJ, Lee JK, Mitchell B. False-positive results for hepatic hemangioma on Tc-99m RBC SPECT caused by a liver metastasis from small-cell lung carcinoma. *Clin Nucl Med* 21:898–899, 1996.

Swayne LC, Diehl WL, Brown TD, et al. False-positive hepatic blood pool scintigraphy in metastatic colon carcinoma. *Clin Nucl Med* 16:630–632, 1991.

Winograd J, Palubinskas AJ. Arterial-portal venous shunting in cavernous hemangioma of the liver. *Radiology* 122:331–332, 1977.

Case 160

Clinical Presentation

31-year-old woman presenting with right upper quadrant fullness. Ultrasound showed a lesion in the posterior aspect of the right hepatic lobe.

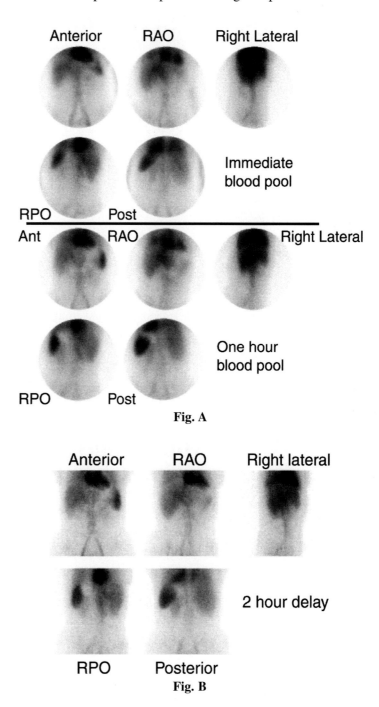

Fig. A

Fig. B

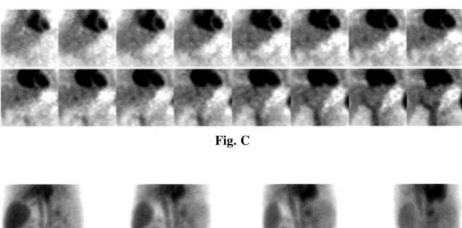

Fig. C

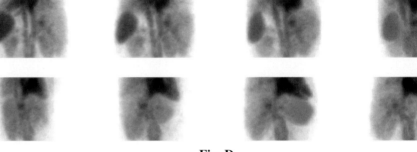

Fig. D

Technique

- 3 cc autologous red blood cells labeled in vitro with 25 mCi technetium-99m.
- Flow images obtained during tracer injection in a 64 × 64 matrix for 1.5 seconds per frame.
- Images obtained in anterior, right anterior oblique, right lateral, posterior, and right posterior oblique views for 500,000 counts each 5 minutes after tracer injection at 1 hour and 2 hours.
- Use a low-energy, all-purpose collimator.
- Single photon emission computed tomography (SPECT) images obtained with a dual-headed gamma camera; 45 images per head; 40 seconds per image.

Image Interpretation

The flow images (not shown) were normal. Figure A shows normal immediate and 1-hour planar blood pool images. Figure B shows normal 2-hour planar blood pool images.

Figure C shows coronal slices reconstructed from SPECT data. Several slices demonstrate a focus of increased tracer activity in the posterior aspect of the right lobe of the liver just below the right ventricle. Figure D shows volume-rendered SPECT images in eight projections that demonstrate the same focus of tracer accumulation.

Differential Diagnosis

- Cavernous hemangioma
- Hepatic angiosarcoma
- Hepatoma

Diagnosis and Clinical Follow-up

CT and ultrasound demonstrated a 2.5-cm lesion consistent with hemangioma in the same location as the focal findings on SPECT. No further follow-up of the lesion was obtained.

Discussion

SPECT has been shown in several small studies to improve the sensitivity of blood pool imaging for cavernous hemangioma, particularly when small lesions of approximately 2 cm are of concern. With the decreased specificity that accompanies the increased sensitivity, it is not surprising that SPECT has falsely identified hemangiomas in several patients. Fortunately, because almost all patients have had other imaging studies, such as ultrasound, CT, and magnetic resonance imaging (MRI), the results of the various studies can be correlated to arrive at a diagnosis that is likely to be more accurate than are the results of any single imaging study.

Suggested Readings

Bonanno N, Baldari S, Cerrito A, et al. Diagnosis of hepatic hemangiomas with 99mTc-labeled red blood cell scanning: Value of SPECT. *J Nucl Biol Med* 35:135–140, 1991.

Brunetti JC, Van Heertum RL, Yudd AP, et al. The value of SPECT imaging in the diagnosis of hepatic hemangioma. *Clin Nucl Med* 13:800–804, 1988.

Kamenjicki E, Stefanovic L, Adic O. Correlation between the blood pool tomoscintigraphy (SPECT) and planar scintigraphy in the diagnostic of the liver hemangioma. *Med Pregl* 46(suppl):60–63, 1993.

Langsteger W, Lind P, Eber B, et al. Diagnosis of hepatic hemangioma with 99mTc-labeled red cells: Single photon emission computed tomography (SPECT) versus planar imaging. *Liver* 9:288–293, 1989.

Case 161

Clinical Presentation

77-year-old female presenting with hepatic lesions noted on abdominal computed tomography (CT).

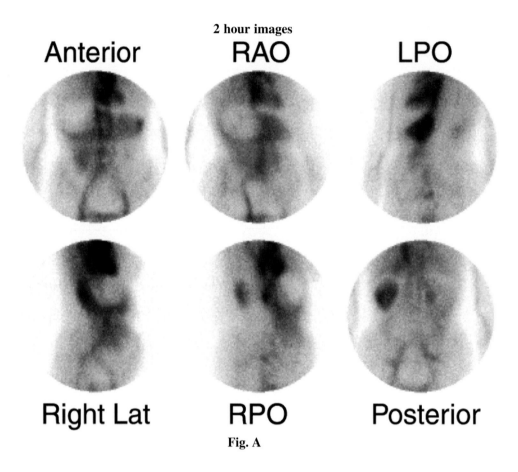

2 hour images

Anterior   RAO   LPO

Right Lat   RPO   Posterior

Fig. A

Technique

- 3 cc autologous red blood cells labeled in vitro with 25 mCi technetium-99m.
- Flow images obtained during tracer injection in a 64 × 64 matrix for 1.5 seconds per frame.
- Images obtained in anterior, right anterior oblique, right lateral, posterior, and right posterior oblique views for 500,000 counts each 5 minutes after tracer injection at 1 hour and 2 hours.
- Use a low-energy, all-purpose collimator.

Image Interpretation

Blood flow images (not shown) demonstrated an area of decreased tracer flow in the right lobe of the liver. Delayed images at 2 hours (Fig. A) show a large area of decreased tracer activity in the right lobe of the liver, with an area of relatively increased activity posteromedially.

Differential Diagnosis

• Cavernous hemangioma
• Hepatic angiosarcoma
• Hepatoma
• Neoplastic disease (primary and metastatic)
• Cyst
• Abscess

Diagnosis and Clinical Follow-up

The large right lobe lesion was a simple cyst. The area of increased activity posteromedially to this was a hepatic cavernous hemangioma.

Discussion

Cavernous hemangiomas are the most common nonmetastatic neoplasm of the liver. They therefore can be serendipitously discovered during the investigation of other hepatic lesions.

Suggested Readings

Harkins LA, Yap HY, Buzdar AU, Blumenschein GR. Benign versus malignant hepatic lesions. A diagnostic dilemma with breast cancer patients. *Cancer* 1983; 52:1308–1311.

Schwartz LH, Gandras EJ, Colangelo SM, Ercolani MC, Panicek DM. Prevalence and importance of small hepatic lesions found at CT in patients with cancer. *Radiology* 1999; 210:71–74.

Section XIV

Pediatric Scintigraphy

Case 162

Clinical Presentation

7-year-old female presenting with a 2-day history of abdominal pain, dysuria, and fever of 102 to 103°F. Physical examination showed right costovertebral angle tenderness. Initial laboratory evaluation included complete blood count (WBC:13.2), urinalysis (20 to 40 WBC and 10 to 20 RBC), blood culture, and urine culture. Technetium-99m–labeled dimercaptosuccinic acid (DMSA) for evaluation of renal involvement and a radionuclide cystography (RNC) for detection of vesicoureteral reflux (VUR) were requested after patient was started on intravenous antibiotics for suspected pyelonephritis.

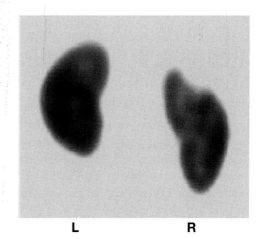

Fig. A

L   R

Technique

DMSA Study

- Technetium-99m DMSA at 0.5 mCi/kg given intravenously. The minimum dose is 0.2 mCi; the maximum dose is 3.0 mCi.
- Use a high- or ultrahigh-resolution, low-energy, parallel hole collimator for single photon emission computed tomography (SPECT) acquisition. Perform planar imaging using a pinhole collimator for young infants.
- Energy window 20% centered at 140 keV.
- Imaging done 4 hours after radiotracer injection. SPECT acquisition is performed with 40 stops per detector or 120 steps with a three-detector imaging system.

RNC Study

- Technetium-99m pertechnetate at a dose of 2 mCi. The patient is asked to urinate prior to the examination. A catheter is placed into the bladder under sterile technique. A 500 ml bag of saline is connected to the catheter. The radiotracer is injected as a bolus into the catheter. The bladder is filled with saline at a pressure of 70-90 cm H_2O.
- High resolution, low energy parallel hole collimator.
- Energy window is 20% centered at 140 Kev.
- Dynamic acquisition is obtained of the filling and voiding. Once the voiding is complete, the computer recording is terminated and the catheter is removed.

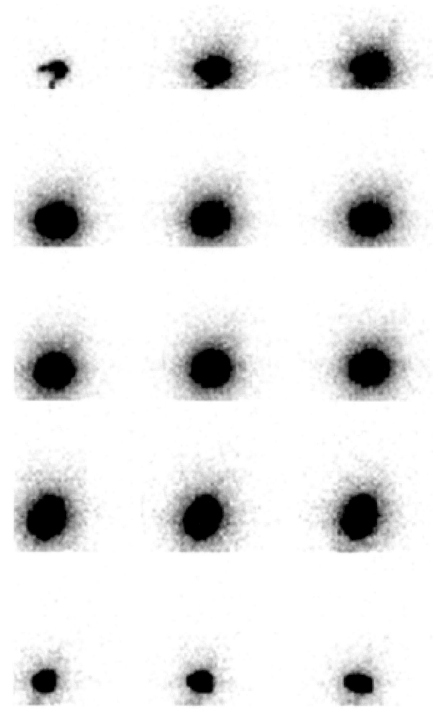

Fig. B

Image Interpretation

A reprojected image of the kidneys (Fig. A) shows a cortical defect in the upper pole of the right kidney. The left kidney is normal. The differential cortical uptake is 52% by the left kidney and 48% by the right kidney.

A radionuclide cystogram (Fig. B) shows no evidence of VUR.

Normal technetium-99m DMSA scan (Fig. C) of a different patient is shown for comparison. There is symmetrical uptake by both kidneys. The contour of both kidneys is smooth with no cortical defects. Normally there is relative lower tracer uptake in the medulla and the collecting systems. The differential cortical uptake is 50% for each kidney.

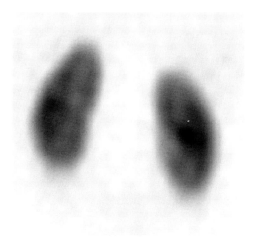

Fig. C

Differential Diagnosis

- Pyelonephritis
- Scarring
- Renal infarction
- Renal trauma
- Vesico-ureteral reflux

Diagnosis and Clinical Follow-up

Urinary tract infection (UTI) was confirmed after urine culture grew >100,000 *Escherichia coli*. The patient was treated for acute pyelonephritis improved on intravenous antibiotics and was discharged after 6 days of hospitalization to finish treatment with oral antibiotics as an outpatient.

Discussion

In the preantibiotic era, UTI was a serious disease with significant mortality. The advent of antibiotics and aggressive diagnostic approaches have reduced the mortality to zero. In the modern era there is still, however, a nonnegligible degree of long term consequences. Of children entering dialysis, 10 to 20% have a history of UTI or reflux, or both.

There are a number of approaches for the diagnostic imaging evaluation of UTI. It is now well-accepted that all children with the first UTI should be evaluated for predisposing factors. The risk factors for the development of scarring related to UTI include (1) obstruction, (2) reflux, (3) young age, (4) delay in treatment, (5) number of pyelonephritic attacks, and (6) unusual bacteria. Technetium-99m DMSA is superior to sonography and to intravenous pyelography (IVP) for the detection of acute pyelonephritis or scar, or both. The number of defects detected on technetium-99m DMSA scintigraphy with repeated episodes of pyelonephritis may increase over time as scarring replaces the renal parenchyma. Abnormalities noted on technetium-99m DMSA scintigraphy are usually seen in one of two recognizable patterns of uptake: (1) generalized decreased uptake or (2) focal decreased uptake with or without loss of volume. It has been reported that DMSA has a sensitivity of 96% and a specificity of 98% for the detection of changes induced by pyelonephritis.

VUR is the most significant host risk factor for the development of UTI and renal scarring, but renal scarring can occur in the absence of VUR in a large percentage of children. Radionuclide cystography is indicated for children diagnosed with UTI for the evaluation of genitourinary reflux. Three degrees of reflux can be recognized with RNC. Grade 1 (Fig. D) corresponds to reflux into the ureter, Grade 2 (Fig. E) corresponds to reflux into the ureter reaching the pelvis that do not appear dilated, and Grade 3 (Fig. F) corresponds to reflux reaching a dilated pelvis, with or without dilated and tortuous ureter.

There is a correlation between the grade of reflux and the severity of scarring detected by technetium-99m DMSA. Higher grades of reflux lead to greater severity of abnormality seen on technetium-99m DMSA.

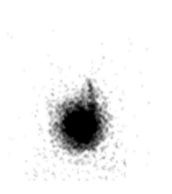
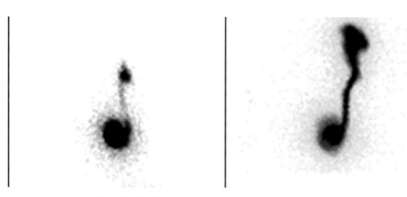

Figs. D, E, F

Suggested Readings

Bjorgvinsson E, Majd M, Eggli K. Diagnosis of acute pyelonephritis in children: Comparison of sonography and 99mTc-DMSA. *AJR Am J Roentgenol* 157:539–543, 1991.

Conway JJ. The role of scintigraphy in urinary tract infection. *Semin Nucl Med* 18:242–243, 1982.

Treves ST, Gelfand M, Willi UV. Vesicoureteric reflux and radionuclide cystography. In: Treves ST, ed. *Pediatric Nuclear Medicine,* 2nd ed. New York: Springer-Verlag, 1995: 411–429.

Kass E, Fink-Bennett D, Cacciarelli A. The sensitivity of renal scintigraphy and sonography in detecting nonobstructive acute pyelonephritis. *J Urol* 148:606–608, 1992.

Sty JR, Wells RG, Schroder BA, Starshak RJ. Diagnostic imaging in pediatric renal inflammatory disease. *JAMA* 256:895, 1986.

Treves ST, Majd M, Kuruc A, Packard AB, Harmon W. Kidneys. In: Treves ST, ed. *Pediatric Nuclear Medicine*, 2nd ed. New York: Springer-Verlag, 1995:339–399.

Case 163

Clinical Presentation

12-year-old boy presenting with a 3-hour history of acute left scrotal pain. The left hemiscrotum was swollen, and the left testicle was tender on palpation. The patient was not sexually active.

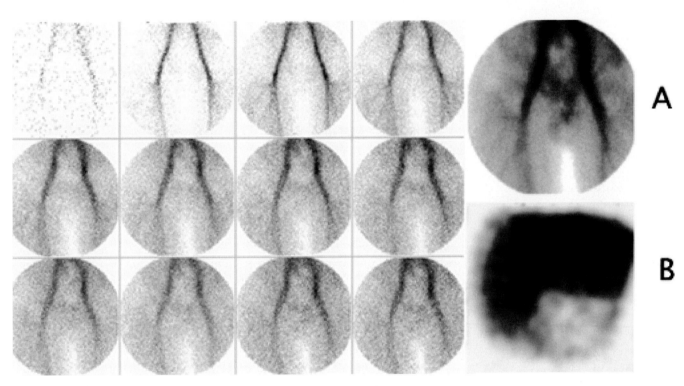

Flow Images

Fig. A, B

Technique

- Technetium-99m pertechnetate 200 μCi/kg given intravenously. Minimum dose is 2 mCi; maximum dose is 15 mCi. A saturated solution of potassium iodide (6 mg/kg) by mouth is recommended to minimize the dose to the thyroid.
- Angiographic images obtained using a high-resolution or converging collimator and a static image should be obtained with a pinhole collimator.
- Energy window 20% centered at 140 keV.
- Imaging time one frame per 3 seconds for 90 seconds. Immediately after this, a 300,000- to 500,000-count anterior static image is obtained. Lead shielding is then placed under the scrotum and an anterior 150,000 count image is obtained using a pinhole collimator. When necessary, an additional anterior pinhole image can be obtained with a cobalt-57 string marker delineating the median raphe.

Image Interpretation

Radionuclide angiogram shows symmetric flow to the scrotum. Tissue phase (Fig. A) and pinhole collimator (Fig. B) images reveal a well-defined area of decreased tracer uptake in the central portion of the left hemiscrotum.

Differential Diagnosis

1. Acute torsion
2. Hydrocele
3. Hematocele
4. Testicular epidermoid cyst

Diagnosis and Clinical Follow-up

The diagnosis was testicular torsion. Following scintigraphy, the patient underwent surgery, at which time acute left testicular torsion was confirmed. The left testicle was found to be viable and bilateral septopexy was performed.

Discussion

From a practical standpoint, the differential diagnosis of the acute scrotum is one of torsion, which is treated by emergency surgery, or of nontorsion, which is treated medically. Torsion generally accounts for 30 to 40% of acute scrotum cases referred for imaging. Epididymitis, orchitis, and torsion of a testicular appendage account for the vast majority of the remaining cases. Scrotal scintigraphy is a reliable means of assessing patients with testicular pain. When performed well and used appropriately, this technique can help avoid the performance of unnecessary surgery without delaying indicated surgery or producing false-negative results.

Normally, testicular torsion is prevented by attachments of the epididymis to the testis and to the posterior scrotal wall. The most common anatomic abnormality predisposing to testicular torsion is high investment of the tunica vaginalis ("bell clapper testis"). Other abnormalities include an elongated mesorchium and separation of the testis and epididymis.

With torsion of the spermatic cord, the vascular supply to the testis is compromised. The likelihood of preserving testicular viability decreases dramatically in a matter of hours after the onset of symptoms. Torsion is treated surgically with immediate detorsion and septopexy when the testicle is viable. Orchiectomy is performed when the testicle is nonviable. Because the "bell clapper" abnormality is typically bilateral, contralateral exploration and septopexy should be routinely performed in boys with testicular torsion.

Physical examination by an experienced clinician is the first and most important component of the evaluation of the acute scrotum. In many cases, the clinical presentation and examination will allow for appropriate management without imaging. In these cases, surgery will not be delayed, and unnecessary imaging will not be performed. The primary role of scintigraphy is to aid in assessing those patients whose diagnosis remains in question after clinical evaluation. When required, scintigraphy must be completed expeditiously and expertly.

Since flow to a normal testicle is virtually imperceptible scintigraphically, angiographic images are interpreted as demonstrating increased or not increased flow to the symptomatic hemiscrotum. Tissue phase images are evaluated for the presence of any regions of decreased tracer uptake. Any photopenic area must be viewed with a high level of suspicion and taken to represent testicular ischemia (or infarction) unless proven otherwise surgically or clinically. A rim of increased tracer uptake surrounding a photopenic area ("bull's-eye sign") is indicative of mid- or late-phase testicular torsion (Fig. C) but does not exclude testicular viability.

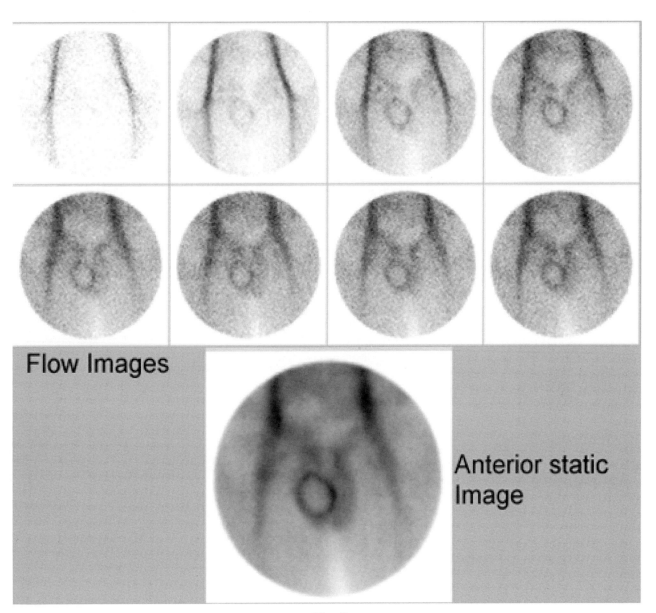

Flow Images

Anterior static Image

Fig. C

Inflammatory conditions, particularly epididymitis and orchitis, typically demonstrate increased blood flow and increased tracer uptake. It is worth noting that this pattern may be seen in cases of spontaneous detorsion, following manual detorsion, and with testicular tumors, which occasionally present with acute scrotal pain or swelling. Clinical history and physical examination are generally sufficient to exclude these possibilities.

Other causes of photopenic areas within the scrotum include hydrocele, hematocele, hernia, testicular hematoma, and abscess.

Over the last decade, color Doppler sonography (CDS) has gained favor for the initial evaluation of patients with acute scrotal pain. This technique permits the simultaneous display of blood flow superimposed on gray scale anatomic images. Advantages of CDS over scintigraphy include easy accessibility, ability to provide structural information, and lack of ionizing radiation.

Suggested Readings

Atkinson GO, Patrick LE, Ball TL, et al. The normal and abnormal scrotum in children: Evaluation with color Doppler sonography. *AJR Am J Roentgenol* 158:613–617, 1992.

Fenner MN, Roszhart DA, Texter JH. Testicular scanning: Evaluating the acute scrotum in the clinical setting. *Urology* 38:237–241, 1991.

Taylor GA, Connolly LP, Treves S. Scrotal scintigraphy. In: Treves S, ed. *Pediatric Nuclear Medicine*, 2nd ed. New York: Springer-Verlag, 1995:400–410.

Thomas WE, Williamson RC. Diagnosis and outcome of testicular torsion. *Br J Surg* 70:213–216, 1983.

Riley TW, Mosbaugh PG, Coles JL, et al. Use of radioisotope scan in evaluation of intrascrotal lesions. *J Urol* 116:472–475, 1976.

Lewis AG, Bukowski TP, Jarvis PD, Wacksman J, Sheldon CA. Evaluation of acute scrotum in the emergency department. *J Pediatr Surg* 30:277–281, 1995.

Mendel JB, Taylor GA, Treves S, et al. Testicular torsion in children: Scintigraphic assessment. *Pediatr Radiol* 15:110–115, 1985.

Case 164

Clinical Presentation

A hepatobiliary scan was requested to help differentiate between biliary atresia and neonatal hepatitis in a 2-week-old infant with extreme lethargy, poor feeding, and a high direct bilirubin. Sepsis and metabolic disorders had been ruled out.

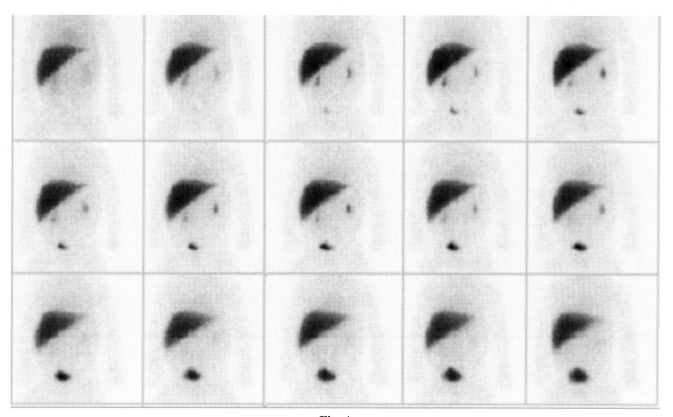

Fig. A

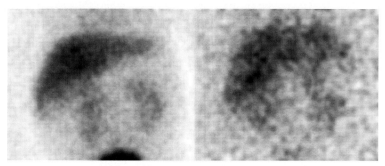

Fig. B—4 & 24 hours

Technique

- 0.05 mCi/kg of technetium-99m disofenin with a minimum dose of 0.25 mCi and a maximum total dose of 3.0 mCi, administered intravenously at the beginning of the acquisition.

- Use a high- or ultrahigh-resolution, low-energy, parallel hole collimator.
- Energy window 20% centered at 140 keV.
- Imaging time for the initial serial 0.5-minute frames is for 60 minutes. Additional images are obtained at 4 and 24 hours.
- Pretreatment with phenobarbital is 2.5 mg/kg twice a day for 3 to 5 days prior to hepatobiliary scintigraphy.

Image Interpretation

Images displayed as 5-minute frames after technetium-99m–labeled disofenin injection (Fig. A) demonstrate prompt hepatic uptake of tracer. The high early liver to background ratio and the clear definition of the liver boundaries indicate that there is good hepatic extraction of technetium-99m disofenin, although the prominent renal excretion suggests a mild degree of hepatic dysfunction. Tracer is not identified in the small intestine.

Images at 4 and 24 hours (Fig. B) show no evidence of tracer in the bowel.

Differential Diagnosis

1. Biliary atresia
2. Severe hepatocellular disease
3. Complete common duct obstruction
4. Intrahepatic cholestasis
5. Ascending cholangitis

Diagnosis and Clinical Follow-up

Hepatoportoenterostomy was performed after an intraoperative cholangiogram confirmed the diagnosis of biliary atresia. The patient improved clinically after surgery and the direct bilirubin normalized.

Discussion

Hyperbilirubinemia in the neonate is very common. In the majority of cases, neonatal hyperbilirubinemia reflects increased indirect bilirubin. This is usually physiological and benign. Direct hyperbilirubinemia, which is less common, has more severe etiologies. The differential diagnosis of direct hyperbilirubinemia includes sepsis, metabolic disorders, biliary atresia, neonatal hepatitis, choledochal cyst, α_1-antitrypsine deficiency, and Alagille syndrome. Differential diagnosis is difficult because these disorders have many common clinical features. Hepatobiliary scintigraphy helps in the differentiation between neonatal hepatitis and biliary atresia.

Biliary atresia has been detected in 1:10,000 live births, and idiopathic neonatal hepatitis has been found in 1:5,000. With either condition, jaundice usually develops at 3 to 6 weeks of age in an otherwise well-appearing, thriving infant, and the stools become acholic. Early surgical intervention is essential in biliary atresia; neonatal hepatitis is managed medically. It has been reported that hepatobiliary scintigraphy is 91% accurate, with 97% sensitivity and 82% specificity for the detection of biliary atresia. Phenobarbital improves the accuracy of hepatobiliary scintigraphy by inducing hepatic enzymes and acting as a choleretic. Tracer uptake is thereby enhanced and its excretion promoted. The recommended dose is 2.5 mg/kg twice a day for 3 to 5 days prior to scintigraphy. Biliary atresia is excluded when hepatobiliary scintigraphy demonstrates tracer excretion into the small intestine. Nonvisualization of tracer within bowel in the presence of efficient hepatic extraction is presumptive evidence of biliary atresia. To make this determination, imaging beyond the first hour is required. We obtain an image at 4 hours. If the bowel is not visualized on that image, we obtain an image at 24 hours. Frequently only the 24-hour image shows tracer in the bowel. Occasionally, because of rapid bowel transit time, tracer in the small intestine will be evident on the 4-hour image but will not be present at 24 hours.

Other etiologies for the pattern of preserved hepatic tracer uptake with nonvisualization of the bowel include bile plug syndrome in patients with cystic fibrosis, severe dehydration, sepsis, prolonged parenteral nutrition, or Alagille syndrome. When hepatic extraction of tracer is poor, a diagnosis of neonatal hepatitis is more likely. Failure to identify tracer excretion in the small intestine, however, prevents exclusion of biliary atresia in cases with both decreased liver extraction and nonvisualization of the small intestine.

Suggested Readings

Gerhold JP, Klingensmith WC, Kuni CC, et al. Diagnosis of biliary atresia with radionuclide hepatobiliary imaging. *Radiology* 146:499–504, 1983.

Hirsig J, Rickham PP. Early differential diagnosis between neonatal hepatitis and biliary atresia. *J Pediatr Surg* 5:159–165, 1980.

Majd M, Reba RC, Altman RP. Effect of phenobarbital on 99mTc-Hida scintigraphy in the evaluation of neonatal jaundice. *Semin Nucl Med* 11:194–204, 1981.

Majd M, Reba RC, Altman RP. Hepatobiliary scintigraphy with Tc-99m PIPIDA in the evaluation of neonatal jaundice. *Pediatrics* 67:140–145, 1981.

Treves ST, Jones AG, Markisz J. Liver and spleen. In: Treves, ST, ed. *Pediatric Nuclear Medicine*, 2nd ed. New York: Springer-Verlag, 1995: 466–495.

Case 165

Clinical Presentation

A 6-year-old girl with a 4-year history of partial complex seizures that had proven refractory to medical treatment was being considered for surgical cortical resection of an epileptogenic focus pending its localization. Computed tomography and magnetic resonance imaging of the brain were within normal limits. Electroencephalography was nonlocalizing. Technetium-99m–labeled bicisate (ECD) single photon emission computed tomography (SPECT) was obtained.

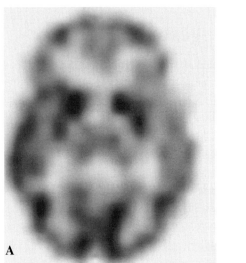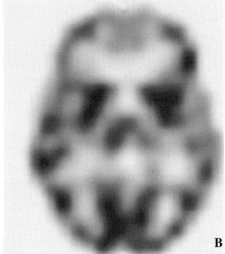

Figs. A, B

Technique

- Technetium-99m bicisate in doses of 0.3 mCi/kg of body weight. The minimum dose is 5 mCi; the maximum dose is 20 mCi.
- Use an ultrahigh-resolution collimator.
- Energy window 20% centered at 140 keV.
- SPECT acquisition on a 128 × 128 matrix with a triple detector system takes approximately 20 minutes. A usual technique includes 40 stops over 360 degrees per detector, 20 to 30 seconds per stop.
- The ictal study performed in an inpatient setting, preferably on an epilepsy monitoring unit. Continuous electroencephalogram (EEG) and videotelemetry are essential to ensure ictal injection of tracer. Venous access is established prior to seizure activity so that radiotracer can be quickly injected at the onset of seizure.

Image Interpretation

Interictal perfusion brain SPECT (Fig. A) demonstrates relative low regional blood flow to the left temporal and posterior frontal regions. Ictal brain SPECT (Fig. B) reveals well-defined increased blood flow to the region of the left

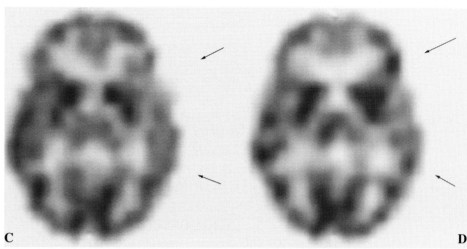

C   D

Figs. C, D

temporal and posterior frontal regions. These correspond to the areas of decreased perfusion on the interictal study. Arrows show the location of the findings on the interictal (Fig. C) and ictal (Fig. D) images.

Differential Diagnosis

- Epilepsy
- Encephalitis
- Tumor
- Luxury perfusion
- Environmental or motor stimulation of cortical activity

Diagnosis and Clinical Follow-up

Subdural grid placement demonstrated abnormal electroencephalographic activity in the posterior frontal and temporal regions, confirming the technetium-99m bicisate SPECT findings. A left temporal and partial frontal lobectomy was performed. The patient has been seizure-free postoperatively.

Discussion

Epilepsy is a recurrent convulsive or nonconvulsive disorder caused by partial or generalized epileptogenic discharge in the cerebrum. It is estimated that seizures become refractory to medical treatment in 10 to 20% of patients with epilepsy. Some patients with medically refractory epilepsy benefit from surgery, with limited cortical resection providing the best results. Identifying the ictal focus and delineating its relationship to language and motor centers is essential in directing cortical resection. This is accomplished with a multimodality approach that includes clinical evaluation, EEG, and imaging. Clinical evaluation alone is extremely inaccurate and scalp EEG has a 10 to 15% rate of false lateralization.

Perfusion brain SPECT has emerged as an important tool in the detection of the seizure focus. Tracers such as technetium-99m bicisate and technetium-99m exametazime, which distribute in the brain proportionately to regional cerebral blood flow, have been used. Interictally, there is often low perfusion in the region of the epileptogenic focus in relation to the normal brain. During an ictus, perfusion to the epileptogenic focus is greater than it is to the normal brain. Its location is more easily identified on ictal than on interictal studies. The sensitivity for detection of the ictal focus has been found to be 97% when tracer is administered ictally. Sensitivity decreases to approximately 50 to 70% if tracer is injected interictally.

Positron emission tomography (PET) has also been used in the workup of patients with intractable seizures. Oxygen use, glucose metabolism, blood flow, and receptor distribution can be mapped and quantified with PET. Fluorine 18–labeled 2-deoxy-D-glucose (^{18}FDG) PET is usually done interictally and shows relatively low metabolism in the region of the epileptogenic focus. Ictal ^{18}FDG PET shows high metabolism in the ictal focus.

Suggested Readings

Krausz Y, Cohen D, Konstantini S, et al. Brain SPECT imaging of temporal lobe epilepsy. *Neuroradiology* 33:274–276, 1991.

Ives JR. Video recording during long-term EEG monitoring of epileptic patients. *Adv Neurol* 46:1–11, 1987.

Harvey AS, Bowe JM, Hopkins IJ, et al. Ictal Tc-99m HMPAO single photon emission tomography in children with temporal lobe epilepsy. *Epilepsia* 34:869–877, 1993.

Ryvlin P, Philippon B, Clinotti L, et al. Functional neuroimaging strategy in temporal lobe epilepsy: A comparative study of F-18 FDG PET and Tc-99m HMPAO SPECT. *Ann Neurol* 31:650–656, 1992.

Packard AB, Roach PJ, Davis RT, et al. Ictal and interictal technetium-99m-bicisate brain SPECT in children with refractory epilepsy. *J Nuc Med* 37:1101–1106, 1996.

Case 166

Clinical Presentation

10-year-old boy presenting with persistent, vague, abdominal pain, fever, decreased appetite, and diarrhea. Abdominal ultrasound and computed tomography revealed a left suprarenal mass.

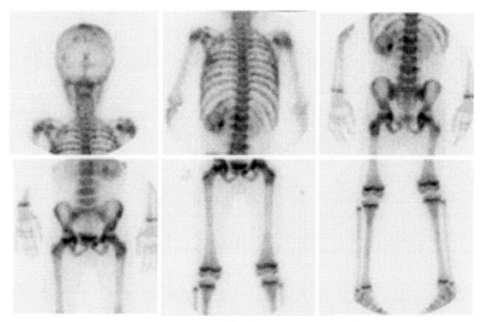

Fig. A

Posterior   Anterior

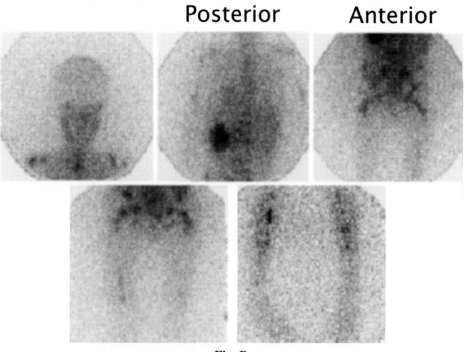

Fig. B

Technique

Technetium-99m Methylene Diphosphonate Bone Scan

- Technetium-99m–labeled methylene diphosphonate (MDP) at 0.2 mCi/kg of body weight given intravenously. The minimum dose is 1 mCi; the maximum dose is 20 mCi.
- Use a high- or ultrahigh-resolution, low-energy, parallel hole collimator. (Supplemental pinhole magnification images may be obtained for improved detail. SPECT is performed for better three-dimensional localization.)
- Planar whole-body or spot views of the entire skeleton obtained 4 hours after tracer injection.

Iodine-123 Metaiodobenzylguanidine Scintigraphy

- Iodine-123 metaiodobenzylguanidine (MIBG) at a dose of 0.2 mCi/kg given intravenously. The minimum dose is 1 mCi, and the maximum dose is 10 mCi.
- Use a high- or ultrahigh-resolution, low-energy, parallel hole collimator.
- Energy window is 20% centered at 159 keV.
- Whole-body images and SPECT are obtained as needed 24 hours after injection.
- Thyroid uptake can be blocked by administration of saturated solution of potassium iodide, 1 drop three times a day, beginning 1 day prior to imaging and continuing for 3 days.

Image Interpretation

Work-up for metastatic disease included technetium-99m MDP bone scan (Fig. A) and iodine-123 MIBG scintigraphy (Fig. B). Technetium-99m MDP scintigraphy shows areas of abnormal tracer uptake in the calvarium, spine, pelvis, ribs, femur and tibia. In addition, tracer is concentrated in the left adrenal mass. Iodine-123 MIBG scintigraphy demonstrates an intense focus of radiotracer uptake in the left upper abdomen and diffuse involvement of the skeleton.

Differential Diagnosis (MIBG uptake)

1. Neuroblastoma
2. Pheochromocytoma
3. Paraganglioma
4. Gastrinoma
5. Insulinoma
6. Medullary thyroid carcinoma
7. Infantile myofibromatosis

Diagnosis and Clinical Follow-up

The presumptive diagnosis was neuroblastoma. Laparotomy with resection of the mass confirmed the diagnosis. Chemotherapy was begun postoperatively.

Discussion

Neuroblastoma, the most common extracranial solid malignancy of childhood, arises from the embryonal neural crest anywhere along the sympathetic nervous system. The most common primary site is the adrenal gland, where 40 to 50% of neuroblastomas originate. Other sites of origin include the paravertebral and presacral sympathetic chains, the organ of Zuckerkandl, the posterior mediastinal sympathetic ganglia, and the cervical sympathetic plexuses. Disseminated disease is present in up to 70% of cases at diagnosis. This most commonly involves cortical bone and bone marrow but also involves liver, skin, and, occasionally, lung. The most characteristic sites of cortical involvement are the calvarium, periorbital facial bones, and the long bones, where a metaphyseal location is typical.

Scintigraphy with MIBG has a sensitivity of greater than 85% for detecting neuroblastoma. At doses used for imaging, cellular uptake of MIBG in neuroblastoma is through a neuronal sodium and energy-dependent transport mechanism. MIBG is labeled with either iodine-131 or iodine-123. Currently only iodine-131 MIBG is available commercially in the United States; iodine-123 is available for investigational use in some pediatric centers. Normal tracer distribution is to the heart, liver, thyroid gland, salivary and lacrimal glands, kidneys, urine, adrenal glands, bowel and muscle. There is no uptake by normal marrow or bone.

In comparison with MIBG, technetium-99m MDP has an equal sensitivity for detecting metastatic disease on a per patient basis but tends to depict the overall extent of disease less accurately. Accurate identification of metastases with skeletal scintigraphy, but not MIBG imaging, frequently requires experience in interpreting pediatric studies. Metaphyseal metastases, which are often symmetrical, may be particularly difficult to detect by less experienced observers.

Suggested Readings

Bousvaros A, Kirks DR, Grossman H. Imaging of neuroblastoma: An overview. *Pediatr Radiol* 16:89–106, 1986.

Brodeur GM, Pritchard J, Berthold F, et al. Revisions of international criteria for neuroblastoma diagnosis, staging, and response to treatment. *J Clin Oncol* 11:1466–1477, 1993.

Connolly LP, Treves ST. *Pediatric Skeletal Scintigraphy with Multimodality Imaging Correlation*. New York: Springer-Verlag, 1997.

Connolly LP, Treves ST, Conway JJ. Pediatric skeletal scintigraphy. In: Henkin RE, Boles MA, Dillehay GL, et al., eds. *Nuclear Medicine*. Philadelphia: Mosby Year Book, 1996:1690–1724.

Farahati J, Mueller SP, Coennen HH, et al. Scintigraphy of neuroblastoma with radioiodinated m-iodobenzylguanidine. In: Treves ST, ed. *Pediatric Nuclear Medicine*, 2nd ed. New York: Springer-Verlag, 1995:528–545.

Gelfand MJ, Elgazzar AH, Kriss VM, et al. Iodine-123-MIBG SPECT versus planar imaging in children with neural crest tumors. *J Nucl Med* 35:1753–1757, 1994.

Krenning EP, Kwekkeboom DJ, Bakker WH, et al. Somatostatin receptor scintigraphy with [In-111-DTPA-D-Phe1] and [123I-Tyr3]-octreotide: The Rotterdam experience with more than 1000 patients. *Eur J Nucl Med* 20:716–731, 1993.

Rufini V, Fisher GL, Shulkin BL, et al. Iodine-123-MIBG imaging of neuroblastoma: Utility of SPECT and delayed imaging. *J Nucl Med* 37:1464–1468, 1996.

Treves ST, Connolly LP, Kirkpatrick JA, et al. Bone. In: Treves ST, ed. *Pediatric Nuclear Medicine*, 2nd ed. New York: Springer-Verlag, 1995:233–301.

Case 167

Clinical Presentation

4-year-old boy presenting with swelling and pain of his left leg for 2 days and fever and a limp for 1 day. There was no history of trauma. Radiographic evaluation of the left leg was within normal limits. Laboratory workup demonstrated a white blood cell count of 13.2 and a sedimentation rate of 48. Blood cultures were obtained.

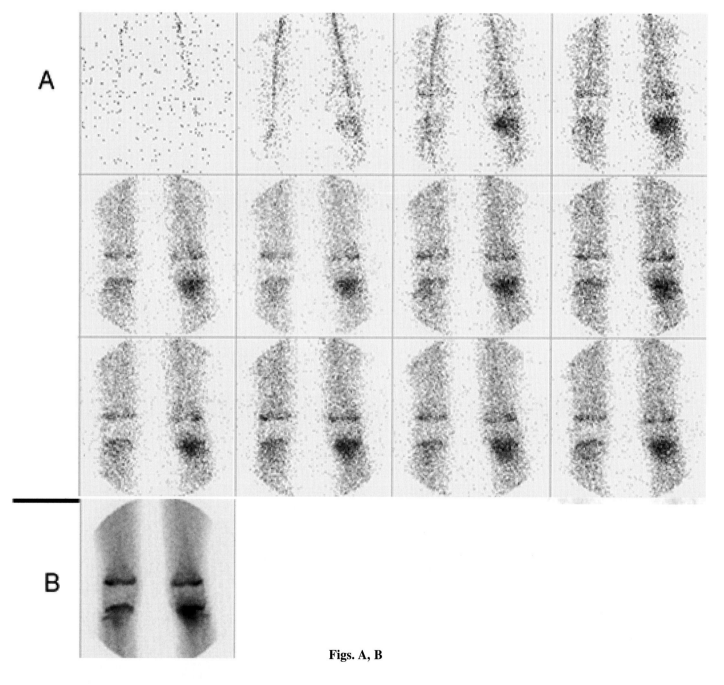

Figs. A, B

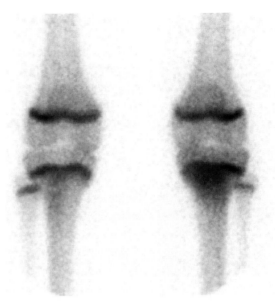

Fig. C

Technique

- Technetium-99m–labeled methylene diphosphonate (MDP) at 0.2 mCi/kg of body weight given intravenously. The minimum dose is 1 mCi; the maximum dose is 20 mCi.
- Use a high- or ultrahigh-resolution, low-energy, parallel hole collimator. Supplemental pinhole magnification images are obtained for improved detail. Single photon emission computed tomography (SPECT) is performed for better three-dimensional localization.
- Imaging time for an initial radionuclide angiogram is 3-second frames for 1 minute. Static blood pool image should be obtained within 5 to 10 minutes of tracer injection. Planar static view of the region of interest should be obtained 4 hours after injection. There should be whole body or spot views of the entire skeleton.

Image Interpretation

Anterior radionuclide angiogram shows increased blood flow to the proximal left tibia (Fig. A). The distribution of increased tracer concentration depicted in the tissue phase imaging corresponds to the area with increased flow demonstrated by radionuclide angiogram (Fig. B). Anterior views of the tibiae (Fig. C) in the skeletal phase reveal abnormal uptake in the proximal left tibial metaphysis.

Differential Diagnosis:

1. Osteomyelitis
2. Soft tissue infection/inflammation
3. Acute trauma
4. Malignancy
5. Sarcoidosis

PEARLS/PITFALLS

- Skeletal scintigraphy in children is best performed with high- or ultrahigh-resolution collimation.

- Pinhole imaging is useful for demonstrating more convincingly or delineating more accurately an abnormality that is identified on planar images. When images of a clinically suspicious area initially appear normal, pinhole images help to confirm the absence of focal abnormalities adjacent to the intensely tracer-avid physis.

- SPECT is often valuable for evaluation of the pelvis.

- Skeletal scintigraphy is the most effective means of screening children with suspected osteomyelitis and normal radiographic evaluation.

- Skeletal phase imaging must encompass the whole body in children with suspected acute osteomyelitis.

- Failure to position the extremities symmetrically and the physes perpendicular to the camera face may mimic or obscure metaphyseal pathology.

- During image processing, care must be taken not to overexpose the epiphyseal-metaphyseal complex. Resultant "blooming" of the image may mimic or obscure metaphyseal pathology.

- An extended pattern of increased localization involving the adjacent physis and bones distal or proximal to an involved metaphysis may be observed. This reflects reactive hyperemia and should not be viewed as evidence of either physeal involvement or multifocal osteomyelitis. *(continued)*

Diagnosis and Clinical Follow-up

Following skeletal scintigraphy, bone biopsy was performed. Cultures grew *Staphylococcus aureus*. Intravenous antibiotic treatment was initiated based on a presumptive diagnosis of acute osteomyelitis. The patient improved on antibiotic treatment and was discharged in good condition after 1 week of hospitalization. Antibiotic treatment course was completed as an outpatient.

Discussion

Acute osteomyelitis is a common pediatric problem. It usually results from hematogenous spread of infection related to transient and often asymptomatic bacteremia. *S. aureus* is the most frequent infective organism.

Approximately 75% of cases involve the long bones, with a metaphyseal location being typical. This metaphyseal predominance reflects high regional vascularity and slow blood flow in looping metaphyseal arterial and venous sinusoidal vessels. The most rapidly growing and larger metaphyses are more commonly involved. Transphyseal vessels allow infection to spread from metaphysis to epiphysis in infants and children prior to 18 months of age. After these vessels are obliterated, the relatively avascular physis serves as a natural barrier to spread of infection. Epiphyseal involvement is, therefore, uncommon between 18 months of age and the time of physeal closure. The flat and irregular bones, such as the pelvis, are involved in approximately 25% of cases. Acute osteomyelitis of the flat and irregular bones characteristically develops in bone adjacent to cartilage.

Early diagnosis of acute osteomyelitis is necessary to prevent significant complications such as sepsis, chronic infection, growth arrest, and bone deformity. Unfortunately, the clinical diagnosis of acute osteomyelitis is difficult in young children who frequently present with only limping or refusal to bear weight. Pain is often not well-localized, and swelling and tenderness are often absent. Fever may be either the only sign or absent in children of all age groups with acute osteomyelitis.

Imaging evaluation usually begins with radiographs. Radiographic diagnosis in the early stages of acute osteomyelitis is difficult, however, because the early radiographic manifestations are neither consistently observed nor specific. In contrast, skeletal scintigraphy, which is typically abnormal within 24 to 48 hours of symptom onset, has proved invaluable in providing prompt early diagnosis of acute osteomyelitis, allowing timely treatment.

As in the adult, scintigraphic evaluation is accomplished with multiphase imaging to help distinguish acute osteomyelitis from cellulitis. A radionuclide angiogram and tissue phase image of the region of highest clinical suspicion and skeletal phase images of the entire skeleton are obtained. The whole body evaluation is important because of the significant incidence of multifocal involvement, particularly in neonates (22% incidence of multifocality), and the frequent absence of localizing signs in young children. Whole body imaging is also valuable in cases in which diseases such as metastatic neuroblastoma and leukemia clinically mimic acute osteomyelitis.

Regionally increased blood flow and localization to the infected bone and adjacent soft tissues are typically revealed on angiographic and tissue phase images. Skeletal phase images usually demonstrate focally increased tracer uptake in an infected bone. Rarely, there is focally decreased to absent uptake that likely reflects regional ischemia caused by vascular tamponade from inflammation and edema.

• *(continued)* The role of magnetic resonance imaging relative to scintigraphy in evaluating suspected acute osteomyelitis has been debated. Although these modalities appear equally sensitive when symptoms are well-localized, poor symptom localization in young children and the incidence of multifocal involvement favor the use of scintigraphy.

Suggested Readings

Applegate KA, Connolly LP, Treves ST. Neuroblastoma presenting clinically as hip osteomyelitis: A signature diagnosis on skeletal scintigraphy. *Pediatr Radiol* 25:S93–S97, 1995.

Asmar BI. Osteomyelitis in the neonate. *Infect Dis Clin North Am* 6:117–132, 1992.

Bressler L, Conway JJ, Weiss SC. Neonatal osteomyelitis examined by bone scintigraphy. *Radiology* 152:685–688, 1984.

Connolly LP, Treves ST. *Pediatric Skeletal Scintigraphy with Multimodality Imaging Correlation.* New York: Springer-Verlag, 1997.

Connolly LP, Treves ST, Conway JJ. Pediatric skeletal scintigraphy. In: Henkin RE, Boles MA, Dillehay GL, et al., eds. *Nuclear Medicine*, Philadelphia: Mosby Year Book, 1996:1690–1724.

Faden H, Grossi M. Acute osteomyelitis in children. *Am J Dis Child* 145:65–69, 1991.

Jones DC, Cady RB. "Cold" bone scans in acute osteomyelitis. *J Bone Joint Surg Br* 63:376–378, 1981.

Mok PM, Reilly BJ, Ash JM. Osteomyelitis in the neonate. *Radiology* 145:677–682, 1982.

Treves ST, Connolly LP, Kirkpatrick JA, et al. Bone. In: Treves ST, ed. *Pediatric Nuclear Medicine*, 2nd ed. New York: Springer-Verlag, 1995:233–301.

Treves S, Khettry J, Broker FH, et al. Osteomyelitis: Early scintigraphic detection in children. *Pediatrics* 57:173–186, 1976.

Case 168

Clinical Presentation

10-year-old boy presenting with a 6-week history of right leg pain after falling while playing football. Radiographs were suggestive of osteosarcoma.

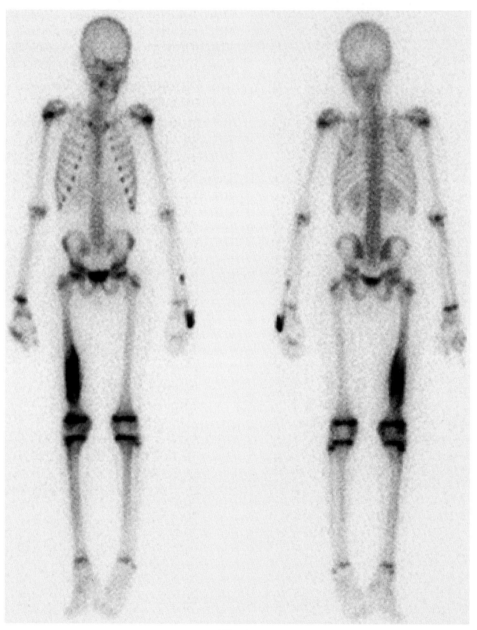

Fig. A

Technique

- Technetium-99m–labeled methylene diphosphonate (MDP) at 0.2 mCi/kg of body weight given intravenously. The minimum dose is 1 mCi; the maximum dose is 20 mCi.

- Use a high- or ultrahigh-resolution, low-energy, parallel hole collimator. Supplemental pinhole magnification images are obtained in addition to the planar images, for improved detail. Single photon emission computed tomography (SPECT) is performed for better three-dimensional localization.
- Imaging time for an initial radionuclide angiogram is 3-second frames for 1 minute. Static blood pool image should be obtained within 5 to 10 minutes following tracer injection. Whole-body or spot views of the entire bony skeleton should be obtained 4 hours after tracer injection. There should be spot planar or SPECT views of the region of interest, as needed.

Image Interpretation

Whole body technetium-99m methylene diphosphonate (MDP) images (Fig. A) demonstrate a focal area of intense increased uptake in the distal diaphyseal region of the right femur. This corresponds to the area of abnormality seen on radiography. No metastatic disease was visualized. Retained tracer is present in the intravenous line of the left hand and wrist.

Differential Diagnosis (solitary site of focal bony tracer uptake):

1. Benign primary tumor
2. Trauma
   a. Accidental
   b. Post-surgical
3. Primary bone malignancy
4. Bony metastasis
5. Osteomyelitis
6. Bony infarct
7. Skin contamination overlying bone structure

Diagnosis and Clinical Follow-up

Biopsy of the primary site proved to be osteosarcoma. Initial metastatic workup was negative. Chemotherapy was initiated, and wide tumoral excision with allograft reconstruction was performed. Follow-up skeletal scintigraphy and chest computed tomography (CT) were obtained at regular intervals for metastatic evaluation. In the fourth year of clinical follow-up, skeletal scintigraphy demonstrated widespread skeletal metastatic disease with soft tissue localization of tracer in pulmonary metastases that was confirmed by CT (Fig. B).

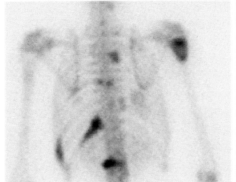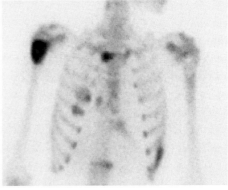

Fig. B

Discussion

Osteosarcoma is the most common primary malignant bone tumor of childhood. The incidence is highest between 10 and 25 years of age. Osteosarcoma is predominantly a lesion of the long bones, where it is typically metaphyseal in location. This case represents a rare case of diaphyseal involvement by the tumor.

Treatment of choice is wide resection and limb-sparing surgery, which is performed in 80% of patients. This treatment approach requires accurate delineation of tumoral extent and assessment of response to preoperative chemotherapy at the primary site as well as identification of metastatic foci, which most commonly involve lung and bone. Survival rates are highest in patients without metastatic disease at presentation whose tumor shows greater than 90 to 95% necrosis prior to resection.

Skeletal scintigraphy typically reveals marked tracer uptake in osteosarcomas, although it is not unusual for regions of decreased uptake to be present as well. Increased tracer uptake in the lesion often extends beyond the pathological margins of the tumor secondary to hyperemia or reactive bone. Assessment of local extent is best based on magnetic resonance imaging (MRI) and thallium-201 imaging, which is especially valuable for estimating tumor viability. Skeletal scintigraphy is the primary means by which skeletal metastases are detected at diagnosis and during follow-up. Skeletal metastases, which appear as areas of increased radionuclide uptake, are often radiographically occult or asymptomatic, or both, at the time of scintigraphic detection. Occasionally, pulmonary metastases accumulate technetium-99m MDP because of osteoid production by the metastatic deposits. There are also rare reports of metastases to other sites, including the liver, kidneys, and lymph nodes, that have been identified with skeletal scintigraphy.

Tumor viability is accurately assessed with thallium-201 scintigraphy; the intense uptake of this tracer in untreated osteosarcoma reflects cellular viability and high metabolic activity. Imaging with thallium-201 is valuable when used in combination with MRI in assessing local disease extent at diagnosis and following chemotherapy and in evaluating response to chemotherapy prior to performing limb-salvage surgery. Thallium-201 uptake in osteosarcoma markedly decreases with a favorable pathological response, which is defined histologically as greater than 90 to 95% necrosis. This can be assessed visually by comparing tumoral and cardiac or background thallium-201 uptake or quantitatively. Various quantitative methods have been proposed, with the optimal method yet to be defined. In another case, shown in Figures C through F, absence of thallium-201 uptake after therapy reflects good response to treatment. Figures C and D show technetium-99m MDP and thallium-201 uptake, respectively, in the bone and tumor prior to therapy. Figures E and F show some post-therapeutic residual technetium-99m MDP irregularity in tracer uptake consistent with expected bony repair and no evidence of abnormal thallium-201 uptake, suggesting no residual viable tumor.

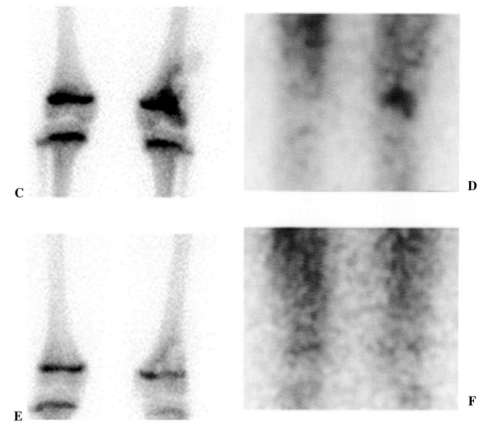

Figs. C, D, E, F

Suggested Readings

Chew FS, Hudson TM. Radionuclide bone scanning of osteosarcoma: Falsely extended uptake patterns. *AJR Am J Roentgenol* 139:49–54, 1982.

Connolly LP, Treves ST. *Pediatric Skeletal Scintigraphy with Multimodality Imaging Correlation*. New York: Springer-Verlag, 1997.

Connolly LP, Treves ST, Conway JJ. Pediatric skeletal scintigraphy. In: Henkin RE, Boles MA, Dillehay GL, et al., eds. *Nuclear Medicine*. Philadelphia: Mosby Year Book, 1996:1690–1724.

Hoefnagel CA, Bruning PF, Cohen P, et al. Detection of lung metastases from osteosarcoma by scintigraphy using ^{99m}Tc-methylene diphosphonate. *Diagnostic Imaging* 50:277–284, 1981.

Kirks DR, Cook TA, Merten DF, et al. The value of radionuclide bone imaging in selected patients with osteosarcoma metastatic to lung. *Pediatr Radiol* 9:139–143, 1980.

Rees CR, Siddiqui AR, duCret R. The role of bone scintigraphy in osteogenic sarcoma. *Skeletal Radiol* 15:365–367, 1986.

Schweil AM, McKillop JH, Milroy R, et al. Mechanism of ^{201}TI uptake in tumours. *Eur J Nucl Med* 15:376–379, 1989.

Thrall JH, Geslein GE, Corcoran RJ, et al. Abnormal radionuclide deposition patterns adjacent to focal skeletal lesions. *Radiology* 115:659–663, 1975.

Treves ST, Connolly LP, Kirkpatrick JA, et al. Bone. In: Treves ST, ed. *Pediatric Nuclear Medicine*, 2nd ed. New York: Springer-Verlag, 1995:233–301.

Vanel D, Henry-Amar M, Lumbrosus J, et al. Pulmonary evaluation of patients with osteosarcoma: Roles of standard radiography, tomography, CT, scintigraphy and tomoscintigraphy. *AJR Am J Roentgenol* 143:519–523, 1984.

Case 169

Clinical Presentation

7-week-old infant male presenting with severe right hydronephrosis detected by a prenatal ultrasonography. Postnatal ultrasonography also demonstrated severe pelvicaliectasis of the right collecting system consistent with right ureteropelvic junction (UPJ) obstruction. Voiding cystourethrography (VCUG) showed no reflux. A technetium-99m–labeled mercaptoacetyltriglycine (MAG-3) study was obtained for evaluation of the presence and severity of obstruction.

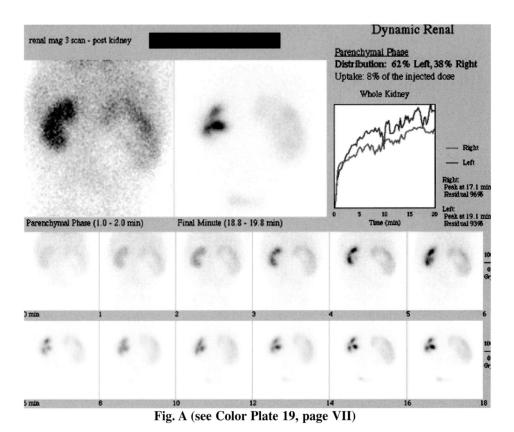

Fig. A (see Color Plate 19, page VII)

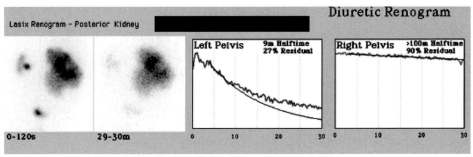

Fig. B (see Color Plate 20, page VII)

Technique

- Technetium-99m MAG-3 at a dose of 0.2 mCi/kg. The minimum dose is 2 mCi; the maximum dose is 10 mCi.
- Use a high- or ultrahigh-resolution, low-energy, parallel hole collimator.
- Energy window 20% centered at 140 keV.
- Dynamic acquisition obtained for a minimum of 20 minutes (or until tracer is seen in the collecting system). For the diuretic phase after Lasix (furosemide) administration (dose: 1 mg/kg; max: 40 mg), dynamic acquisition obtained for 30 minutes.
- Bladder catheterization and intravenous access established prior to injection of radiotracer.

Image Interpretation

The parenchymal phase (Fig. A) shows an enlarged right kidney with a central area of decreased tracer uptake representing the dilated collecting system. The relative uptake of radiotracer is 38% by the right kidney and 62% by the left kidney. The cortical transit time, defined as the time between injection of the tracer and the first appearance of tracer into the collecting system is greater than 20 minutes for the right side and 4 to 5 minutes for the left. There is marked retention of tracer in the right collecting system prior to diuretic administration.

Thirty minutes after administration of furosemide (Fig. B) 91% residual radiotracer remains in the right pelvis, and a half-time of greater than 100 minutes is noted. These findings indicate a right UPJ obstruction. Tracer washout from the left kidney is augmented by furosemide, indicating no obstruction.

Differential Diagnosis:

1. Obstructed urinary collecting system
2. Urinoma
3. Ureterocele
4. Surgical diversion of the urinary collecting system overlying the kidney

Diagnosis and Clinical Follow-up

The patient underwent a right pyeloplasty. A follow-up technetium-99m MAG-3 obtained after surgery (Fig. C) shows a cortical transit time of 4 to 5 minutes bilaterally. The relative uptake of tracer by the right kidney is 49% and by the left is 51%. Drainage remains slow from the dilated right renal pelvis. There is spontaneous drainage of the left kidney.

Following administration of furosemide (Fig. D), there is prompt and near complete washout from the right renal pelvis (half-time = 4 minutes and residual in right renal pelvis = 7%). This nonobstructive response to furosemide indicates a favorable surgical result. The left kidney shows normal diuretic response.

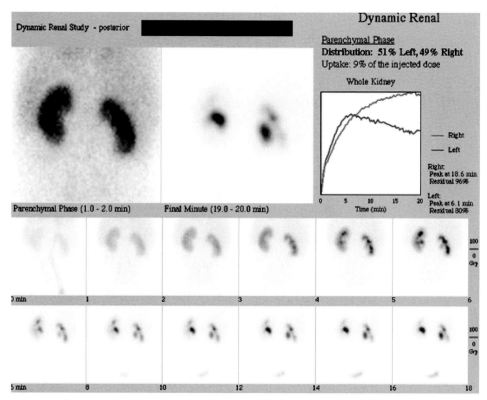

Fig. C (see Color Plate 21, page VIII)

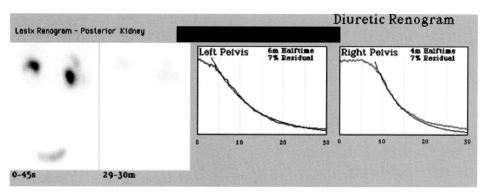

Fig. D (see Color Plate 22, page VIII)

Discussion

Urinary tract obstruction is defined as any restriction to urinary flow that, if left untreated, will cause progressive renal deterioration. The likelihood of functional impairment is determined by the degree, site, and etiology of obstruction, coexistence of reflux, compliance of the renal pelvis, presence of infection, and age of the patient.

Nuclear medicine plays an important role in the evaluation, therapy planning, and monitoring of patients with hydronephrosis. Radiotracers that are rapidly eliminated by the kidneys such as technetium-99m MAG-3, technetium-99m diethylenetriamine pentaacetic acid (DTPA), and technetium-99m glucoheptonate may be used for the evaluation of obstruction. We favor technetium-99m MAG-3 because of the higher kidney to background ratio and the rapid excretion, which provides good temporal resolution.

Studies performed to assess suspected renal obstruction most often consist of standard parenchymal imaging from 1 to 2 minutes after injection of tracer, drainage phase imaging through 20 minutes post-injection, and, when spontaneous drainage is not observed, dynamic post-furosemide imaging. An alternative method entails administering furosemide 15 minutes prior to tracer administration (F-15 diuretic renography).

The interpretation of a dynamic renal scan includes evaluation of the parenchymal phase, the cortical transit time, and the drainage phase. In children with suspected obstruction, the parenchymal phase provides important information regarding differential renal function and renal morphology. The diuretic phase includes calculation of the washout half-time and the percentage of initial activity remaining in the collecting system at 30 minutes after diuretic administration.

The diuretic half-time is calculated in our institution using a monoexponential interpolation between two points; one point during early diuresis and another point before the curve changes from monotonic decay. In addition, a 30-minute post-diuretic residual is calculated. In cases of obstruction, there is large residual radiotracer in the renal pelvis at 30 minutes after administration of furosemide. In the case presented, a half-time greater than 100 minutes and a 90% residual are indicative of obstruction.

In the newborn infant, the renal uptake of the radiotracer, cortical transit time, and excretion may be physiologically delayed. Technetium-99m MAG-3, however, has been found reliable in this age group for the detection of obstruction.

Suggested Readings

Koff SA, Thrall JH, Keyes JW. Assessment of hydronephrosis in children using diuretic radionuclide renography. *J Urol* 123:531–534, 1980.

Thrall JH, Koff SA, Keyes JW. Diuretic radionuclide renography and scintigraphy in the differential diagnosis of hydroureteronephrosis. *Semin Nucl Med* 11:89–104, 1981.

Treves ST. The ongoing challenge of diagnosis and treatment of urinary tract infection, vesicoureteral reflux and renal damage in children. *J Nucl Med* 35:1608–1611, 1994.

Treves ST, ed. *Pediatric Nuclear Medicine.* New York: Springer-Verlag, 1995.

Wong JC, Rossleigh MA, Farnsworth RH. Utility of technetium-99m MAG3 diuretic renography in the neonatal period. *J Nucl Med* 36:2214–2219, 1995.

Index